Infection and Immunity

Infection and Immunity

Editors

Jon S Friedland MA PhD FRCP FRCPE
Reader and Honorary Consultant
Department of Infectious Diseases
Imperial College London
Hammersmith Hospital
Du Cane Road
London

Liz Lightstone MA PhD FRCP
Senior Lecturer and Honorary Consultant Renal Physician
Faculty of Medicine
Imperial College London
Hammersmith Hospital
Du Cane Road
London

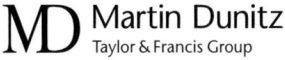
Martin Dunitz
Taylor & Francis Group

© 2003 Martin Dunitz, an imprint of the Taylor & Francis Group plc

First published in the United Kingdom in 2003
by Martin Dunitz, an imprint of the Taylor & Francis Group plc, 11 New Fetter
Lane, London EC4P 4EE

Tel.: +44 (0) 20 7583 9855
Fax.: +44 (0) 20 7842 2298
E-mail: info@dunitz.co.uk
Website: http://www.dunitz.co.uk

Although every effort has been made to ensure that all owners of copyright
material have been acknowledged in this publication, we would be glad to
acknowledge in subsequent reprints or editions any omissions brought to our
attention.

A CIP record for this book is available from the British Library.

ISBN 1 84184 373 3

Distributed in the USA by
Fulfilment Center
Taylor & Francis
10650 Toebben Drive
Independence, KY 41051, USA
Toll Free Tel.: +1 800 634 7064
E-mail: taylorandfrancis@thomsonlearning.com

Distributed in Canada by
Taylor & Francis
74 Rolark Drive
Scarborough, Ontario M1R 4G2, Canada
Toll Free Tel.: +1 877 226 2237
E-mail: tal_fran@istar.ca

Distributed in the rest of the world by
Thomson Publishing Services
Cheriton House
North Way
Andover, Hampshire SP10 5BE, UK
Tel.: +44 (0)1264 332424
E-mail: salesorder.tandf@thomsonpublishingservices.co.uk

Composition by Tek-Art, Croydon, Surrey.
Printed and bound in Spain by Grafos, S. A.

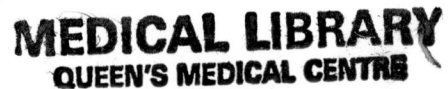

Contents

Contributors

Daniel M Altmann
Transplantation Biology Group
MRC Clinical Sciences Centre
ICSM
Hammersmith Hospital
Du Cane Road
London W12 0NN, UK

Ilaria Bellantuono
Imperial College School of Medicine
Hammersmith Hospital
Du Cane Road
London W12 0NN, UK

Rosemary J Boyton
Transplantation Biology Group
MRC Clinical Sciences Centre
ICSM
Hammersmith Hospital
Du Cane Road
London W12 0NN, UK

Menna R Clatworthy
The Cambridge Institute for Medical Research
and the Department of Medicine
University of Cambridge School of Clinical
Medicine
Cambridge
UK

Andrew P Cope
Senior Lecturer in Rheumatology
Kennedy Institute of Rheumatology
ICSM
Charing Cross Hospital
Fulham Palace Road
London W6 RF, UK

Kevin A Davies
Professor of Medicine
Brighton and Sussex Medical School
University of Brighton at Falmer
Brighton BN1 9PH, UK

Stephan Ellmerich
Transplantation Biology Group
MRC Clinical Sciences Centre
ICSM
Hammersmith Hospital
Du Cane Road
London W12 0NN, UK

Jon S Friedland
Department of Infectious Diseases
Faculty of Medicine
Imperial College of Science, Technology and
Medicine
London, UK

David W Holden
Centre for Molecular and Microbiology and
Infection
Armstrong Road
Imperial College London
London SW7 2AZ, UK

Shiou Chih Hsu
Imperial College School of Medicine
Hammersmith Hospital
Du Cane Road
London W12 0NN, UK

Jeremy Hull
University Lecturer and Honorary Consultant
Paediatrician
University Department of Paediatrics
John Radcliffe Hospital
Oxford OX3 9DU, UK

Babak Javid
MRC Clinical Fellow
Wellcome Trust Centre for Molecular
Mechanisms in Disease
Addenbrooke's Hospital
Hills Road
Cambridge CB2 2XY, UK

Paul J Lehner
Wellcome Trust Senior Clinical Fellow
Cambridge Institute for Medical Research
Wellcome Trust Centre for Molecular
Mechanisms in Disease
Addenbrooke's Hospital, Hills Road
Cambridge CB2 2XY, UK

Nicholas M Price
MRC Training Fellow
Department of Infectious Diseases
Imperial College School of Medicine
Du Cane Road
London W12 0NN, UK

Francisco Ramirez
Imperial College School of Medicine
Hammersmith Hospital
Du Cane Road
London W12 0NN, UK

Robert C Read
Division of Genomic Medicine
Infectious Diseases Unit, E Floor
Royal Hallamshire Hospital
University of Sheffield
Sheffield S10 2GF, UK

Kenneth GC Smith
The Cambridge Institute for Medical Research
and the Department of Medicine
University of Cambridge School of Clinical
Medicine
Cambridge
UK

Sunil Shaunak
Reader in Infectious Diseases
Faculty of Medicine
Imperial College School of Medicine
Hammersmith Hospital
Du Cane Road
London W12 0NN, UK

Hans J Stauss
Reader
Department of Immunology
Imperial College School of Medicine
Hammersmith Hospital
Du Cane Road
London W12 0NN, UK

Bernd M Spriewald
Institute for Clinical Immunology
Department of Medicine III
Friedrich-Alexander-University
Erlangen-Nürnberg, Germany

Kate E Unsworth
Centre for Molecular and Microbiology
and Infection
Armstrong Road
Imperial College London
London SW7 2AZ, UK

Kathryn J Wood
Professor of Immunology
Nuffield Department of Surgery
University of Oxford
John Radcliffe Hospital
Oxford OX3 9DU, UK

David Wyllie
Clinical Lecturer in Microbiology
Nuffield Department of Clinical Laboratory
Sciences
University of Oxford
John Radcliffe Hospital
Oxford OX3 9DU, UK

Preface

Infection and immunity is in the news. A look at the science news confirms that research on transplantation and novel treatments for cancer or killer diseases such as HIV or tuberculosis has been moving forward at an explosive pace. It remains critical to link these developments in basic science with the realities of medicine and the needs of patients. Similarly there is a real need to develop true clinical scientists trained primarily either as clinicians or as scientists but who still have an interest in and understanding of both clinical practice and basic science. It is with these clinical scientists in mind that we have designed this book.

This volume is divided into two sections focusing on immunity and infection. Each chapter explores a rapidly evolving area of clinical science and aims to highlight not only current areas of acute research interest, but how the specific basic science connects to the patient. Many genetic and environmental elements contribute to the development of autoimmunity. In the first three immunity chapters of section one, the role of MHC genes, cytokine networks and B-cells are considered respectively by Danny Altmann, Andrew Cope and Ken Smith. Kevin Davies, editor of the series of which this book is one volume, contributes a chapter on current thinking in complement biology, an important link between innate and adaptive immunity. In the final two chapters of section one, Katherine Wood tackles transplantation and issues of peripheral tolerance whilst Hans Stauss takes a closer look at tumour immunology, both areas where recent insights into molecular and cellular mechanisms have led to novel therapeutic approaches.

The second section of the book starts with a chapter by Jeremy Hull on the genetics of infection, which looks at the building blocks on which host defence is based. In general, whether or not a person succumbs to an infection depends on a battle between the host immune system and the armamentarium of particular viruses or bacteria. The host response to infection is the focus of two chapters. The first co-authored by David Wyllie and Robert Read reviews toll-like receptors that activate innate immune responses to bacteria and the second, co-authored by Nick Price and one of the editors, focuses on how matrix metalloproteinase secretion may lead to tissue destruction in infection. In some cases pathogens try to harness the immune system for their own ends and, in one example of this, Sunil Shaunak looks at chemokines in the context of HIV infection. The emphasis of the final two chapters then switches to the pathogen. Babak Javid and Paul Lehner examine how viruses avoid the immune system whilst Kate Unsworth and David Holden consider bacterial pathogenesis and the key role of pathogenicity islands.

Each chapter is a distinct invitation to think about key research problems in the exciting areas of infection and immunity. We are hoping that this slim volume will appeal both to scientists curious about the clinical application of research and also to clinicians wondering whether academic medicine might be the way forward. If this book succeeds in catching your interest and imagination, and particularly if it galvanises you to think about, and get involved in, some aspect of clinical science, then it will have been a success.

Jon S. Friedland
Liz Lightstone

To Jo and Ian

Section A

Immunity

1

Human leucocyte antigen (HLA) transgenic mice for the analysis of autoimmune disease

Daniel M Altmann, Stephan Ellmerich, Rosemary J Boyton

Objectives • Overview • Introduction • Human leucocyte antigen disease associations • Human leucocyte antigen transgenic mice • Conclusions • Glossary • References

OBJECTIVES

(1) To review the rationale for generating human leucocyte antigen (HLA) transgenic mice as a tool to elucidate mechanisms predisposing to autoimmunity.

(2) To define how studies of HLA transgenic mice have contributed to identifying autoimmune T-cell epitopes.

OVERVIEW

Multiple genes are involved in susceptibility to autoimmune and infectious diseases. However, the human leucocyte antigen (HLA) immune response genes frequently contribute one of the strongest effects. This is the case for many of the diseases believed to have an autoimmune aetiology, including ankylosing spondylitis, which is strongly associated with particular HLA class I alleles, and Type 1 diabetes, associated with specific HLA class II alleles. The normal role of the HLA gene products in binding antigen and presenting it to T-lymphocytes offers clues as to the possible mechanisms underlying these disease associations. However,

> 30 years after the initial associations were first noted, we still lack definitive models to explain these disease mechanisms or to use as the basis for the design of rational, specific therapies. The impact of gene cloning and transgenesis technologies in this field allows the expression of disease-predisposing genes in transgenic mice in the hope of creating better disease models. Transgenic mice expressing HLA genes and other disease-associated molecules, including T-cell receptors and co-stimulatory molecules, can be used to explore models of disease susceptibility. These transgenics can thus be used for approaches that would be impossible using either cultured cells from human patients or normal laboratory mice. HLA-restricted epitopes can be defined from antigens implicated in the activation of pathogenic T-lymphocytes. Furthermore, the conditions leading to HLA-dependent induction of autoimmune disease can be dissected, leading to the design of specific therapies which are capable of blocking pathogenic immune responses without causing global immuno-suppression. This approach has been used to

investigate models of several diseases including ankylosing spondylitis, multiple sclerosis and Type 1 diabetes. As Human Genome Project initiatives offer further candidate disease genes of known or unknown function to be tested, these transgenic disease models should form an important starting baseline for experiments to build a composite picture of genetic susceptibility.

1. INTRODUCTION

For many diseases considered to have an autoimmune aetiology, alleles of the human leucocyte antigen (HLA) immune response genes are the strongest markers of genetic susceptibility.[1–6] Such observations, originally made > 30 years ago on the basis of serological tissue typing, have been borne out by genotypic analysis of HLA polymorphic sequences and subsequently by full genome scans. Although these diseases clearly involve multiple genes, as well as environmental factors, the major risk appears to be conferred within the HLA region. The diseases within this group include not just the classical antibody-mediated diseases such as Grave's disease and myasthenia gravis, but also diseases such as Type 1 diabetes and multiple sclerosis (MS) in which T-cells are implicated in the pathogenic effector mechanisms.

Immunology has excellent tools for probing the molecular mechanisms that underlie these diseases. Over the past 15 years or so, the impact of molecular biology and improved T-cell culture techniques have fuelled optimism that disease mechanisms would be elucidated and rational, specific therapies developed. At the centre of this view is the belief that a common factor underlying these diverse conditions is that the disease-predisposing HLA allele presents a peptide derived from the target self-tissue to self-reactive T-lymphocytes, triggering the subsequent disease process. While this view is clearly an oversimplification of these complex and polygenic diseases, the strong HLA associations lend credence to the hypothesis and suggest that therapies targeted at a central peptide/major histocompatibility complex (MHC)/T-cell receptor (TCR) interaction could

be effective. The murine models of these diseases, including Type 1 diabetes in the non-obese diabetic (NOD) mouse and experimental allergic encephalomyelitis (EAE; a murine model for MS), also constitute complex and poorly understood phenotypes, and yet can be successfully treated by homing in on the central interaction.[7–9] Application of this approach to human diseases assumes some knowledge of the key components in the disease process. Which are the disease-associated HLA products and what is the mechanism by which they confer disease risk? Which proteins within the tissue constitute the primary targets of attack and which peptides from these are the dominant T-cell epitopes? Which are the populations of T-cells that recognize these HLA/peptide complexes and do they show particular characteristics, e.g. with respect to cytokine profile or TCR usage?

Faced with a spectrum of poorly understood autoimmune diseases, the best place to start would seem to be with one of the strongest and most indisputably reliable observations, the enhanced susceptibility among individuals carrying particular HLA alleles. Several groups have taken the view that since the HLA gene products confer enhanced disease risk, it is sensible to express the disease-related genes in transgenic mice and thus investigate mechanisms of susceptibility.[10] Since the HLA genes confer enhanced risk rather than acting as disease genes *per se*, it is not normally anticipated that HLA transgenic mice would spontaneously develop a disease associated with that allele. Indeed, that would be a misleading and unphysiological result: while many Type 1 diabetes patients have the DQ8 allele, most DQ8 individuals do not have Type 1 diabetes.[11] The goal of HLA transgenic experiments is to create laboratory strains that can better mimic the molecular interaction giving rise to the human disease and create a mouse showing enhanced susceptibility to the induction of disease compared with a non-transgenic or an HLA transgenic carrying an irrelevant allele.

Transgenic mice can be readily generated by cloning the gene of interest along with appropriate regulatory DNA sequences and microinjecting this construct into the pronucleus of a fertilized, single-cell embryo. Human genes are extremely variable in length, from tens to hundreds of kilobases (kb), encompassing a few or several exons. Cloning the gene of interest with respect to a given disease can therefore itself present a significant challenge. Many different cloning vectors derived from bacteria or yeast have been developed to allow the manipulation of isolated fragments of human DNA. Most of the HLA genes can be isolated within a stretch of 30–40 kb of DNA. The clone must encompass not just the coding exons but also the flanking, regulatory DNA regions. It is these regions of DNA that will bind specific DNA transcription factors in the nucleus of the cell, determining, for example, whether a particular HLA gene is strongly or weakly expressed in activated B-lymphocytes. In considering associations of HLA genes with disease, it is frequently overlooked that it is not just the protein-encoding DNA sequences that are polymorphic but also, in many cases, the upstream regulatory sequences, termed promoters. Thus, one cannot exclude the possibility that particular associations are observed because of regulatory features of a gene causing it to be strongly activated in a particular tissue during inflammation. This makes it important to try and work with genes that encompass all the flanking, regulatory DNA sequences, as they were organized in the human genome. Such constructs are referred to generically as genomic clones.

While many of the transgenic mice that have been generated use this approach, an alternative approach is to splice gene segments into multi-purpose cassettes. This approach is considerably easier but also has a number of drawbacks. A complementary DNA (cDNA) clone is synthesized by reverse-transcribing the messenger RNA from a human cell expressing the HLA gene of interest. Because this transcript contains only the information for making the protein from the RNA, all regulatory information from the flanking DNA sequences is lost and, along with it, all information on where and how to turn on transcription of the gene. This problem is solved by inserting the cDNA into an expression cassette, placing it alongside a stretch of

promoter sequence from a related, relevant gene, such as a murine MHC class II gene. In this way, one can generate transgenic mice with a pattern of gene expression which, in general, is reminiscent of MHC class I or class II patterns, although any specific variation resulting from promoter differences will have been lost. Furthermore, because cassettes of this type supply only a limited stretch of regulatory DNA, transgene constructs of this type are more prone to yielding lines with problems of low or inappropriate expression. Once the cloned human DNA has been produced and characterized, it is highly purified for microinjection into the oocytes. A proportion of the resulting offspring are born with the human sequence incorporated into the germline, generally as multiple copies integrated at a single, random site.

What can be achieved with such transgenic mice that cannot be achieved by studying patients' T-cell immune responses? HLA transgenics can be used to map the epitopes of candidate target antigens from self-tissues (or indeed from microbial and tumour antigens) recognized in the context of particular HLA alleles. The issue of disease susceptibility can be addressed by attempting to see if transgenic mice can be induced to develop pathology which is dependent on the expression of the gene associated with the human disease. In this way, transgenic mice can be used to evaluate the candidacy of supposedly disease-associated alleles. Transgenic models of this type can also be developed to encompass the inclusion of other implicated gene products, from human TCR to candidate genes identified in genome scans.

Many of these approaches have now been applied to the field of autoimmunity and other immunological diseases for some 15 years. The aim of this chapter is to review some of the transgenic experiments and assess their contribution to the unravelling of disease mechanisms.

2. HUMAN LEUCOCYTE ANTIGEN (HLA) DISEASE ASSOCIATIONS

An important (though sometimes overlooked) starting point for transgenic studies to model the role of HLA genes in disease is to obtain a firm idea of the specific, implicated genes. During the mid-1980s the advent of polymerase chain reaction (PCR) technology and automated DNA sequencing led to an explosion of information on HLA alleles.[12] This involved both the identification of hundreds of new alleles as well as attempts to determine which alleles were significantly overrepresented or underrepresented in particular disease groups compared with healthy, ethnically matched controls. Many diseases showed distinct HLA associations in different ethnic groups.[13,14] Associations of hundreds of diseases with the HLA region were identified, some of these probably fortuitous and some likely to be informative. Disease associations, weakly indicated by typing for broad serological HLA types, were strengthened and found to indicate association with a specific allelic sequence, a DNA sequence motif shared between a number of alleles or a gene linked to the serological marker.[15] For many years, the possibility remained that the observed HLA associations would turn out to indicate a primary association with some other, nearby, unidentified gene. However, the HLA region has now been entirely sequenced and, although the functions of many of the genes in the region are still unknown, the likelihood of finding new genes to explain old disease associations is much reduced.

For some HLA-associated diseases there is a high degree of confidence that a gene has been identified which has a causal role in susceptibility. In other cases, data point to a number of possible candidates in the HLA region but no specific culprit has been identified. Different regions of the HLA complex have been implicated in various diseases. Early studies often showed associations with HLA class I products, mainly because these were the serological specificities that could be tested. While some of the associations, such as those in Type 1 diabetes and immunoglobulin (Ig) A nephropathy, turned out to indicate associations with linked HLA class II genes, some diseases show clear associations with class I alleles. An example of this is the association of the spondyloarthropathies, specifically ankylosing spondylitis (AS), with HLA-B27.[16] Studies on HLA alleles in

the inflammatory arthritides consistently show a strong HLA-B27 effect, with relative risks of around 150. Because of the common role of specific infections such as *Klebsiella* and *Yersinia* in the aetiology of these diseases, much work has been done on the possibility of some form of preferential interaction between HLA-B27 and components of the infectious agents. Another hypothesis proposed molecular mimicry between components of these organisms and HLA-B27/peptide complexes. These possibilities remain open, as does a more recent model suggesting that the role of HLA-B27 in these diseases is a direct consequence of novel features of its folding and presentation at the cell surface.[17] Strong associations with HLA class I alleles are also seen, for example, in Behçets's syndrome (with HLA-B51) and chorioretinopathy (with HLA-A29).

Of the HLA class II molecules expressed at the cell surface, DP, DQ and DR, the majority of disease associations have been identified for the latter two products. It is unclear why relatively few diseases should be associated with HLA-DP, despite the facts that these products show a relatively high degree of polymorphism and act as presenting molecules for human CD4 T-cells. Linkage disequilibrium between HLA-DR and HLA-DQ can often make it difficult to verify whether a disease shows a primary association with one or other locus. For example, the vast majority of HLA-DR15 (formerly DR2) Caucasians are also DQ6, making it hard to determine whether susceptibility is likely to be conferred by some effect of the DR or DQ product.[18] There are three well-known associations with this DR15–DQ6 region: MS, Goodpasture's disease and narcolepsy.[18–20] There is also a strong negative association with Type 2 diabetes.[11] Of these, Goodpasture's disease is believed to involve a primary association with HLA-DR. This was surmised from comparison of sequence motifs in positively and negatively associated HLA-DR alleles.[19] The negative association in Type 1 diabetes is believed to be with the DQ locus on similar grounds.[11] MS has been more difficult to unravel: while the vast majority of T-cell clones against myelin components isolated from patients are DR15 restricted,[21] genetic studies consistently show a slight increase of DQ6 over DR15, implicating the DQ locus in the primary association.[18,22] This paradox highlights both the value and the pitfalls of designing genetically relevant transgenic experiments to investigate mechanisms in HLA-associated disease. This point is made even more compellingly by narcolepsy, a disease showing an overwhelming association with DQ6 which confers a relative risk of around 40, yet without good evidence for immune pathology and therefore lacking a strong hypothesis of disease susceptibility to test.[20] Rheumatoid arthritis (RA) shows a moderate association of around 4–9 with some of the subtypes of DR4.[23,24] It has been proposed that in this case the mechanism may involve the presentation to HLA-DQ-restricted T-cells of peptide from the hypervariable sequence of the DRβ chain itself. However, this model is difficult to reconcile with the lack of any primary association with HLA-DQ alleles.[25] The skin disease pemphigus vulgaris is also noteworthy in the context of HLA-DQ-1 and -DR-associated disease: the disease, which involves a relatively focused pathology caused by autoantibodies to skin desmoglein, is associated with either HLA-DR or HLA-DQ in different ethnic groups.[26–28]

The association of Type 1 diabetes with HLA-DQ has been the subject of much investigation. It has been proposed that the ranking of positively and negatively associated HLA-DQ alleles indicates a correlation whereby the positively associated alleles have a serine or valine at position 57 in the DQβ chain and the negatively associated alleles have an aspartamate.[11] Analysis of HLA class II crystals showed this amino acid residue to be critical for formation of a salt bridge with the DQα chain, this in turn determining the accessibility of the peptide-binding groove. An additional aspect of susceptibility to Type 1 diabetes is the enormously enhanced risk conferred by heterozygosity for DQB1*0302 and DQB1*0201, particularly in juvenile-onset disease.[29] A possible explanation for this is that there is formation of a disease-predisposing mixed heterodimer, generated in heterozygous individuals by pairing of the DQα chain from one haplotype with the DQβ chain from the other.[2]

It will be clear from the above that hopes of using HLA transgenic mouse models to elucidate simple disease pathways, whereby an implicated HLA allele automatically presents a self-peptide to self-reactive T-cells and so accounting for disease susceptibility, may be over optimistic. However, support for a simple relationship between the implicated HLA allele and disease comes from the study of coeliac disease.[30] While driven by the dietary antigen gluten, and thus not formally autoimmune, this intestinal disorder is T-cell mediated and associated with HLA-DQ2. HLA-DQ is strongly expressed at sites of tissue damage and abundant DQ2-restricted T-cells recognizing epitopes of gluten can be identified. At present, this represents the prototypic HLA-associated disease, having a strong genetic association and demonstrable T-cells restricted by that product and presumed to be pathogenic.

3. HUMAN LEUCOCYTE ANTIGEN (HLA) TRANSGENIC MICE

During the mid-1980s, advances in mammalian gene cloning, along with refinements in the techniques for making transgenic mice, made HLA transgenic mice possible. Initial experiments reflected the availability of the particular genes that had been cloned rather than the testing of any specific disease hypothesis. Thus, the first xenogeneic MHC transgenic experiment demonstrated expression of porcine MHC in a mouse.[31] Shortly after this, various HLA class I molecules were expressed in mice. The basic rules of expression were similar to other transgenic lines: the level of gene expression was correlated with the number of gene copies integrated into the genome, faithful tissue expression was largely dependent on the inclusion of upstream and downstream DNA regulatory sequences, and a proportion of transgene-positive founders turned out to be infertile or not to express the protein.

Early experiments with HLA class I and class II transgenic mice aimed to establish the usefulness of these mice for studying 'humanized' responses. Key questions were, whether the human molecules could function to present peptides to murine T-cells, whether this would depend on a species-matched interaction with CD4 or CD8, and whether the murine TCR repertoire and its plasticity would allow responses of similar specificity to the human HLA-restricted responses.[32–43] In general, HLA products function normally in the murine immune system and responses may be improved in the context of a species-matched CD4 or CD8 interaction but are not dependent on them. Where experiments were done to investigate whether the specificity of murine HLA-restricted responses showed similarities to the responses of humans carrying those HLA alleles, similarities were found.[36–39]

3.1 Mapping of HLA-restricted epitopes

An important foothold in understanding the pathogenesis of any autoimmune disease could be obtained by identifying those peptides from an implicated target antigen that constitute immunodominant T-cell epitopes. This has often proved difficult to achieve in patients due to several factors, including heterogeneity of genetic background and disease state. In some diseases, such as Type 1 diabetes, it may be that by the time the patient presents, much of the target tissue (in this case the pancreatic β-cells) has been destroyed and with it the antigen trigger-driving T-cell stimulation. In the case of MS, many myelin proteins have been considered as targets in disease, including myelin basic protein (MBP), proteolipoprotein (PLP), myelin oligodendrocyte glycoprotein (MOG) and αB-crystallin. Clearly, it would be of great value to know which are the HLA-DR15-presented immunodominant epitopes from these proteins, since these responses could then be investigated for their possible role in the events leading to MS. In fact, while many thousands of patients' T-cell responses have been investigated and some dominant responses identified, such as the DR15-restricted response to MBP 83–104,[21] it has been difficult to assemble any consensus.

HLA transgenic mice have now been extensively used for mapping HLA-restricted epitopes in infectious diseases such as tuberculosis, measles, hepatitis C and malaria, and in responses to self-antigens.[37,38,43–46] Responses to peptides spanning the amino acid sequence of self-antigens have been investigated for antigens including insulin and glutamic acid decarboxylase 65 (both implicated in Type 1 diabetes), and type II collagen and human cartilage glycoprotein-39 (HCgp-39) (both implicated in RA).[44,47–50] These studies are greatly helped by using HLA transgenic mice carrying a knockout mutation for endogenous MHC class II genes. Some groups have adopted the approach of immunizing mice with whole protein for the self-antigen, preparing T-cell hybridomas from the primed cells and then screening these for the frequency of clones recognizing specific peptides from the protein sequence.[44,48,50] Another approach is to immunize mice with pools of peptides covering the sequence of the antigen in question and then screen the response of *ex vivo* T-cells to each individual peptide. Several DQ8-restricted epitopes from GAD65 have been identified by these approaches and shown to overlap with the immunodominant epitopes recognized by patients with Type 1 diabetes expressing this allele.[51–53] The same approach used in DR4 transgenic mice identified different epitopes from this protein, restricted by HLA-DR4.[44] These HLA-DR4 transgenic mice were also used to identify epitopes from the HCgp-39 antigen implicated as a candidate autoantigen in RA.[50] Nine epitopes were identified, of which three were considered immunodominant. Most of the epitopes were recognized by T-cells from DR4+ RA patients and, on the whole, did not elicit responses from DR4+ or DR4– healthy controls.

3.2 Disease studies in HLA transgenics

This chapter opened with a discussion of autoimmune diseases as multifactorial in aetiology with HLA genes contributing one predisposing effect, albeit a strong one. It was therefore not anticipated that HLA transgenics would (or should) spontaneously develop autoimmune disease. It was thus a surprise when rats carrying a high-copy number of

HLA-B27 were found to develop pathology including inflammatory peripheral arthritis, inflammatory and fibrotic spinal lesions, and gastrointestinal inflammation.[54] Various experiments with HLA-B27 transgenic mice had failed to show any enhanced disease susceptibility. Since some models of arthritis, including adjuvant arthritis and streptococcal cell-wall arthritis, are more readily induced in rats, it was reasoned that rat transgenic models would be more useful than the mice. There were initial concerns that disease may be some form of non-physiological, transgene-integration artefact, since disease required the presence of some 40 or more copies of the transgene to be incorporated into the genome. However, the model withstands scrutiny since various high-copy number B27 transgenics develop disease while HLA-B7 controls do not.[55] This highlights the value of comparing an allele strongly associated with the human disease with another that is not, a point missed by many other studies. The subsequent application of the HLA-B27 transgenic rats to investigate the factors contributing to disease demonstrates some of the potential benefits of a transgenic approach for elucidating disease mechanisms. Rats that have been derived into a specific pathogen-free environment do not develop disease, allowing for the reintroduction of individual organisms to look at their effect.[56] Altering the rat strain background genes is also protective. Disease is transferable by bone-marrow-derived cells but is not dependent on transgenic expression in the thymus, suggesting a role for peripheral antigen presentation and T-cell responses, although not necessarily for thymic positive or negative selection.[57] Furthermore, overloading the transgenic HLA-B27 molecules with influenza peptide reduces the level of disease, suggesting that the HLA contribution to disease is indeed likely to be through conventional presentation of peptide.[55] Spontaneous inflammatory disease is seen also in HLA-A29 transgenic mice, which spontaneously develop a disease resembling chorioretinopathy.[58] In humans, this disease is strongly HLA-A29 associated, about 96% of patients carrying this allele compared with 7% of controls.

Among HLA class-II-associated disease, the well-documented association of Type 1 diabetes with DQ8 (encoded by the *DQB1*0302* gene) has made this interaction a subject of transgenic studies. Several groups analysed DQ8 transgenic mice that, unlike the examples described above, did not develop spontaneous autoimmune disease, irrespective of the genetic background used. It has been shown that the mice could be used to map the epitopes recognized in candidate target islet antigens, such as glutamic acid decarboxylase, and that patterns of recognition resembled those in DQ8 patients. T-cell lines specific for some GAD epitopes were able to transfer insulitis to recipient mice if the islets had been mildly damaged by pretreatment with suboptimal doses of the β-cell-damaging drug streptozotocin.[59] The idea that disease induction requires expression of the appropriate HLA molecule as well as some other stimulatory event is supported by a further study in HLA-DQ8 transgenic mice. These mice are not in themselves susceptible to spontaneous disease and nor are mice with transgenic expression of the co-stimulatory molecule B7-1 targeted to pancreatic β-cells. However, when the two lines are crossed, >80% of mice develop diabetes by 8 months of age.[60] This phenotype is not seen when the control allele, DQB1*0601, is used.

In MS, the association with HLA-DR15, -DQ6 and the need to establish whether central nervous system (CNS) damage could be due to the frequently observed response to MBP 83–104 or some other myelin candidate antigen such as MOG or αB-crystallin, have been a trigger for transgenic studies. A recurrent conundrum in studies using this approach is the interpretation of experiments that lean on the modulation of pre-existing, experimentally induced mouse models. The mouse model for MS is EAE. This model depends on injecting susceptible inbred mouse strains, such as SJL or B10.PL, with two doses of myelin antigen in adjuvant, followed by doses of pertussis toxin. The model has been invaluable for the basic principles of autoimmune disease that have been learnt from it. At the same time, there are concerns about the histopathological verity of the model alongside the human CNS changes.

Experiments in which details of the experimental disease profile are altered by superimposing the effect of an HLA transgene on the mouse model can be difficult to interpret in the context of the human disease.

In murine models of autoimmunity, spontaneous disease can be observed in transgenic mice that have been made transgenic for expression of a TCR derived from autoreactive T-cells. This approach has been applied by various groups to investigate spontaneous disease in double HLA and TCR humanized transgenics. Mice were made that expressed HLA-DR15 as well as an MS T-cell-derived TCR specific for MBP 84–102 presented by DR15.[61] A minority of mice developed spontaneous CNS lesions, although disease could be efficiently induced by injection of peptide and pertussis toxin. These effects can be seen in mice strains that are usually resistant to EAE.

4. CONCLUSIONS

Hundreds of diseases have been reported to show associations with specific HLA alleles. In some cases, the effects can be very pronounced, such that an individual with one allele carrying 50 or 100 times the disease risk of an individual with another allele. In an attempt to define some of the molecular and cellular events that may underpin these associations, the HLA genes implicated in many diseases have been cloned and expressed in transgenic mice. These HLA genes function normally within the murine immune system and can thus be used to identify the immunodominant epitopes within candidate target antigens that may be recognized during the pathogenic, autoimmune response. The approach can then be used to study disease susceptibility *in vivo* and the other factors that may contribute to it. However, from genome scans, it is clear that HLA genes may constitute only one region (albeit the strongest) out of 10–20 genetic regions contributing to overall disease susceptibility. The other autoimmunity-predisposing genes may include polymorphic variants of cytokine genes and co-stimulatory molecules, as well as currently unknown genes. Transgenic, humanized disease models offer an

exciting possibility for building up a composite picture of each of the genes contributing to a complex disease process, and thereby designing new therapies that will be able to selectively suppress the pathogenic process without causing widespread immunosuppression.

GLOSSARY

Allele	The variant sequence of a gene carried at a particular, polymorphic locus.
Complementary DNA (cDNA)	A gene construct which has been synthesized by translating messenger RNA into the complementary DNA sequence, thus containing only protein-coding sequences, in the absence of any regulatory DNA sequences.
Genome scan	Analysis of genomic DNA from disease-affected families using polymorphic markers distributed across all the chromosomes to identify regions associated with disease.
Human leucocyte antigen (HLA) class II	The region within the HLA complex containing the cell-surface expressed heterodimers, HLA-DP, -DQ and -DR that are involved in peptide presentation to CD4 T-lymphocytes. The region also contains intracellular molecules involved in peptide processing and presentation such as HLA-DM and LMP2.
Human leucocyte antigen (HLA) disease associations	The observations that some diseases show a positive or negative association with particular HLA alleles.
Human leucocyte antigen (HLA)-DQ	An HLA class II heterodimer, poorly expressed compared to

HLA-DR, but implicated in susceptibility to a number of diseases including Type 1 diabetes and coeliac disease.

Human leucocyte antigen (HLA)-DR An HLA class II heterodimer used for antigenic peptide presentation to CD4 T-cells and implicated in susceptibility to a number of diseases including rheumatoid arthritis and Goodpasture's disease.

Knockout mouse Mouse strain mutated to lose expression of a specific protein through targeted disruption of the corresponding gene.

Linkage disequilibrium The co-inheritance of genes which are near each other in the genome and between which recombination rarely occurs.

Major histocompatibility complex (MHC) Generic term for the genetic region containing the class I, class II, class III and other immune-response genes. Known in humans as the HLA region and in mice as the H-2 region.

Polymorphism The existence of multiple alleles at a particular locus, thus giving rise to genetic variability.

Promoter DNA sequence found upstream of the part encoding the protein itself and which carries sites responsible for turning on and regulating expression of the protein in appropriate tissues.

T-cell epitope The peptidic sequences from within the sequence of a protein found to be recognized by T-lymphocytes.

T-cell receptor (TCR) The clonotype-specific, heterodimeric receptor (formed either by an αβ pair or by a γδ pair) used by the kT-cell to recognize antigenic peptides presented in the context of MHC molecules.

Transgenic mouse Mouse strain that expresses a new protein or proteins due to the integration of a foreign DNA sequence in the germline.

REFERENCES

Scientific papers

1. Altmann DM, Sansom D, Marsh SG. What is the basis for HLA-DQ associations with autoimmune disease? *Immunol Today* 1991; **12**: 267–70.
2. Nepom GT, Erlich H. MHC class-II molecules and autoimmunity. *Annu Rev Immunol* 1991; **9**: 493–525.
3. Altmann DM. HLA-DQ associations with autoimmune disease. *Autoimmunity* 1992; **14**: 79–83.
4. Todd JA, Acha-Orbea H, Bell JI et al. A molecular basis for MHC class II–associated autoimmunity. *Science* 1988; **240**: 1003–9.
5. Thorsby E, Lundin KE, Ronningen KS et al. Molecular basis and functional importance of some disease-associated HLA polymorphisms. *Tiss Antigens* 1989; **34**: 39–49.
6. Thorsby E. Invited anniversary review: HLA associated diseases. *Hum Immunol* 1997; **53**: 1–11.
7. Wicker LS, Todd JA, Peterson LB. Genetic control of autoimmune diabetes in the NOD mouse. *Annu Rev Immunol* 1995; **13**: 179–200.
8. Sundvall M, Jirholt J, Yang, HT et al. Identification of murine loci associated with susceptibility to chronic experimental autoimmune encephalomyelitis. *Nature Genet* 1995; **10**: 313–7.
9. Nicholson LB, Greer JM, Sobel RA et al. An altered peptide ligand mediates immune deviation and prevents autoimmune encephalomyelitis. *Immunity* 1995; **3**: 397–405.
10. Schwartz BD. HLA class II transgenic mice: the chance to unravel the basis of HLA class II associations with disease. *J Exp Med* 1994; **180**: 11–13.
11. Todd JA, Bell JI, McDevitt HO. HLA-DQ beta gene contributes to susceptibility and resistance

to insulin-dependent diabetes mellitus. *Nature* 1987; **329**: 599–604.

12. Marsh SG. 1998 HLA class II region sequences. *Tiss Antigens* 1998; **51**: 467–507.

13. Todd JA, Mijovic C, Fletcher J et al. Identification of susceptibility loci for insulin-dependent diabetes mellitus by trans-racial gene mapping. *Nature* 1989; **338**: 587–9.

14. Marrosu MG, Murru MR, Costa G et al. DRB1–DQA1–DQB1 loci and multiple sclerosis predisposition in the Sardinian population. *Hum Molec Genet* 1998; **7**: 1235–7.

15. Vartdal F, Sollid LM, Vandvik B et al. Patients with multiple sclerosis carry DQB1 genes which encode shared polymorphic amino acid sequences. *Hum Immunol* 1989; **25**: 103–10.

16. Brown M, Wordsworth P. Predisposing factors to spondyloarthropathies. *Curr Opin Rheumatol* 1997; **9**: 308–14.

17. Allen RL, Bowness P, McMichael A. The role of HLA-B27 in spondyloarthritis. *Immunogenetics* 1999; **50**: 220–7.

18. Spurkland A, Ronningen KS, Vandvik B et al. HLA-DQA1 and HLA-DQB1 genes may jointly determine susceptibility to develop multiple sclerosis. *Hum Immunol* 1991; **30**: 69–75.

19. Phelps RG, Rees AJ. The HLA complex in Goodpasture's disease: a model for analyzing susceptibility to autoimmunity. *Kidney Int* 1999; **56**: 1638–53.

20. Mignot E, Tafti M, Dement WC, Grumet FC. Narcolepsy and immunity. *Adv Neuroimmunol* 1995; **5**: 23–37.

21. Ota K, Matsui M, Milford EL et al. T-cell recognition of an immunodominant myelin basic protein epitope in multiple sclerosis. *Nature* 1990; **346**: 183–7.

22. Serjeantson SW, Gao X, Hawkins BR et al. Novel HLA-DR2-related haplotypes in Hong Kong Chinese implicate the DQB1*0602 allele in susceptibility to multiple sclerosis. *Eur J Immunogenet* 1992; **19**: 11–9

23. Fugger L, Svejgaard A. Association of MHC and rheumatoid arthritis. HLA-DR4 and rheumatoid arthritis: studies in mice and men. *Arthritis Res* 2000; **2**: 208–11.

24. Holmdahl R, Andersson EC, Andersen CB et al. Transgenic mouse models of rheumatoid arthritis. *Immunol Rev* 1999; **169**: 161–73.

25. Fugger L, Svejgaard A. HLA-DQ7 and -DQ8 associations in DR4-positive rheumatoid arthritis patients. A combined analysis of data available in the literature. *Tiss Antigens* 1997; **50**: 494–500.

26. Sinha AA, Brautbar C, Szafer F et al. A newly characterized HLA DQ beta allele associated with pemphigus vulgaris. *Science* 1988; **239**: 1026–9.

27. Scharf SJ, Freidmann A, Steinman L et al. Specific HLA-DQB and HLA-DRB1 alleles confer susceptibility to pemphigus vulgaris. *Proc Natl Acad Sci USA.* 1989; **86**: 6215–19.

28. Miyagawa S, Amagai M, Niizeki H et al. HLA-DRB1 polymorphisms and autoimmune responses to desmogleins in Japanese patients with pemphigus. *Tiss Antigens* 1999; **54**: 333–40.

29. Caillat-Zucman S, Garchon HJ, Timsit J et al. Age-dependent HLA genetic heterogeneity of type 1 insulin-dependent diabetes mellitus. *J Clin Invest* 1992; **90**: 2242–50.

30. Sollid LM. Molecular basis of celiac disease. *Annu Rev Immunol* 2000; **18**: 53–81.

31. Frels WI, Bluestone JA, Hodes RJ et al. Expression of a microinjected porcine class I major histocompatibility complex gene in transgenic mice. *Science* 1985; **228**: 577–80.

32. Kalinke U, Arnold B, Hammerling GJ. Strong xenogeneic HLA response in transgenic mice after introducing an alpha 3 domain into HLA B27. *Nature* 1990; **348**: 642–4.

33. Engelhard VH, Lacy E, Ridge JP. Influenza A-specific, HLA-A2.1-restricted cytotoxic T lymphocytes from HLA-A2.1 transgenic mice recognize fragments of the M1 protein. *J Immunol* 1991; **146**: 1226–32.

34. Vitiello A, Marchesini D, Furze J et al. Analysis of the HLA-restricted influenza-specific cytotoxic T lymphocyte response in transgenic mice carrying a chimeric human-mouse class I major histocompatibility complex. *J Exp Med* 1991; **173**: 1007–15.

35. Kievits F, Ivanyi P, Krimpenfort P et al. HLA-restricted recognition of viral antigens in HLA transgenic mice. *Nature* 1987; **329**: 447–9.

36. Man S, Ridge JP, Engelhard VH. Diversity and dominance among TCR recognizing HLA-A2.1+ influenza matrix peptide in human MHC class I transgenic mice. *J Immunol* 1994; **153**: 4458–67.

37. Shirai M, Arichi T, Nishioka M et al. CTL responses of HLA-A2.1-transgenic mice specific for hepatitis C viral peptides predict epitopes for CTL of humans carrying HLA-A2.1. *J Immunol* 1995; **154**: 2733–42.

38. Blum-Tirouvanziam U, Servis C, Habluetzel A et al. Localization of HLA-A2.1-restricted T cell epitopes in the circumsporozoite protein of *Plasmodium falciparum*. *J Immunol* 1995; **154**: 3922–31.

39. Wentworth PA, Vitiello A, Sidney J et al. Differences and similarities in the A2.1-restricted cytotoxic T cell repertoire in humans and human leukocyte antigen-transgenic mice. *Eur J Immunol* 1996; **26**: 97–101.

40. Yamamoto K, Fukui Y, Esaki Y et al. Functional interaction between human histocompatibility leukocyte antigen (HLA) class II and mouse CD4 molecule in antigen recognition by T cells in HLA-DR and DQ transgenic mice. *J Exp Med* 1994; **180**: 165–71.

41. Altmann DM, Douek DC, Frater AJ et al. The T cell response of HLA-DR transgenic mice to human myelin basic protein and other antigens in the presence and absence of human CD4. *J Exp Med* 1995; **181**: 867–75.

42. Woods A, Chen HY, Trumbauer ME et al. Human major histocompatibility complex class II-restricted T cell responses in transgenic mice. *J Exp Med* 1994; **180**: 173–81.

43. Tishon A, LaFace DM, Lewicki H et al. Transgenic mice expressing human HLA and CD8 molecules generate HLA-restricted measles virus cytotoxic T lymphocytes of the same specificity as humans with natural measles virus infection. *Virology* 2000; **275**: 286–93.

44. Patel SD, Cope AP, Congia M et al. Identification of immunodominant T cell epitopes of human glutamic acid decarboxylase 65 by using HLA-DR(alpha1*0101,beta1*0401) transgenic mice. *Proc Natl Acad Sci USA* 1997; **94**: 8082–7.

45. Geluk A, Taneja V, van Meijgaarden KE et al. Identification of HLA class II-restricted determinants of *Mycobacterium tuberculosis*-derived proteins by using HLA-transgenic, class II-deficient mice. *Proc Natl Acad Sci USA* 1998; **95**: 10,797–802.

46. Geluk A, van Meijgaarden KE, Franken KL et al. Identification of major epitopes of *Mycobacterium tuberculosis* AG85B that are recognized by HLA-A*0201-restricted CD8+ T cells in HLA-transgenic mice and humans. *J Immunol* 2000; **165**: 6463–71.

47. Andersson EC, Hansen BE, Jacobsen H et al. Definition of MHC and T cell receptor contacts in the HLA-DR4 restricted immunodominant epitope in type II collagen and characterization of collagen-induced arthritis in HLA-DR4 and human CD4 transgenic mice. *Proc Natl Acad Sci USA* 1998; **95**: 7574–9.

48. Congia M, Patel S, Cope AP et al. T cell epitopes of insulin defined in HLA-DR4 transgenic mice are derived from preproinsulin and proinsulin. *Proc Natl Acad Sci USA* 1998; **95**: 3833–8.

49. Wicker LS, Chen SL, Nepom GT et al. Naturally processed T cell epitopes from human glutamic acid decarboxylase identified using mice transgenic for the type 1 diabetes-associated human MHC class II allele, DRB1*0401. *J Clin Invest* 1996; **98**: 2597–603.

50. Cope AP, Patel SD, Hall F et al. T cell responses to a human cartilage autoantigen in the context of rheumatoid arthritis-associated and nonassociated HLA-DR4 alleles. *Arthritis Rheum* 1999; **42**: 1497–507.

51. Herman AE, Tisch RM, Patel SD et al. Determination of glutamic acid decarboxylase 65 peptides presented by the type I diabetes-associated HLA-DQ8 class II molecule identifies an immunogenic peptide motif. *J Immunol* 1999; **163**: 6275–82.

52. Boyton RJ, Lohmann T, Londei M et al. Glutamic acid decarboxylase T lymphocyte responses associated with susceptibility or resistance to type I diabetes: analysis in disease discordant human twins, non-obese diabetic mice and HLA-DQ transgenic mice. *Int Immunol* 1998; **10**: 1765–76.

53. Liu J, Purdy LE, Rabinovitch S et al. Major DQ8-restricted T-cell epitopes for human GAD65 mapped using human CD4, DQA1*0301, DQB1*0302 transgenic IA(null) NOD mice. *Diabetes* 1999; **48**: 469–77.

54. Hammer RE, Maika SD, Richardson JA et al. Spontaneous inflammatory disease in transgenic rats expressing HLA-B27 and human β2m: an animal model of HLA-B27-associated human disorders. *Cell* 1990; **63**: 1099–112.

55. Taurog JD, Maika SD, Satumtira N et al. Inflammatory disease in HLA-B27 transgenic rats. *Immunol Rev* 1999; **169**: 209–23.

56. Taurog JD, Richardson JA, Croft JT et al. The germfree state prevents development of gut and joint inflammatory disease in HLA-B27 transgenic rats. *J Exp Med* 1994; **180**: 2359–64.

57. Breban M, Hammer RE, Richardson JA, Taurog JD. Transfer of the inflammatory disease of HLA-B27 transgenic rats by bone marrow engraftment. *J Exp Med* 1993; **178**: 1607–16.

58. Szpak Y, Vieville JC, Tabary T et al. Spontaneous retinopathy in HLA-A29 transgenic mice. *Proc Natl Acad Sci USA* 2001; **98**: 2572–6.

59. Wen L, Wong FS, Burkly L et al. Induction of insulitis by glutamic acid decarboxylase peptide-specific and HLA-DQ8-restricted CD4(+) T cells from human DQ transgenic mice. *J Clin Invest* 1998; **102**: 947–57.

60. Wen L, Wong FS, Tang J et al. *In vivo* evidence for the contribution of human histocompatibility leukocyte antigen (HLA)-DQ molecules to the development of diabetes. *J Exp Med* 2000; **191**: 97–104.

61. Madsen LS, Andersson EC, Jansson L et al. A humanized model for multiple sclerosis using HLA-DR2 and a human T-cell receptor. *Nature Genet* 1999; **23**: 343–7.

2

Manipulating cytokine networks in autoimmunity

Andrew P Cope

Objectives • Overview • Introduction • Historical background • Classification of cytokines and their receptors • Cytokine biology • Cytokines in immunity and host defence • Evaluating the role of cytokines in autoimmunity • Manipulating cytokine networks in autoimmunity as illustrated through tumour necrosis factor blockade • Use of other biologicals to manipulate cytokine networks in rheumatoid arthritis • Conclusions • References

OBJECTIVES

(1) To review the biology of cytokines and how they influence immune function in health and disease.

(2) To demonstrate how cytokine networks are controlled in the prototypic inflammatory disease, rheumatoid arthritis (RA); in particular to show how a single cytokine, tumour necrosis factor-alpha, may contribute to a cascade of pathological events in RA.

OVERVIEW

Cytokine biology has made significant advances over the past two decades. The achievements have come about through a combination of new technologies and rigorous experimentation, culminating in the development and subsequent marketing of a new generation of therapeutics. Understanding the molecular basis of cytokine networks in the context of chronic inflammatory and autoimmune diseases is perhaps best illustrated by the recent successes of targeting proinflammatory cytokines in the prototypic chronic inflammatory disease, rheumatoid arthritis. On the one hand, the clinical response to this therapeutic approach has challenged current concepts of cytokine function, hierarchies and redundancy, while on the other hand it has provided unique opportunities for investigators to explore cytokine networks and their role in health and disease directly in humans.

1. INTRODUCTION

To begin to understand the complexities of soluble messenger molecules such as cytokines in human biology requires a broad knowledge not only of innate and acquired immunity, but of the specific interactions between the two. Since the immune system has evolved primarily to combat the universe of foreign pathogens, it comes as no surprise that the same defence systems should be deployed during the evolution and resolution of inflammatory diseases.

Indeed, the overlap, in histopathological terms, between infection and inflammation is well documented. Nevertheless, the real issue has become not what switches on and sustains the inflammatory process, so much as what mechanisms, in a non-susceptible host, turn an acute inflammatory process off. If we can understand in depth the molecular mechanisms of homeostasis, then we will have made significant progress towards solving the defects of the host immune system when things go wrong.

Manipulating cytokine networks has a lot to do with understanding the balance between proinflammatory and anti-inflammatory mediators. The specific diseases themselves matter less, since the players are pretty much the same. To begin to study this stimulating field of medical research, it is worth exploring how cytokines were first identified, how cytokine and receptor families have expanded and evolved, and how structure and function account for the unique biological characteristics of these cell messenger molecules, as distinct from hormones. Understanding the role of cytokines and their expression profiles in host defence provides insight into the pathogenesis of chronic inflammation. Analysis of patterns of cytokine expression in the laboratory, and manipulation of their expression *in vitro* and *in vivo*, have become the tools of the trade.

Finally, to illustrate the complexities of cytokine networks in humans described in some depth herein are the processes of experimentation through which tumour necrosis factor-alpha (TNF-α) was identified as a therapeutic target in rheumatoid arthritis (RA), and how the 'definitive' experiments were subsequently carried out in controlled clinical trials in patients. Readers are encouraged to go on to sample some of the excellent reviews published to date which describe the progress made in exploring cytokine networks in other autoimmune diseases, such as multiple sclerosis and Type 1 diabetes.

2. HISTORICAL BACKGROUND

Although the term cytokine was first coined by Cohen in 1974[1], cell-derived soluble factors were appreciated as far back as the early 1960s, when immunologists demonstrated the presence of lymphocyte-derived factors whose specific *in vitro* characteristics generated their initial descriptive names. In response to mitogen, and in subsequent studies the mixed lymphocyte reaction or antigen stimulation, lymphocytes produced newly synthesized mitogenic and blastogenic factors [lymphocyte mitogenic factor (LMF) and blastogenic factor (BF), respectively] which promoted cell growth,[2] and cytotoxins which induced cell death.[3] During the 1970s, the term lymphokine was first introduced to describe these soluble lymphocyte-derived factors. Soon after these initial reports, experiments revealed that non-lymphoid cells, such as monocytes and macrophages, produced factors with specific functions, e.g. lymphocyte activation factor (LAF) *in vitro*[4] and endogenous pyrogen (EP) activity *in vivo*.[5] From 1979, the generic term interleukin (IL) was subsequently introduced to classify these factors (reviewed in Oppenheim and Gery[6]). BF/LMF were found to include IL-2 and the endogenous pyrogen IL-1. Other soluble factors were soon identified, including the colony-stimulating factors (CSF) and interferons (IFN), but these cytokines kept their names.

The 1980s, the era of molecular cloning, brought with it a huge expansion in the molecular characterization of cytokines including the IFN,[7-9] the first receptors, including IL-2Rα,[10] cytokines with suppressive functions such as TGF-β[11] and IL-10,[12] and the neutrophil chemoattractants or chemokines, NAP-1 and IL-8.[13,14] Following initial high-performance liquid chromatography (HPLC) purification and sequencing, the molecular cloning of these factors made it possible to group cytokines according to structural homology, as well as by function. In more recent years these families have expanded through the identification of homologues encoded not only by mammalian genes but also by viruses (reviewed in MacFadden et al[15]).

It soon became clear that large families of such factors existed. As such, these factors came to be defined as soluble extracellular proteins that act locally to regulate innate and adaptive immunity through effects on cell activation and growth, differentiation and repair processes. Many functions could be ascribed to restoring homeostasis and, as such, formed an integral component of host defence. This definition has changed little, although it has become appreciated that there exist a significant number of cytokines which function as cell-surface molecules and, in a few instances, as intracellular ligands.

3. CLASSIFICATION OF CYTOKINES AND THEIR RECEPTORS

To facilitate discussion, examples of cytokine and receptor families are included, listed according to structure and/or function for cytokines in Table 2.1, and illustrated according to homology for receptors in Figure 2.1.

4. CYTOKINE BIOLOGY

Well over 150 cytokines have been characterized, each structurally distinct on the one hand, while sharing receptors and signalling pathways on the other. This large number raises several important questions which have puzzled immunologists for decades. Do cytokines contribute to physiological processes in a unique way or is there redundancy? This can best be appreciated with an understanding of cytokine structure and function, as well as an analysis of specific characteristics that distinguish groups of cytokines from other mediators.[16,17]

4.1 Structure and biological activity

Cytokines can exist as small molecules, e.g. such as chemokines of 8–10 kDa molecular weight, or may exist as larger oligomers, such as IFN-γ, IL-8 and IL-10, which are homodimers. In contrast, TNF-α is active as a homotrimer, while lymphotoxin (LT) exists as both homotrimers (LT-α_3) and heterotrimers (LT-$\alpha_1\beta_2$). Higher oligomers may also exist, such as platelet factor-4 and IL-16. Many cytokines are glycosylated and may be produced by many cells of both haematopoietic and non-haematopoietic origin. They are pleiotropic in that they interact with a broad range of cellular targets and may exert multiple

Table 2.1 Examples of cytokine families according to structure and/or function

IL-1 family	TNF family	IL-6 family
IL-1α	TNF-α	IL-6
IL-1β	LTα, β	IL-11
IL-1Ra	FasL	oncostatin M
IL-18	CD27L	CT-1
	CD30L	
Interferons	CD40L	Growth and
	TWEAK	angiogenic factors
IFN-α	RANKL	
IFN-β	APRIL	TGF-β
IFN-γ	TRAIL	BMPs
	LIGHT	PDGF
		VEGF

Immunomodulatory	Chemokines	
IL-2	CXC	CC and CX3C
IL-4	MGSA/Gro	MCP-1-5
IL-7	ENA-78	RANTES
IL-9	IL-8	I-309
IL-10	GCP-2	MIP-1α, β, γ
IL-12	CTAP III	eotaxin 1 and 2
IL-13	βTG	TARC
IL-15	NAP-2	SLC
IL-16	IP-10	ELC
IL-17	MIG	Lymphotactin
	SDF-1	Fractalkine

Haematopoetic factors		
IL-3	GM-CSF	
IL-5	CSF-1	
EPO	G-CSF	

effects. The spectrum of cytokines produced by a single cell type will depend not only on the stimulus but also on the state of the cell, whether it is in a resting or activated state, and the phase of the cell cycle. The presence of other factors, either soluble or bound to the cell surface of neighbouring cells signalling through

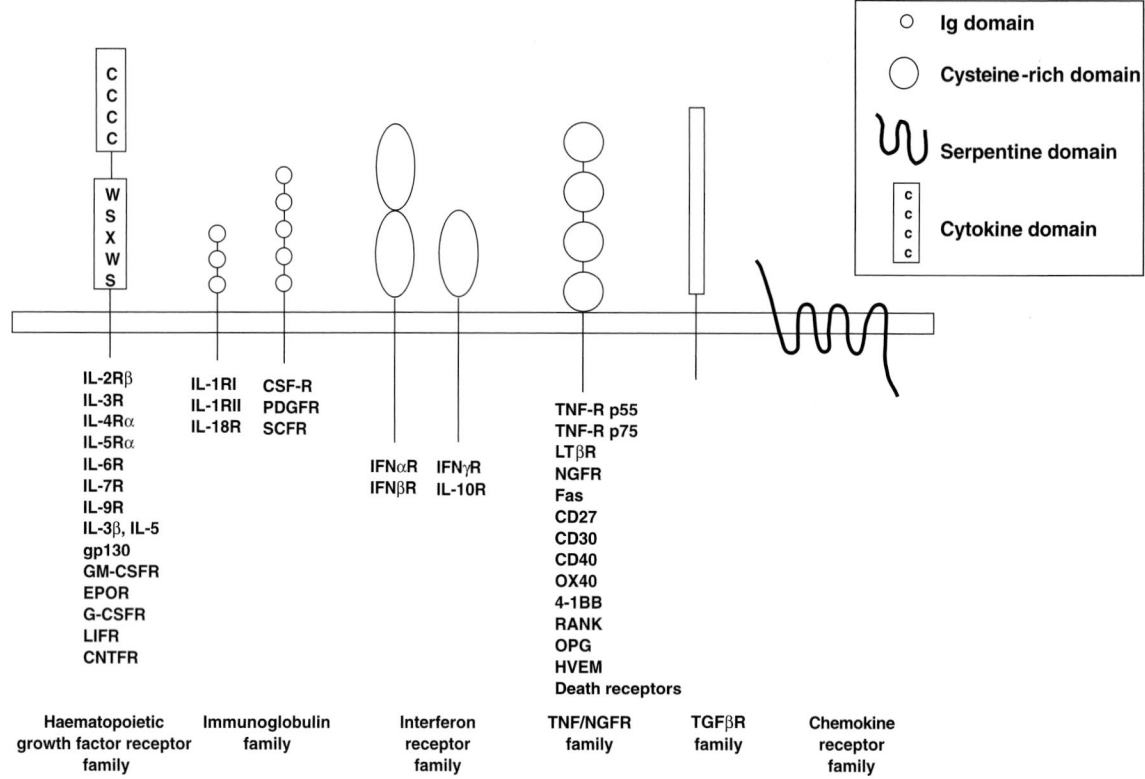

Fig. 2.1 Cytokine receptor families. There are six main families of cytokine receptor, based upon structural homology of the extracellular domains.

cell to cell (juxtacrine) mechanisms, is also important. Extensive analysis of cytokine expression *in vitro* and, more importantly, *in vivo* has revealed that, with few exceptions, cytokines are expressed during physiological responses over periods of hours, while chronic sustained expression is characteristic of pathological disease states. In other words, cytokine expression is inducible rather than constitutive.

Another key characteristic is that cytokines act locally (either in an autocrine or paracrine fashion) and, with few exceptions, are inactive in serum or plasma. This is due in part to their relatively short half-life. Their highly specific biological activity is facilitated by their expression at nmol–fmol concentrations *in vivo*, by their binding to specific receptors at high affinity [dissociation constant (K_d) nmol–fmol], and by their ability to signal biological responses at low receptor occupancy (e.g. ~ 10%). Together, these characteristics distinguish the majority of cytokines from hormones. The differences are summarized in Table 2.2. Exceptions to these trends are haematopoietic growth factors, including IL-6, CSF and EPO, which share characteristics with both cytokines and hormones. Recently, it has become more apparent that a subset of cytokines and growth factors are maintained in tissues through binding to extracellular matrix proteins either on the cell surface or in the extracellular compartment. These may become activated or processed following a stimulus such as trauma. This appears to provide another means whereby the host can respond rapidly to its environment. Critically, cytokine expression and their responses are tightly regulated. This avoids sustained expression and the potential for aberrant signalling and the promotion of pathological responses such as chronic inflammation.[18]

Table 2.2 Biological characteristics that distinguish cytokines from hormones

	Cytokines	Hormones
Site of action	Local	Distant
Cell source	Many cell types	Specialized cells
Biosynthesis	Inducible, transient	Constitutive, sustained
Half-life	Short (minutes)	Long (hours to days)
Activity in serum/plasma	Inactive	Active

4.2 Analysis of cytokine expression *in vitro* and *in vivo*

Within a very short time of the molecular cloning and identification of cytokines, workers developed assays to measure the expression of cytokines *in vitro* and *in vivo* with the aim of developing greater understanding of pathological processes.[18] Indeed, data soon suggested that expression levels might correlate with a disease state, or the stage and progression of a particular disease. If expression was anomalous, this provided potential therapeutic targets for evaluation. Since cytokines had not conventionally been detected at significant levels in the body fluids or tissues of healthy individuals, huge effort was made to develop highly sensitive techniques for studying gene and protein expression.

Table 2.2 lists some of the experimental approaches that, in many laboratories, have become routine. In general, the bioassay has become the gold standard, being much more sensitive, though less specific, than an immunoassay. More recently, the development of real-time polymerase chain reaction (PCR)-

Table 2.3 Analysis of cytokine expression

Cytokine detection

1. Biological fluids (serum, cerebrospinal fluid, bronchoalveolar lavage fluid, synovial fluid)
   - immunoassays (e.g. ELISA, RIA)
   - bioassays (e.g. proliferation, cytotoxicity, chemotaxis, induction of protein expression)

2. Cells or cell cultures (primary cells or cell lines – *ex vivo* or *in vitro*)
   - secreted factors   ELISA, RIA, ELISPOT
   - cell surface factors   flow cytometry
   - intracellular factors   flow cytometry, Northern analysis, RPA, *in situ* hybridization, RT-PCR, real-time PCR and microarrays for cytokine profiling

3. Tissue
   - immunohistochemistry
   - immunoblotting from tissue homogenates
   - mRNA (see above)

ELISA, enzyme linked immunoadsorbent assay; RIA, radioimmunoassay; RPA, ribonuclease protection assay; RT-PCR, reverse transcriptase polymerase chain reaction.

based assays has vastly improved sensitivity and quantification at the mRNA level. For protein, intracellular assays for cytokine expression can be analysed by flow cytometry, providing opportunities to identify unequivocally the cell source of the factor under study – particularly important where the number of cells derived from tissues may be limiting. For more details, refer to Oppenheim and Feldmann.[17]

5. CYTOKINES IN IMMUNITY AND HOST DEFENCE

Cytokines are pleiotropic. This means that they have multiple targets and can have multiple effects on different cells. Therefore, it is not surprising that as a group of soluble factors they can influence fundamental biological processes such as cell growth and differentiation, and programmed cell death (known as apoptosis), as well as play key roles in haematopoiesis, inflammation, angiogenesis, fibrosis and repair. On the one hand, many of these effects are beneficial, contributing to host defence to foreign pathogens, targeting infected cells, mounting an efficient effector response and orchestrating repair of damaged tissue. On the other hand, there exists great potential for inducing tissue damage if these processes become uncontrolled. This is perhaps best illustrated in the context of host immunity.

5.1 Role of cytokines in innate immunity

Cytokines provide an essential effector arm to combat infection, and are secreted in conjunction with other soluble and cellular components of the innate immune system. Their expression is induced by microbial products, perhaps the best characterized being lipopolysaccharide (LPS), a component of bacterial cell walls.[19] Indeed, LPS is one of the most potent inducers of inflammatory cytokines such as IL-1β, TNF-α and IL-6 following activation of macrophages.[20] The cytokine expression profile has direct clinical correlates. For example, expression of IL-1β, TNF-α, IL-6 and IFN-γ in the systemic circulation contributes to fever, myalgia, arthralgia, anorexia and anaemia,[21] while in severe infections, such as septic shock, their expression can

lead to hypotension, ischaemia and tissue necrosis.[22] Cytokines of the IL-6 family, such as IL-6 itself, oncostatin M, LIF and IL-11, are thought to be major players in the induction of an acute phase response, where proteins such as C-reactive protein (CRP) are overproduced.[23] Animal models have played an important role in identifying the soluble factors that coordinate these pathophysiological processes and have been central to exploring the efficacy of blocking cytokine activity *in vivo*.[24]

5.2 Role of cytokines in acquired immunity

The acquired or adaptive immune system contributes to host defence through the induction of highly specific responses to foreign proteins or antigens, with increased speed of onset and magnitude of responses with subsequent exposure to the foreign protein. The principal effector responses are mediated through the actions of antibodies produced by B-lymphocytes and of lymphocyte-derived cytokines (lymphokines), such as IFN-γ, produced by T-cells. The outcome of antigen-specific stimulation of lymphocytes via specific antigens is greatly influenced by the local cytokine microenvironment, produced by both lymphocytes and inflammatory cells. This microenviroment can determine the programme of lymphocyte differentiation, proliferation and effector responses, which follows antigen-specific stimulation.

The process of differentiation has been studied extensively and has led to a paradigm where activation and differentiation of particular T-cell and B-cell subsets leads to quite distinct patterns of effector response, depending on the profile of cytokines expressed.[25] For example, T-cells which produce IL-2, IFN-γ and LT are designated type 1 helper T-cells (Th1). Th1 play a role in defence against intracellular pathogens. T-cells producing IL-4, IL-5 and IL-13, designated type 2 helper T-cells (Th2) drive B-cell antibody-mediated responses. While the specific subsets of T-cell effectors that are generated are useful for purposes of discussion and experimentation, it is the overall cytokine profile, rather than a particular T-cell subset and surface-membrane phenotype, which dictates the nature of the immune response. Nevertheless, the model has proved useful for exploring the extent to which T-cell responses become polarized in different diseases, and the mechanisms of initiation, commitment and gene transcription which characterize Th polarization. The role of subset specific transcription factors such as GATA-3, T-bet and the nuclear factor for activating of T-cells (NFAT) are of particular importance (Figure 2.2). Indeed, this model has led to some conditions being labelled as Th1 diseases (e.g. Type 1 diabetes, RA, Hashimoto's thyroiditis) or Th2 diseases (e.g. atopy and asthma). From a therapeutic viewpoint, Th1 and Th2 responses are reciprocally regulated, opening up ways to divert the immune response away from one that might be detrimental to the host (Fig. 2.2). There is also great interest in the

transcriptional regulation, as well as the genetic basis, of Th differentiation.[26,27] In particular, the possibility that functional polymorphisms of genes directly involved in exaggerated, or inappropriately skewed, immune responses towards Th1 (IL-12 and IL-12R) or Th2 (IL-4R) responses could provide a molecular basis for the pathogenesis of complex polygenic diseases. Asthma and autoimmunity are perhaps the best examples.[28,29]

6. EVALUATING THE ROLE OF CYTOKINES IN AUTOIMMUNITY

Historically, an experimental approach to elucidate a role for cytokines in chronic inflammatory diseases has evolved with the assumption that expression of and/or responses to cytokines are different in disease, and that this

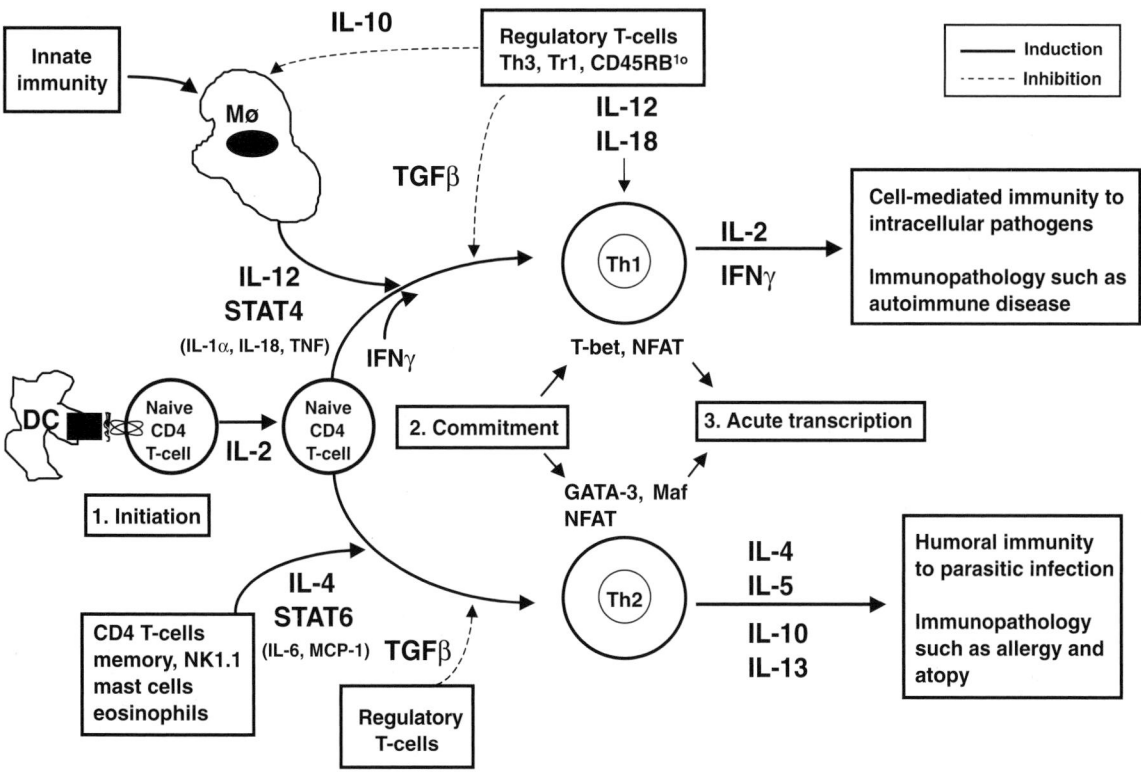

Fig. 2.2 A model of T-helper (Th) cell differentiation. Current models propose that naive CD4+ T-cells undergo three phases – an initiation, a commitment and a gene transcription phase. The cytokines and transcription factors implicated at each stage are indicated. STAT, signal transducer and activator of transcription. Cross-regulatory networks are indicated by the dotted arrows.

difference may be genetically determined. In an attempt to identify candidate cytokines which may be responsible for promoting a disease process, two difficulties arise at the outset. Firstly, since multiple cytokines are involved in pathological processes, how does one set about identifying the dominant player or players? This is especially challenging considering that cells are literally bathed in multiple soluble factors that signal at the cell surface. Secondly, the primary role of cytokines is to maintain homeostasis in the context of cell growth and development. Therefore, how is it possible to discriminate between cytokines which are beneficial and those which are pathogenic? According to these criteria, overexpression of a particular cytokine is insufficient evidence in its own right to implicate such a factor in the pathogenic process.

As technology has advanced, so too has the level of sophistication used to address these questions. In the 1980s, purified, and subsequently recombinant, cytokines were used to test cellular responses to challenge *in vitro*. A useful tool to determine the effects of endogenous cytokine activities was cytokine neutralization with specific polyclonal and monoclonal antibodies. The commonly used markers of responsiveness were cell activation, growth or cytotoxicity, but the relationship between these responses and autoimmunity were far from clear. Towards the end of the 1980s, several spontaneous and induced rodent models of autoimmunity had been characterized (reviewed in Sakaguchi[30]), and these became essential vehicles for studying the effects of recombinant cytokines and of blocking their function *in vivo*. By the 1990s, transgenic and knockout technology (both unconditional and conditional) were routine in many laboratories, and these provided unique opportunities for defining the pathological effects of overexpression in selected tissues, and the physiological functions of cytokines by gene deletion.[31,32] Conditional knockouts have provided investigators with another level of sophistication where cytokine genes can be inactivated in specific tissues or cell lineages. In some cases, the phenotype of mutant mice has turned out to

be unexpected,[33] and has prompting a search for analogous functional mutations in the human genome in populations of patients with relevant disease characteristics. In others, spontaneous disease in mouse strains have led to the identification of natural mutations,[34–36] prompting similar probing of the human gene for novel polymorphisms which co-segregate with a particular disease phenotype.[37] Regardless of these results, this experimental approach cannot be undertaken in humans. Consequently, the ultimate test of the role for a specific cytokine in the pathogenesis of disease in humans is the controlled clinical trial.

It will now be illustrated how, over a period of more than a decade, these technologies have been utilized to explore the role of proinflammatory cytokines in a prototypic chronic inflammatory disease in humans.

6.1 RA – the prototypic chronic inflammatory autoimmune disease

There are relatively few diseases where there is sufficient evidence for a definitive role of cytokines in disease pathogenesis. One exception is RA.[18] RA is a chronic inflammatory disease characterized by inflammation of the synovial joint lining layer, erosion and destruction of underlying cartilage and bone. The prevalence of the disease is 0.5–1.0%, with a clear female preponderance (~ 3:1). More recently, it has been recognized that for patients with severe, chronic and active disease there is a significant increase in mortality, as well as morbidity, with survival curves comparable to those of four-vessel coronary artery disease or stage III Hodgkin's lymphoma. The histopathological features of inflamed RA synovium extend throughout the synovial joint. They comprise an increase in thickness of the lining layer of six to eight cells due to infiltration with synoviocyte cells of fibroblast and macrophage lineage, and significant increases in the thickness of the sublining layer through infiltration with mononuclear cell populations, predominantly T-lymphocytes and macrophages, and to a lesser extent B-lymphocytes and dendritic cells. In a subset of patients, follicular lymphoid aggregates predominate, reminiscent of secondary lymphoid organs. These are organized around blood vessels and neovascularization is evident. The principal site of immuno-inflammatory activity is the junction where the synovial tissue (or pannus) encroaches upon the cartilage.

It was soon appreciated that synovial mononuclear cells expressed activation markers on their cell surface, providing evidence for local chronic immune activation.[38] This led to models of disease pathogenesis which implicate cognate interactions between multiple cell types, including cartilage antigen-specific T-cells and professional antigen-presenting cells,[39] B-cells, the production of autoantibodies including rheumatoid factor,[40] and the proliferation of synovial fibroblasts.[41] These interactions initiate and sustain a cascade of cytokine and proteinase production which ultimately leads to cartilage destruction and bone resorption.[18,42]

The prediction from this model is that many of the cytokines expressed following engagement between cells of the adaptive immune system would be expressed at the site of local synovial inflammation. Initial approaches by some laboratories focused on expression of cytokines in serum and synovial fluid. This approach has its limitations because cytokines are expressed locally, many have a short half-life and few spill over in to the systemic circulation. Indeed, multiple mechanisms provide a means to neutralize cytokine bioactivity to prevent aberrant expression at sites distant from the inflammatory process. Nevertheless, there are some exceptions, perhaps IL-6 being the best. Synovial fluid, on the other hand, is local to the inflamed tissue but is viscous, hard to manipulate, and is rich in proteoglycans (PG), neutrophils (PMN), serum proteins and proteinases, all of which could inhibit the function of, or degrade, cytokine activity. Expression of synovial fluid cytokines is not reproducible and it is not possible to define a normal range, since the volume, protein and cell content of fluid is too variable to make the levels of expression meaningful, let alone comparable, between samples.

As an alternative, many laboratories studied the expression of secreted cytokines in cultures of dissociated cells from inflamed synovial membrane tissue.[18] This has been complemented by immunohistochemical and *in situ* hybridization analysis of frozen synovial tissue sections. Together, it has been possible to apply most of the techniques discussed above (see Table 2.3). Although there is sampling bias towards late disease, this approach has revealed that there exists a vast array of cytokines whose pattern of expression varies little between patients. Based on a large amount of data from many laboratories, these can be subgrouped according to broad function (Table 2.4). The data reveal that there exist both pro-inflammatory and anti-inflammatory cytokines, haematopoietic growth factors, chemotactic factors and fibroblast growth factors at levels sufficient to signal.[18] The profile of expression is not dissimilar to that found in osteoarthritis (OA), though the levels are much higher in RA. In summary, all the ingredients required to sustain the inflammatory response are present but, importantly, macrophage-derived products by far outweigh the expression of T-cell-derived cytokines. The finding of relatively low level expression of IL-2, IFN-γ and, especially, IL-4 at the protein and mRNA level has puzzled investigators for many years, and has challenged the hypothesis that the autoimmune process in inflamed synovial joints is driven by activated T-cells.[43,44] This topic is still hotly debated.

Given that cytokine expression is tightly regulated through multiple mechanisms that aim to maintain homeostasis, the finding that these cytokines are expressed and secreted by synovial cells at high levels, and for prolonged periods, is all the more striking in the absence of exogenous stimuli. This is quite different to peripheral blood cells, in which cytokine expression is very low and often not detectable in the absence of a stimulus, such as a mitogen or LPS. Indeed, even in the presence of mitogen, cytokine mRNA expression is transient rather than sustained.[45] The data suggest that endogenous factors drive the response in RA. This key observation has provided a molecular framework for exploring the mechanisms that drive the inflammatory response *in vivo*.

Table 2.4 Cytokine expression in inflamed rheumatoid synovial joints		
Pro-inflammatory	Mixed function	Anti-inflammatory
IL-1α, β	IL-6	IL-4
IL-8	IFN-γ	IL-10
IL-12	IL-16	IL-11
IL-15	TGF-β	IL-13
IL-17		
IL-18	Functional inhibitors	Chemokines
TNF-α		IL-8
GM-CSF	IL-1Ra	Groα
M-CSF	sIL-1R	MIP-1
LIF	sTNF-R	ENA-78
IFN-α, β	IL-18BP	RANTES
Growth factors		
bFGF		
PDGF		
VEGF		

6.2 Evidence for cytokine networks in RA

The data above raise several questions that have important implications for defining therapeutic targets. Is there redundancy or does each cytokine have unique pathophysiological functions that promote inflammation? Is there hierarchy, with some cytokines driving the expression of others in what amounts to a cytokine cascade? What endogenous factors sustain expression *in vivo*? To address these and related questions, laboratories have focused on the components of the disease process which lead to target organ damage, namely cartilage erosion and bone destruction. The experimental approach was determined to some extent by the observation that IL-1 (also termed catabolin) was by far the most potent inducer of cartilage matrix degradation, based on its effects on PG synthesis and GAG production in cartilage explants.[46] In addition, the activities of IL-1 on synovial fibroblasts explained many of the pathological features of RA.[47]

Strategies to identify which factors upregulated IL-1 production in RA synovial cultures were based on previous evidence, indicating that the most potent inducers were LPS, IL-1 itself, TNF and IFN-γ. Since LPS and IFN-γ were unlikely candidates in RA joints, attempts were made to compare the effects of TNF and IL-1 in regulating the cytokine cascade, since they shared many inflammatory properties and expression of both cytokines were upregulated in the RA joints. Using neutralizing rabbit polyclonal antibodies to TNF, Brennan et al[48] demonstrated that sustained IL-1 production was dramatically attenuated in cultures of dissociated RA synovial cells incubated with anti-TNF, compared to those cultured with anti-LT as a control. In parallel experiments, studies revealed that TNF also regulated the production of IL-6, IL-8, granulocyte–macrophage colony-stimulating factor (GM-CSF) and IL-10 (reviewed in Feldmann et al[7]). In contrast, neutralizing IL-1 activity with the IL-1 receptor antagonist, IL-1ra, had much less of an effect on TNF expression in this experimental system. The data provided the first clear evidence of a hierarchy of cytokine expression and implicated TNF as a factor involved at a more proximal stage of the cytokine cascade, which could drive inflammatory cytokine expression in joints. The approach also provided strong evidence for the existence of cytokine networks, involving complex cross-regulation, which could be manipulated by neutralizing one component.

6.3 Evidence for immunoregulatory networks in inflamed joints

Thus far, the discussion has focused on the candidate proinflammatory cytokines expressed in inflamed synovial tissue. The data documented a predominance of macrophage-derived cytokines, with a relative paucity of T-cell cytokines. In the light of these observations, what evidence, if any, is there to suggest the existence of factors involved in maintaining homeostasis? Our current understanding is that such homeostasis is achieved to a significant extent through the expression of anti-inflammatory cytokines (e.g. IL-4, IL-13, IL-10, IL-11 and

TGF-β), many of which are known to be products of activated CD4+ T-cells, hence the term immunoregulatory T-cells.

While IL-4 is rarely detected, if ever, in synovial T-cells, IL-13 is expressed.[49] However, like IL-10, which is more abundant in joints,[50] IL-13 is also expressed by natural killer (NK) cells and B-cells, suggesting that, since synovial T-cells are generally hyporesponsive, these anti-inflammatory factors are likely to be derived from other cell types. As a group, these anti-inflammatory cytokines have overlapping effects, sharing some with TGF-β, one of the most potent immunosuppressive cytokines documented to date. Thus, there is good evidence for immunoregulatory cytokine networks in RA. While the effects on proinflammatory cytokine expression of adding recombinant cytokines such as IL-10 or neutralizing mAb to synovial cell cultures confirm their anti-inflammatory function,[50] this approach has also provided clear evidence that the activity of immunoregulatory factors present in synovial joints is insufficient to switch off the inflammatory process.

6.4 TNF – a good target in chronic inflammatory disease?

Data gathered over the last decade have characterized the biology of TNF *in vitro* and *in vivo*. Its pleiotropy is in part related to the widespread expression of two high-affinity receptors, the 55 (p55) and 75 kDa (p75) TNF receptors (TNFR). Based on this knowledge, and the paradigm of disease pathogenesis for RA, it is easy to see that many of the effects of TNF, like those of IL-1, could contribute to the perpetuation of the inflammatory process *in vivo* (reviewed in Feldmann et al,[18] Fig. 2.3). Several of these biological properties are worthy of mention. First, TNF is a growth factor when lymphocytes are stimulated at the same time as antigen receptor ligation, and is a potent activator of macrophages and endothelial cells. Activation of endothelium and upregulation of ICAM-1 and VCAM-1 are critical steps in leucocyte trafficking, where cells roll, prior to adhering and transmigration across endothelium. This latter step is further facilitated not only by its chemoattractant properties for neutrophils but also through induction of expression of chemokines by TNF

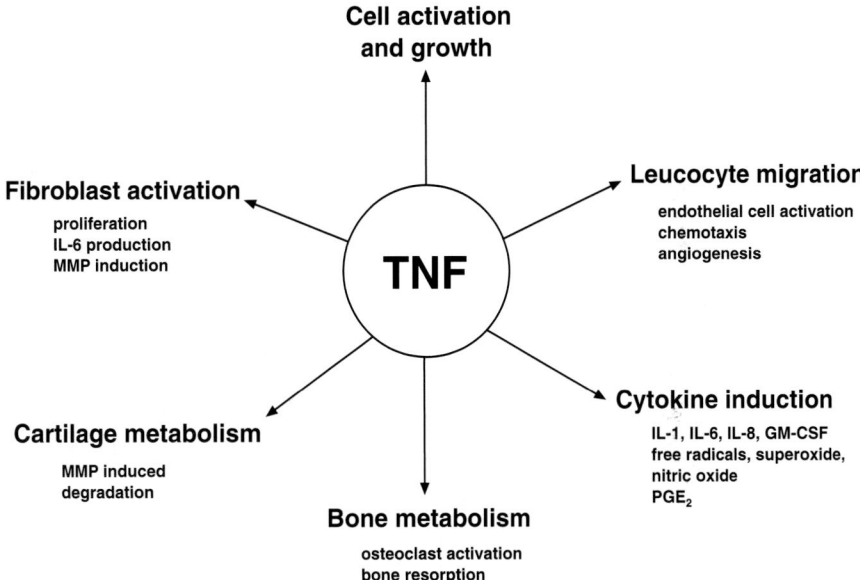

Fig. 2.3 The pleiotropic effects of tumour necrosis factor (TNF) in inflamed synovial joints. TNF targets many cell types and induces multiple proinflammatory activities by signalling through TNF-R expressed on mononuclear, cartilage and bone-derived cell lineages. MMP, matrix metalloproteinase.

and other cytokines. This is an especially important step in the adhesion of lymphocytes and monocytes to activated endothelial cells, since it leads to structural changes in the conformation of integrins required for efficient binding to cognate ICAM-1 receptors. Another process thought to be of importance in sustaining the inflamed synovium is angiogenesis, an event common to both physiological as well as pathological conditions, whereby vascular endothelial tubes are generated and permeate through the tissues. The principal drivers of this process are not clear but likely include physicochemical properties of the environment such as pH and oxygen tension, in addition to a growing family of angiogenic factors. One factor is vascular endothelial growth factor (VEGF), produced by endothelial cells and macrophages, whose expression is also regulated by TNF.[51]

Second, cells resident in the joint, such as fibroblast-like synoviocytes (FLS) are also responsive to TNF. Engagement of TNFR on these cells leads to upregulation of other cytokines, including IL-6 and the fibroblast growth factors (FGF), basic FGF and platelet-derived growth factor (PDGF), both of which are potent growth factors for FLS.[41] IL-6 may contribute to B-cell activation and immunoglobulin production. In addition, TNF and IL-1 induce the production of a panel of matrix metalloproteinases (MMP),[52] whose targets include extracellular matrix components such as aggrecan (aggrecanases), collagen (collagenase, MMP1), stromelysin (MMP3) and fibronectin (many MMP). These enzymes are thought to be the key effectors and mediators of cartilage matrix destruction. Other components likely to be of importance, some of which are also induced by TNF, include the generation of nitric oxide and reactive oxygen species. These and other free radicals may well contribute to the phenotype of the 'stressed' synovium, in part through the activation of stress sensor signal transduction pathways, including NF-κB and mitogen-activated protein kinase (MAPK) signalling pathways.[53] In turn, these lead to a defined programme of transcription of other inflammatory cytokine genes, and to the synthesis of lipid mediators such as prostaglandins.

Third, in addition to RANK ligand, another TNF cytokine family member, TNF also activates osteoclasts through signalling pathways similar to those in monocytes.[54] Osteoclast activation is an essential step towards bone resorption. It should be noted that many of the biological effects of TNF are shared with other cytokines expressed in synovial joints, including IL-1, IL-6, CSF and chemokines. Nevertheless, the data show that TNF is a pivotal cytokine in the pathogenesis of RA.

6.5 Experimental models of TNF dysregulation

Cytokine expression is regulated at multiple levels which can be viewed as a series of checkpoints that prevent sustained overexpression. Regulation of TNF provides good examples of these checkpoints (Figure 2.4), which include transcription and post-transcriptional/post-translational processes,[55–57] cleavage of the cell-surface TNF precursor by the proteinase TNF-α converting enzyme (TACE)[58] and internalization of surface TNFR or shedding of surface TNFR (reviewed in Feldmann et al[18] and Wallach et al[59]).

This latter process has the combined effect of reducing surface expression while generating a natural TNF inhibitor capable of neutralizing TNF and recruiting signalling molecules that may silence or attenuate TNFR signals.[59] If TNF overexpression is an important factor in the generation of chronic inflammation such as arthritis, one would predict that manipulation and dysregulation of these processes might, in their own right, lead to inflammatory disease.

Compelling data supporting this prediction came first from the laboratory of Kollias and colleagues in 1991,[60] who had been studying the role of the 3' untranslated region (UTR) of mRNA. Since TNF, like other genes including c-myc, GM-CSF, IFN-γ and COX, carries reiterative AUUUA sequences in the 3' UTR (AU-rich elements (ARE)] thought to contribute to mRNA instability,[57] Kollias and colleagues generated transgenic mice expressing mutant mouse or human TNF transgenes.[60] In these constructs, the 3' ARE sequence was replaced with a rabbit β-globin intron (hence, TNF-globin transgenic mice). As a consequence, TNF was

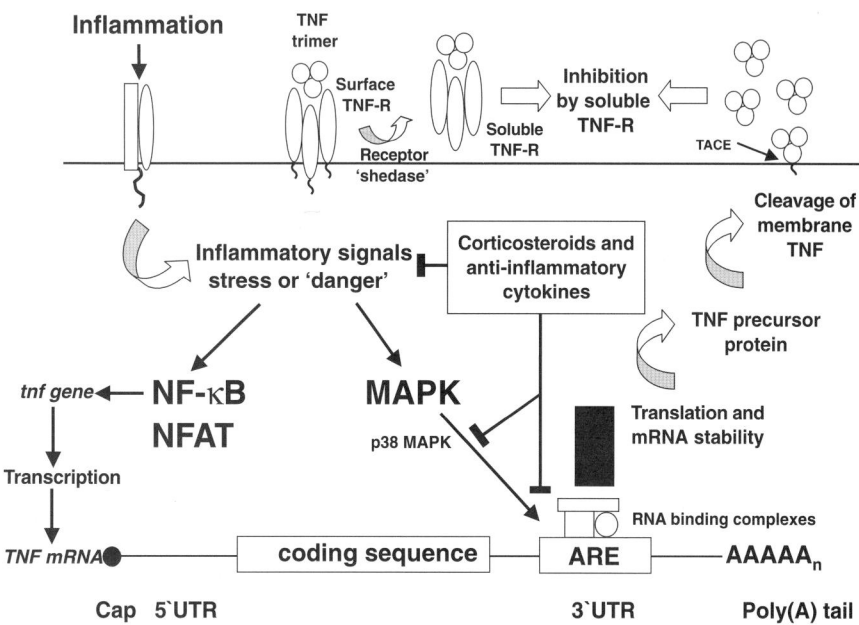

Fig. 2.4 Checkpoints in the regulation of tumour necrosis factor (TNF) expression. Inflammatory or 'danger' signals activate several intracellular signal transduction pathways, the most important being NF-κB and the MAPK pathways. Of these, the p38 MAPK pathway plays a dominant role in post-transcriptional regulation by modifying the RNA binding complexes that regulate inflammatory gene mRNA stability at the 3'UTR. The anti-inflammatory effects of corticosteroids and cytokines may arise through the interruption of TNF gene expression at this level. MAPK, mitogen-activated protein kinase; UTR, untranslated region; ARE, AU-rich element; TACE, TNF-α converting enzyme; NFAT, nuclear factor for activation of T-cells.

overexpressed and sustained *in vivo*. With 100% penetrance, mice developed a chronic inflammatory disease of joints, characterized by inflamed synovium or pannus, cartilage erosion and bone destruction. By 6–8 weeks of age, the architecture of the joint was completely destroyed; anti-TNF treatment from birth completely inhibited the arthritic process.

The same group refined these models in a number of ways, including mutating the membrane proximal cleavage site of the TNF-globin construct. This generates TNF that is fixed in the plasma membrane; the phenotype is similar. Other groups have targeted TNF to the pancreatic islets.[61] This leads to intense insulitis, but diabetes only develops when the transgene is expressed in diabetes-prone strains of mice or when additional co-stimulatory molecules are coexpressed in the β-islets.[62] Kollias and colleagues[68] have also generated knockin mice

where the endogenous TNF gene has been replaced with genomic sequence lacking 69 base pairs of ARE rich repeats, in order to define more precisely the sequences within the 3' of the TNF gene responsible for TNF dysregulation. Strikingly, these TNF ΔARE mice develop not only arthritis but also inflammatory bowel disease resembling human Crohn's disease. These elegant experiments in mice provide compelling evidence to support the notion that sustained overexpression of TNF is sufficient to induce chronic inflammatory disease.

6.6 Evidence for TNF dysregulation in humans

There now exists plentiful evidence for prolonged, sustained expression of TNF and other proinflammatory cytokines in RA in humans.[18] The finding that TNF expression can be detected in unstimulated synovial joint cell cultures, as well as in synovial tissue sections is only part of the picture. More precisely, TNF bioactivity depends on the balance between the expression of cognate TNFR on target cells and the relative abundance of the naturally occurring TNF inhibitors, which are generated through proteolytic cleavage of both cell-surface receptors. In RA synovial joints, both p55 and p75 TNFR are upregulated on T-cells, macrophages and FLS.[64] Furthermore, by immunoassay it has been possible to demonstrate upregulation of soluble p55 and p75 TNFR (sTNFR) in culture supernatants.[65] Both TNF inhibitors are preferentially upregulated in synovial fluid compared to serum, and levels correlate with disease activity. In RA, increased sTNFR levels are presumably insufficient to completely neutralize TNF *in vivo*, while in OA TNF bioactivity is difficult to detect, suggesting that this inhibitory mechanism is effective in OA but not in RA.[65] The same could be said for the expression of other cytokines with anti-inflammatory properties that are known, at least *in vitro*, to downregulate TNF and IL-1 production (see section 6.3). These data provide further support for the notion that it is the relative balance of cytokines, their cognate receptors and their inhibitors, that determine the outcome of the inflammatory process, rather than the absolute expression of each component. Indeed, analogous to TNF and soluble TNFR, correlations between IL-1 and IL-1Ra expression have been shown to predict outcome from inflammatory and infectious diseases.[66]

The search for genetic polymorphisms which might contribute to the dysregulation of pro-inflammatory cytokines in patients with chronic inflammatory diseases such as RA has been the subject of intense research. The results of such analyses are far from conclusive but there are suggestions that such genetic factors may play a role. For example, several polymorphisms in the TNF promoter region have been reported,[67] and great effort has been made to determine whether these single nucleotide polymorphisms (SNP) confer disease susceptibility or severity independently of the human leucocyte antigen (HLA) class II region, since the TNF/LT locus is

encoded within the major histocompatibility complex (MHC) class IV region.[68] These SNPs could contribute as independent factors as part of an extended MHC haplotype, where multiple genotypes contribute to disease susceptibility and/or severity. For the human *tnf* gene, SNPs have been identified at base positions −308, −238, −376, −163, +70 and +489 from the transcription start site, but their functional relevance remains to be determined. IL-10 polymorphisms have also been described, and one set of IL-10 promoter SNPs studied in the context of patients with neuropsychiatric SLE.[69] In RA there has also been considerable interest in IFN-γ gene polymorphisms.[70]

One of the more exciting findings of recent years has been the identification of the genetic basis for a series of periodic fever syndromes, related to familial Mediterranean fever (FMF). McDermott et al[71] identified a series of mutations in the coding region of the p55 TNFR gene in a series of families with a similar clinical syndromes comprising periodic fever, serositis, rash, lymphadenopathy and a non-deforming arthritis. These mutations map to different parts of the receptor; some could influence shedding of the p55 TNFR, while others may influence the capacity for the TNFR to cluster and signal upon ligand interaction. Either way, the defects may enhance TNFR signalling responses. Regardless of the specific mechanisms, these studies demonstrate at the molecular level, the importance of this ligand/receptor pathway in the development of inflammatory disease in humans.

6.7 What drives TNF expression *in vivo*

The discussion above would predict that there are many potential mechanisms through which the expression of proinflammatory cytokines is upregulated. Much is known about factors that can induce TNF production *in vitro*, but the mechanisms involved in driving TNF production in RA are less clear. Table 2.5 lists some of these and illustrates the diversity of intracellular pathways that induce TNF production. Similarly, many factors are capable of switching off TNF expression or biological activity.

Table 2.5 Inducers of TNF expression	
Agent	**Example**
bacterial products	LPS, staphylococcal exotoxin, mycobacterial antigens
viruses	Sendai virus, HIV
parasites	malarial antigens
cytokines	IFN-γ, GM-CSF, IL-1 and TNF
pharmacologic	phorbol esters, phosphatase inhibitors
radiation	UV, γ irradiation
others	complement (C5a)

Table 2.6 Suppressors of TNF production	
Agent	**Example**
cytokines	IL-4, IL-10, IL-11, IL-13, TGFβ
viruses	Epstein Barr virus
pharmacologic	phosphodiesterase inhibitors, thalidomide, cyclosporin A, dexamethasone, Vit D3, ethanol, adenosine, oestradiol, progesterone, chlorpromazine, leflunomide

Table 2.6 lists some of the better known factors whose mechanism of action has been studied in the belief that more refined targeting of TNF blockade could be developed in the longer term. These include pharmacological agents that have a long track record in suppressing inflammation in the clinic, including corticosteroids.

A few drugs are worthy of mention in the context of antirheumatic agents. Gold and aspirin have been reported to interfere with the activation of the transcription factor NF-κB, a potent activator of multiple proinflammatory and stress genes.[72,73] Corticosteroids are perhaps the gold standard anti-inflammatory agents and would be used more widely, and at higher dosages, were it not for their profound side effects on metabolism in liver and bone. There are multiple intracellular targets of steroid action, including, importantly, inhibition of adaptor protein (AP)-1 and NF-κB activation,[74,75] and of p38 MAPK activation.[76] Another important mechanism is the capacity for steroids to deacetylate histones,[77] which would have the effect of altering chromatin structure, thereby attenuating the accessibility of transcription factor complexes to DNA consensus elements in the promoters of inflammatory genes. Together, these data indicate that clinicians have been manipulating cytokine networks for decades, if not for centuries!

7. MANIPULATING CYTOKINE NETWORKS IN AUTOIMMUNITY AS ILLUSTRATED THROUGH TUMOUR NECROSIS FACTOR (TNF) BLOCKADE

7.1 Lessons from the mouse

Spontaneous or induced models of autoimmunity in rodents have been extremely useful for validating hypotheses based on *in vitro* studies of cytokine expression in inflammation. The effects of TNF blockade in murine autoimmune disease models other than arthritis have been reviewed elsewhere.[78] The initial experience with polyclonal anti-TNF antiserum came largely from studies of the attenuation of septic shock.[24] Subsequently, neutralizing mAb were tested in murine collagen-induced arthritis, an acute inflammatory joint disease with features of RA in humans.[79] The advantage of this model is that therapy can be instituted before, at the onset or after the inflammatory disease has become clinically apparent. While preventive regimens with anti-TNF completely blocked paw swelling and joint damage, treatment at the time of onset of arthritis was also very effective. The regimens adopted were administered over short periods of time of up to 1 week, and so the effects of neutralizing a key component of the innate immune response over prolonged periods were never explored in depth.

7.2 Lessons from the clinic

It was the results of studies documenting the effects of neutralizing anti-TNF mAb in established collagen-induced arthritis, and the dosing regimens used, which provided the major incentive for the first clinical trial of anti-TNF therapy in a cohort of patients with RA (reviewed in Feldmann and Maini[80]). At about this time, a chimeric (mouse × human) antibody, cA2 (infliximab, Remicade) became available for study. This mAb is approximately 75% human sequence and is a high-affinity IgG1 mAb (1.8×10^{-9} kDa). Subsequent pharmacokinetic analyses revealed that at high doses (10 mg/kg) it is still detectable in serum 10–12 weeks after a single infusion, and preclinical studies showed it to be safe in healthy volunteers. One major concern raised by this strategy was whether prolonged neutralization of a cytokine with important effects in multiple processes would be safe in patients. Sustaining the integrity of host defence to foreign pathogens was a particular concern, especially since patients with severe, active, chronic RA are prone to infection, regardless of their immunosuppressive treatment.

The first cohort of 20 patients was studied in an open-label trial.[81] After a 1-month washout period, patients who had failed conventional disease-modifying drugs and who had persistent active, erosive disease received a total of 20 mg/kg in two to four intravenous infusions spread over a period of 2 weeks. Rapid improvement in all indices were observed, including swollen and tender joint scores, pain, early morning stiffness, locomotor function and global assessment of disease activity, as well as laboratory parameters, such as measurements of the acute phase response (ESR and CRP). Maximum improvement was seen in the first 4 weeks, but up to 60–70% improvement was maintained for a median of 12 weeks. Importantly, the treatment was well tolerated and there were no serious adverse events. Anti-TNF (Remicade) is now licensed for use with methotrexate, while the equally effective p75 TNFR-IgG fusion protein (Enbrel) is also available in combination or alone.[82]

This initial promising outcome prompted a randomized, double-blind, multicentre, placebo-controlled trial (RCT) of ~ 70 patients, recruited throughout Europe in 1994,[83] and subsequently the ATTRACT trial, whose 2-year outcome data have recently been published.[84] These studies, which addressed dosing and frequency of infusions, as well as progression of radiographic evidence of joint disease, have been reviewed in depth elsewhere. However, several specific points are worthy of mention here. First, the high frequency of responders (up to ~ 70%) indicated that TNF was an important mediator of the chronic inflammatory process in a significant proportion of patients. This heterogeneous population of patients recruited from all over the world is quite distinct in genetic and phenotypic terms in comparison with inbred strains of mice. Second, the data provided unequivocal evidence to refute the idea that cytokine function was redundant, and supported the notion that cytokine cascades and networks not only existed but were amenable to therapeutic manipulation, to the benefit of patients. In this regard, there was no statistically significant increase in severe infections in patients receiving anti-TNF, although there understandably remains considerable concern over this potential complication, particularly with respect to an increased risk of tuberculosis (TB). Third, within the constraints of ethical clinical research, it was possible to begin to dissect how anti-TNF exerted its potent anti-inflammatory effects in humans.

7.3 Mechanisms of action

In general terms, the effects of TNF, or its inhibition, on induction of inflammatory cytokines, cell activation and growth, and, in particular, its effects on endothelial cell activation and leucocyte trafficking *in vitro*, have been substantiated in patients. It is likely that there are at least four principal mechanisms to account for the majority of effects. These have been reviewed in detail recently by Feldmann and Maini[80] and are as described below.

7.3.1 Attenuation of the cytokine cascade
Through an analysis of serum levels of cytokines and their soluble receptors, it has been shown that anti-TNF downregulates the expression of IL-1, IL-6 and IL-8. The effects are

rapid, as illustrated by the dramatic falls in IL-6 levels, which closely parallel changes in the acute phase response.

7.3.2 Downregulation of cell trafficking to synovial joints

This has been tested in a number of ways. First, levels of the chemokines IL-8 and MCP-1 detectable in serum fall with treatment. Second, levels of a subset of soluble adhesion molecules, which may reflect endothelial expression *in vivo*, were also reduced. These include soluble E-selectin and ICAM-1, but not VCAM-1. Consistent with these findings, there is a concomitant rise in the number of circulating T-lymphocytes detectable within days of commencing therapy. Perhaps more striking are the changes observed in serial synovial tissue biopsies taken from knee joints prior to and 2 weeks after the first infusion. These show dramatic reductions in infiltrating leucocytes, as well as in the thickness of the lining layer.[85]

7.3.3 Angiogenesis

Synovial tissue analysis, in combination with serum VEGF levels, suggests that the active process of angiogenesis in inflamed joints is slowed.[51]

7.3.4 Joint protection

Anti-TNF treatment reduces expression of MMP1 and MMP3,[86] which in turn predicts that cartilage breakdown will be reduced. On the basis of serial radiographs taken over a period of 2 years, the ATTRACT study recently reported almost complete halting of progression of joint damage based on established radiographic scores, determined by independent radiologists blinded to the treatment.[84] This was suggested after 1 year of starting treatment but was sustained at 2 years. Interestingly, even in those patients who had a relatively poor clinical response to anti-TNF it was possible to demonstrate evidence of joint protection. The implication of this observation is that there exists some dissociation between inflammation and cartilage and bone damage.

There still remain unanswered questions, particularly with respect to how anti-TNF therapy influences the immune system. As mentioned, there is no clear detrimental effect of prolonged TNF blockade on the incidence of infections, although there is a trend to more frequent mild upper respiratory tract infections and TB. What is of potential importance is the finding that T-cell and proliferative cytokine responses are dramatically enhanced with anti-TNF treatment.[87,88] This is in accord with extensive *in vitro* and *in vivo* mouse studies that implicated chronic TNF overexpression in the attenuation of T-cell reactivity in RA,[89] but also in several models of autoimmunity in the mouse. This has been discussed in more detail elsewhere.[78] Of particular note are the findings that TNF protects lupus mice from disease. TNF blockade exacerbates the disease, and even in non-susceptible strains it has been possible to detect spontaneous production of autoantibodies. Based on these data, therefore, it was not so surprising that up to 8% of patients developed IgM anti-nuclear antibodies (ANA).[90] Isolated cases of drug-induced lupus have also been documented, associated in rare cases with an isotype switch of ANA from IgM to IgG and IgA. A more recent observation is that in a very small proportion of patients there have been reported episodes of what appear to be demyelinating disease, a finding in agreement with acceleration of autoimmune encephalomyelitis in TNF-deficient mice (discussed in Cope[78]). While these data suggest that TNF blockade improves immune function, perhaps resetting the immune system by restoring the function of immunoregulatory T-cell subsets, they also demonstrate that such immune boosting can, in susceptible individuals, have pathological sequelae. Nevertheless, these findings may also explain the low incidence of infection in patients treated with anti-TNF for ≥ 2 years.

8. USE OF OTHER BIOLOGICALS TO MANIPULATE CYTOKINE NETWORKS IN RHEUMATOID ARTHRITIS (RA)

It can be seen that there exist multiple potential targets for manipulating cytokine networks in chronic inflammatory disease. It is of some interest that the same candidates have been considered for different diseases, such as Crohn's disease. In RA, clinical trials have been broadly focused on neutralizing proinflammatory cytokines (e.g. TNF, IL-1 and IL-6) or reconstituting immunoregulatory networks with anti-inflammatory cytokines such as IL-10 and IL-11. In addition to blocking TNF, there is now considerable experience with IL-1 blockade, with increasing experience for IL-6 blockade. For IL-1 blockade, the receptor antagonist IL-1Ra has been used,[91] while both anti-IL-6 and anti-IL-6R modalities are in trial;[92] the rationale for both has been outlined above. Other strategies to block proinflammatory cytokine production include IL-18 blockade (anti-IL-18 and an IL-18 binding protein), where differentiation of Th1 cells could be perturbed, are in development. It is likely that this, together with anti-IL-12-directed treatments, will be tested in other Th1-driven diseases.

Finally, recombinant IL-10 has been shown to be effective in patients with RA (reviewed in Keystone et al[93]). The effects are likely to be due in part to inhibition of IL-1, TNF, IL-6 and IFN-γ production, as well as increases in endogenous soluble TNFR expression. On balance, these strategies have proven beneficial in RA, but the effects are short-lasting and not as striking as those observed for TNF, IL-1 or IL-6 blockade.

9. CONCLUSIONS

Advances in cytokine biology have transformed studies from the test tube to the clinic. Two major hurdles have been overcome. The first relates to the concern that there exists considerable redundancy within cytokine networks. This concern appears to be unfounded. The second hurdle is that, at least in the short term, cytokine blockade has a safety profile which may outweigh the risks of persistent active disease, at least for some diseases. This appears to be especially true for host defence against foreign pathogens. Although manipulating cytokine networks in humans is now a reality, the next major challenge is for government agencies and hospital trusts to evaluate cytokine-targeted therapies in terms of direct health care costs and benefits. At one extreme, £8,000 per annum seems a considerable sum to pay for 1 year's treatment for one patient with arthritis. At the other extreme, the Human Rights Act puts a different flavour on a patient's accessibility to treatment and 'postcode prescribing' practice, in which treatment is withheld despite evidence for improved quality (and perhaps prolongation) of life.

REFERENCES

Websites

- http://arthritis-research.com.
- http://www.academicpress.com/cytokinereference.

Scientific papers

1. Cohen S, Bigazzi PE, Yoshida T. Similarities of T cell function in cell-mediated immunity and antibody production. *Cell Immunol* 1974; **12**: 150–9.
2. Kasakura S, Lowenstein L. A factor stimulating DNA synthesis derived from the medium of leucocyte cultures. *Nature* 1965; **208**: 794–5.
3. Ruddle NH, Waksman BH. Cytotoxic effects of lymphocyte–antigen interaction in delayed hypersensitivity. *Science* 1967; **157**: 1060–2.
4. Gery I, Gershon RK, Waksman BH. Potentiation of cultured mouse thymocyte responses by factors released by peripheral leucocytes. *J Immunol* 1971; **107**: 1778–80.
5. Rosenwasser LJ, Dinarello CA, Rosenthal AS. Adherent cell function in murine T lymphocyte antigen recognition. IV Enhancement of murine T-cell antigen recognition by human leukocyte pyrogen. *J Exp Med* 1979; **150**: 70–9.
6. Oppenheim JJ, Gery I. From lymphodrek to IL-1. *Immunol Today* 1993; **3**: 119.
7. Taniguchi T, Ohno S, Fuji-Kuritama Y, Muratmatsu M. The nucleotide sequence of human fibroblast interferon cDNA. *Gene* 1980; **10**: 11–15.
8. Nagata S, Taira H, Hall A et al. Synthesis in *E. coli* of a polypeptide with human leukocyte interferon activity. *Nature* 1980; **284**: 316–20.
9. Gray PW, Leung DW, Pennica D et al. Expression of human immune interferon cDNA in *E. coli* and monkey cells. *Nature* 1982; **285**: 503–8.
10. Leonard WJ, Depper JM, Crabtree GR et al. Molecular cloning and expression of cDNAs for the human interleukin-2 receptor. *Nature* 1984; **311**: 626–31.

11. Derynck R, Jarrett JA, Chen EY et al. Human transforming growth factor-beta complementary DNA sequence and expression in normal and transformed cells. *Nature* 1985; **316**: 701–5.

12. Moore K, Viera P, Fiorentino DF et al. Homology of cytokine synthesis inhibitory factor (IL-10) to Epstein-Barr versus gene BCRF1. *Science* 1990; **248**: 1230–4.

13. Matsushima K, Morishita K, Yoshimura T et al. Molecular cloning of cDNA for a human monocyte derived neutrophil chemotactic factor (MDNCF) and the induction of MDNCF mRNA by interleukin 1 and tumor necrosis factor. *J Exp Med* 1988; **167**: 1883–93.

14. Larsen CG, Anderson AO, Appella E et al. Indentity of chemotactic cytokine for T-lymphocytes with neutrophil activating protein (NAP-1): a candidate interleukin 8. *Science* 1989; **243**: 1464–6.

15. MacFadden G, Graham K, Opgenorth A. Poxvirus growth factors. In: MacFadden G (ed), *Viroreceptors, Virokines and Related Immune Modulators Encoded by DNA Viruses.* Austen, TX: RG Landes & Co, 1995.

16. Vilcek J. The cytokines: an overview. In: *The Cytokine Handbook*. Thompson AW, ed. New York: Academic Press, 1998.

17. Oppenheim JJ, Feldmann M. *Cytokine Reference*. New York: Academic Press, 2000.

18. Feldmann M, Brennan FM, Maini RN. Role of cytokines in rheumatoid arthritis. *Annu Rev Immunol* 1996; **14**: 397–440.

19. Carswell EA, Old LJ, Kassel RL et al. An endotoxin-induced serum factor that causes necrosis of tumors. *Proc Natl Acad Sci USA* 1975; **72**: 3666–70.

20. Beutler B, Cerami A. The biology of cachectin/TNF – a primary mediator of the host response. *Annu Rev Immunol* 1989; **7**: 625–55.

21. Tracey KJ, Wei H, Manogue KR et al. Cachectin/tumor necrosis factor induces cachexia, anemia, and inflammation. *J Exp Med* 1988; **167**: 1211–27.

22. Cerami A, Beutler B. The role of cachectin/TNF in endotoxic shock and cachexia. *Immunol Today* 1988; **9**: 28–31.

23. Taga T, Kishimoto T. Gp130 and the interleukin-6 family of cytokines. *Annu Rev Immunol* 1997; **15**: 797–819.

24. Beutler B, Milsark IW, Cerami AC. Passive immunization against cachectin/tumor necrosis factor protects mice from lethal effect of endotoxin. *Science* 1985; **229**: 869–71.

25. Mosmann TR, Coffman RL. TH1 and TH2 cells: different patterns of lymphokine secretion lead to different functional properties. *Annu Rev Immunol* 1989; **7**: 145–73.

26. Avni O, Rao A. T cell differentiation: a mechanistic view. *Curr Opin Immunol* 2000; **12**: 654–9.

27. Rogge L, Bianchi E, Biffi M et al. Transcript imaging of the development of human T helper cells using oligonucleotide arrays. *Nature Genet* 2000; **25**: 96–101.

28. Caggana M, Walker K, Reilly AA et al. Population-based studies reveal differences in the allelic frequencies of two functionally significant human interleukin-4 receptor polymorphisms in several ethnic groups. *Genet Med* 1999; **1**: 267–71.

29. Morahan G, Huang D, Ymer SI et al. Linkage disequilibrium of a type 1 diabetes susceptibility locus with a regulatory IL12B allele. *Nature Genet* 2001; **27**: 218–21.

30. Sakaguchi S. Animal models of autoimmunity and their relevance to human diseases. *Curr Opin Immunol* 2000; **12**: 684–90.

31. Kollias G. What can we learn from transgenic mice? In: Feldmann M, Brennan FM, eds. *Cytokines in Autoimmunity* Austin TX: RG Landes, 1996.

32. Cope A. What can we learn from 'gene knockout' mice? In: Feldmann M, Brennan FM, eds. *Cytokines in Autoimmunity* Austin, Tex: RG Landes 1996.

33. Makris C, Godfrey VL, Krahn-Senftleben G et al. Female mice heterozygous for IKK gamma/NEMO deficiencies develop a dermatopathy similar to the human X-linked disorder incontinentia pigmenti. *Mol Cell* 2000; **5**: 969–79.

34. Watanabe-Fukunaga R, Brannan CI, Copeland NG et al. Lymphoproliferation disorder in mice explained by defects in Fas antigen that mediates apoptosis. *Nature* 1992; **356**: 314–17.

35. Takahashi T, Tanaka M, Brannan CI et al. Generalized lymphoproliferative disease in mice, caused by a point mutation in the Fas ligand. *Cell* 1994; **76**: 969–76.

36. Ho AM, Johnson MD, Kingsley DM. Role of the mouse ank gene in control of tissue calcification and arthritis. *Science* 2000; **289**: 265–70.

37. Nurnberg P, Thiele H, Chandler D et al. Heterozygous mutations in ANKH, the human ortholog of the mouse progressive ankylosis gene, result in craniometaphyseal dysplasia. *Nature Genet* 2001; **28**: 37–41.

38. Cush JJ, Lipsky PE. Phenotypic analysis of synovial tissue and peripheral blood lymphocytes isolated from patients with rheumatoid arthritis. *Arthritis Rheum* 1988; **31**: 1230–8.

39. Dayer JM, Burger D. Cytokines and direct cell contact in synovitis: relevance to therapeutic intervention. *Arthritis Res* 1999; **1**: 17–20.

40. Weyand CM, Goronzy JJ, Takemura S, Kurtin PJ. Cell–cell interactions in synovitis. Interactions between T cells and B cells in rheumatoid arthritis. *Arthritis Res* 2000; **2**: 457463.

41. Pap T, Muller-Ladner U, Gay RE, Gay S. Fibroblast biology. Role of synovial fibroblasts in the pathogenesis of rheumatoid arthritis. *Arthritis Res* 2000; **2**: 361–7.

42. Ritchlin C. Fibroblast biology. Effector signals released by the synovial fibroblast in arthritis. *Arthritis Res* 2000; **2**: 356–60.

43. Firestein GS, Zvaifler NJ. How important are T cells in chronic rheumatoid synovitis? *Arthritis Rheum* 1990; **33**: 768–73.

44. Firestein GS, Xu WD, Townsend K et al. Cytokines in chronic inflammatory arthritis. I. Failure to detect T cell lymphokines (interleukin 2 and interleukin 3) and presence of macrophage colony-stimulating factor (CSF-1) and a novel mast cell growth factor in rheumatoid synovitis. *J Exp Med* 1988; **168**: 1573–86.

45. Buchan G, Barrett K, Turner M et al. Interleukin-1 and tumour necrosis factor mRNA expression in rheumatoid arthritis: prolonged production of IL-1 alpha. *Clin Exp Immunol* 1988; **73**: 449–55.

46. Saklatvala J, Sarsfield SJ, Townsend Y. Pig interleukin 1: purification of two immunologically different leukocyte proteins that cause cartilage resorprtion, lymphocyte activation, and fever. *J Exp Med* 1985; **162**: 1208–122.

47. Dayer JM, Graham R, Russell, G, Krane SM. Collagenase production by rheumatoid synovial cells: stimulation by a human lymphocyte factor. *Science* 1977; **195**: 181–3.

48. Brennan FM, Chantry D, Jackson A et al. Inhibitory effect of TNF alpha antibodies on synovial cell interleukin-1 production in rheumatoid arthritis. *Lancet* 1989; **2**: 244–7.

49. Isomaki P, Luukkainen R, Toivanen P, Punnonen J. The presence of interleukin-13 in rheumatoid synovium and its anti-inflammatory effects on synovial fluid macrophages from patients with rheumatoid arthritis. *Arthritis Rheum* 1996; **39**: 1693–702.

50. Katsikis PD, Chu CQ, Brennan FM et al. Immunoregulatory role of interleukin 10 in rheumatoid arthritis. *J Exp Med* 1994; **179**: 1517–27.

51. Paleolog EM, Young S, Stark AC et al. Modulation of angiogenic vascular endothelial growth factor by tumor necrosis factor alpha and interleukin-1 in rheumatoid arthritis. *Arthritis Rheum* 1998; **41**: 1258–65.

52. Dayer JM, de Rochemonteix B, Burrus B et al. Human recombinant interleukin 1 stimulates collagenase and prostaglandin E2 production by human synovial cells. *J Clin Invest* 1986; **77**: 645–8.

53. Schett G, Tohidast-Akrad M, Steiner G, Smolen J. The stressed synovium. *Arthritis Res* 2001; **3**: 80–6.

54. Gravallese EM, Galson DL, Goldring SR, Auron PE. The role of TNF-receptor family members and other TRAF-dependent receptors in bone resorption. *Arthritis Res* 2001; **3**: 6–12.

55. Tsai EY, Yie J, Thanos D, Goldfeld AE. Cell-type-specific regulation of the human tumor necrosis factor alpha gene in B cells and T cells by NFATp and ATF-2/JUN. *Mol Cell Biol* 1996; **16**: 5232–44.

56. Falvo JV, Uglialoro AM, Brinkman BM et al. Stimulus-specific assembly of enhancer complexes on the tumor necrosis factor alpha gene promoter. *Mol Cell Biol* 2000; **20**: 2239–47.

57. Clark A. Post-transcriptional regulation of pro-inflammatory gene expression. *Arthritis Res* 2000; **2**: 172–4.

58. Black RA, Rauch CT, Kozlosky CJ et al. A metalloproteinase disintegrin that releases tumour-necrosis factor-alpha from cells. *Nature* 1997; **385**: 729–33.

59. Wallach D, Varfolomeev EE, Malinin NL et al. Tumor necrosis factor receptor and Fas signaling mechanisms. *Annu Rev Immunol* 1999; **17**: 331–67.

60. Keffer J, Probert L, Cazlaris H et al. Transgenic mice expressing human tumour necrosis factor: a predictive genetic model of arthritis. *Eur Molec Biol Org J* 1991; **10**: 4025–31.

61. Picarella DE, Kratz A, Li CB et al. Transgenic tumor necrosis factor (TNF)-alpha production in pancreatic islets leads to insulitis, not diabetes. Distinct patterns of inflammation in TNF-alpha and TNF-beta transgenic mice. *J Immunol* 1993; **150**: 4136–50.

62. Green EA, Flavell RA. The temporal importance of TNFalpha expression in the development of diabetes. *Immunity* 2000; **12**: 459–69.

63. Kontoyiannis D, Pasparakis M, Pizarro TT et al. Impaired on/off regulation of TNF biosynthesis in mice lacking TNF AU-rich elements: implications for joint and gut-associated immunopathologies. *Immunity* 1999; **10**: 387–98.

64. Brennan FM, Gibbons DL, Mitchell T et al. Enhanced expression of tumor necrosis factor receptor mRNA and protein in mononuclear cells isolated from rheumatoid arthritis synovial joints. *Eur J Immunol* 1992; **22**: 1907–12.

65. Cope AP, Aderka D, Doherty M et al. Increased levels of soluble tumor necrosis factor receptors in the sera and synovial fluid of patients with rheumatic diseases. *Arthritis Rheum* 1992; **35**: 1160–9.

66. Miller LC, Lynch EA, Isa S et. al. Balance of synovial fluid IL-1 beta and IL-1 receptor antagonist and recovery from Lyme arthritis. *Lancet* 1993; **341**: 146–8.

67. Verweij CL, Huizinga TW. Tumour necrosis factor alpha gene polymorphisms and rheumatic diseases. *Br J Rheumatol* 1998; **37**: 923–6.

68. van Krugten MV, Huizinga TW, Kaijzel EL et al. Association of the TNF +489 polymorphism with susceptibility and radiographic damage in rheumatoid arthritis. *Genes Immunol* 1999; **1**: 91–6.

69. Rood MJ, Keijsers V, van der Linden MW et al. Neuropsychiatric systemic lupus erythematosus is associated with imbalance in interleukin 10 promoter haplotypes. *Ann Rheum Dis* 1999; **58**: 85–9.

70. Khani-Hanjani A, Lacaille D, Hoar D et al. Association between dinucleotide repeat in non-coding region of interferon-gamma gene and susceptibility to, and severity of, rheumatoid arthritis. *Lancet* 2000; **356**: 820–5.

71. McDermott MF, Aksentijevich I, Galon J et al. Germline mutations in the extracellular domains of the 55 kDa TNF receptor, TNFR1, define a family of dominantly inherited autoinflammatory syndromes. *Cell* 1999; **97**: 133–44.

72. Yoshida S, Kato T, Sakurada S et al. Inhibition of IL-6 and IL-8 induction from cultured rheumatoid synovial fibroblasts by treatment with aurothioglucose. *Int Immunol* 1999; **11**: 151–8.

73. Alpert D, Vilcek J. Inhibition of IkB kinase activity by sodium salicylate *in vitro* does not reflect its inhibitory mechanism in intact cells. *J Biol Chem* 2000; **275**: 10,925–9.

74. Auphan N, DiDonato JA, Rosette C et al. Immunosuppression by glucocorticoids: inhibition of NF-kB activity through induction of I kappa B synthesis. *Science* 1995; **270**: 286–90.

75. Yang-Yen HF, Chambard JC, Sun YL et al. Transcriptional interference between c-Jun and the glucocorticoid receptor: mutual inhibition of DNA binding due to direct protein-protein interaction. *Cell* 1990; **62**: 1205–15.

76. Lasa M, Brook M, Saklatvala J, Clark AR. Dexamethasone destabilizes cyclooxygenase 2 mRNA by inhibiting mitogen-activated protein kinase p38. *Mol Cell Biol* 2001; **21**: 771–80.

77. Ito K, Barnes PJ, Adcock IM. Glucocorticoid receptor recruitment of histone deacetylase 2 inhibits interleukin-1β-induced histone H4 acetylation on lysines 8 and 12. *Mol Cell Biol* 2000; **20**: 6891–903.

78. Cope AP. Regulation of autoimmunity by proinflammatory cytokines. *Curr Opin Immunol* 1998; **10**: 669–76.

79. Williams RO, Feldmann M, Maini RN. Anti-tumor necrosis factor ameliorates joint disease in murine collagen-induced arthritis. *Proc Natl Acad Sci USA* 1992; **89**: 9784–8.

80. Feldmann M, Maini RN. Anti-TNFa therapy of rheumatoid arthritis: what have we learned? *Annu Rev Immunol* 2001; **19**: 163–96.

81. Elliott MJ, Maini RN, Feldmann M et al. Treatment of rheumatoid arthritis with chimeric monoclonal antibodies to tumor necrosis factor alpha. *Arthritis Rheum* 1993; **36**: 1681–90.

82. Moreland LW, Baumgartner SW, Schiff MH. Treatment of rheumatoid arthritis with a recombinant human tumor necrosis factor receptor (p75)–Fc fusion protein. *N Engl J Med* 1997; **337**: 141–7.

83. Elliott MJ, Maini RN, Feldmann M et al. Randomised double-blind comparison of chimeric monoclonal antibody to tumour necrosis factor alpha (cA2) versus placebo in rheumatoid arthritis. *Lancet* 1994; **344**: 1105–10.

84. Lipsky PE, van der Heijde DM, St Clair EW et al. Infliximab and methotrexate in the treatment of rheumatoid arthritis. Anti-Tumor Necrosis Factor Trial in Rheumatoid Arthritis with Concomitant Therapy Study Group. *N Engl J Med* 2000; **343**: 1594–602.

85. Taylor PC, Peters AM, Paleolog E et al. Reduction of chemokine levels and leukocyte traffic to joints by tumor necrosis factor alpha blockade in patients with rheumatoid arthritis. *Arthritis Rheum* 2000; **43**: 38–47.

86. Brennan FM, Browne KA, Green PA et al. Reduction of serum matrix metalloproteinase 1 and matrix metalloproteinase 3 in rheumatoid arthritis patients following anti-tumour necrosis factor-alpha (cA2) therapy. *Br J Rheumatol* 1997; **36**: 643–50.

87. Cope AP, Londei M, Chu NR et al. Chronic exposure to tumor necrosis factor (TNF) *in vitro* impairs the activation of T cells through the T cell receptor/CD3 complex; reversal *in vivo* by anti-TNF antibodies in patients with rheumatoid arthritis. *J Clin Invest* 1994; **94**: 749–60.

88. Berg L, Lampa J, Rogberg S et al. Increased peripheral T cell reactivity to microbial antigens

and collagen type II in rheumatoid arthritis after treatment with soluble TNFa receptors. *Ann Rheum Dis* 2001; **60**: 133–39.

89. Cope AP, Liblau RS, Yang XD et al. Chronic tumor necrosis factor alters T cell responses by attenuating T cell receptor signaling. *J Exp Med* 1997; **185**: 1573–84.

90. Charles PJ, Smeenk RJ, De Jong J et al. Assessment of antibodies to double-stranded DNA induced in rheumatoid arthritis patients following treatment with infliximab, a monoclonal antibody to tumor necrosis factor alpha: findings in open-label and randomized placebo-controlled trials. *Arthritis Rheum* 2000; **43**: 2383–90.

91. Bresnihan B, Alvaro-Gracia JM, Cobby M et al. Pavelka K, Rau R, Rozman B, Watt I, Williams B, Aitchison R, McCabe D, Musikic P. Treatment of rheumatoid arthritis with recombinant human interleukin-1 receptor antagonist. *Arthritis Rheum* 1998; **41**: 2196–204.

92. Yoshizaki K, Nishimoto N, Mihara M, Kishimoto T. Therapy of rheumatoid arthritis by blocking IL-6 signal transduction with a humanized anti-IL-6 receptor antibody. *Springer Semin Immunopathol* 1998; **20**: 247–59.

93. Keystone E, Wherry J, Grint P. IL-10 as a therapeutic strategy in the treatment of rheumatoid arthritis. *Rheum Dis Clin N Am* 1998; **24**: 629–39.

3

B-cells and autoimmune disease

Menna R Clatworthy, Kenneth GC Smith

Objectives • Overview • B-cells and the immune response • B-cell tolerance and its breakdown • B-cells, autoantibody and disease • Diseases with directly pathogenic autoantibody • Diseases associated with immune-complex-mediated inflammation • Diseases in which B-cells play an uncertain role • Conclusions • References

OBJECTIVES

(1) To review the biology of B-cell functions, in particular how B-cell tolerance is maintained and broken down.
(2) To explore the role of B-cells in autoimmune disease and how autoantibodies can contribute directly to pathogenesis, how they can mediate disease through immune complex formation and to review the autoimmune diseases in which B-cells play an uncertain role.

OVERVIEW

Autoantibodies have been described in most autoimmune diseases, yet the precise role played by antibody and the B-cell in most of these diseases is not clear. In a number of diseases these antibodies are known to be pathogenic but in others their significance is unknown. In addition, the role of the B-cell in autoimmunity may well extend beyond that of antibody secretion. The importance of delineating the contribution of different cell types to the development of disease lies in the targeting of

treatment. Anti-T-cell immunosuppression, e.g. cyclosporin, is not effective in many autoimmune diseases [such as systemic lupus erythematosus (SLE) or vasculitis] in which broad spectrum immunosuppression is currently required. Defining the pathogenic contribution of other cell types will encourage targeting of treatment to them, potentially increasing effectiveness whilst reducing toxicity. Here we will discuss the role of B-cells and of autoantibody in the pathogenesis of autoimmunity. We will first provide background information on the B-cell immune response, then on the maintenance and breakdown of B-cell tolerance. In the final section we will discuss evidence for the involvement of B-cells in individual autoimmune diseases.

1. B-CELLS AND THE IMMUNE RESPONSE

1.1 B-cell and antibody function

The immune system responds in two broad ways to invading microorganisms: the innate response, consisting of phagocytic cells and complement, and the acquired or adaptive response, in which antigen-specific B- and T-cells are central players. B-cells secrete antibodies which mediate the elimination of microorganisms and present antigen to T-cells.[1]

Antibodies consist of two heavy chains and two light chains which are held together by disulphide bonds (Fig. 3.1). The N-terminal of each chain possesses a variable region that contributes to the antigen binding site. The constant region defines the isotype of the antibody [immunoglobulin (Ig) IgM, IgG, IgA, IgE, IgD] and determines if the light chain is of the κ or λ type (Table 3.1).[2]

IgM is the first antibody isotype produced. It tends to be of low affinity but exists in pentameric form, and is therefore able to bind simultaneously to multivalent antigens, thus binding with high avidity. The large size of these pentamers means that IgM is usually confined to the circulation. The other antibody isotypes exist as monomers (IgG, IgE, IgD) or as dimers (IgA) and can diffuse out of the blood stream into tissues. IgG is the principal isotype in blood and extracellular fluid, and IgA is found primarily in mucosal secretions.[1,2]

Antigen-specific antibody binds to invading microbes, neutralizing their effects directly or facilitating other mechanisms of disposal. Antibody-coated pathogens may be recognized by Fcγ receptor III (FcγRIII) on natural killer (NK) cells triggering the release of cytotoxins (antibody-dependent cell-mediated cytotoxicity; ADCC). Antibody can bind to FcR on phagocytic cells such as macrophages and neutrophils (PMN), facilitating phagocytosis (a process known as opsonization). Alternatively, antibodies may activate the complement system causing direct lysis of the pathogen or further enhancing opsonization (Table 3.2).[1,3,4]

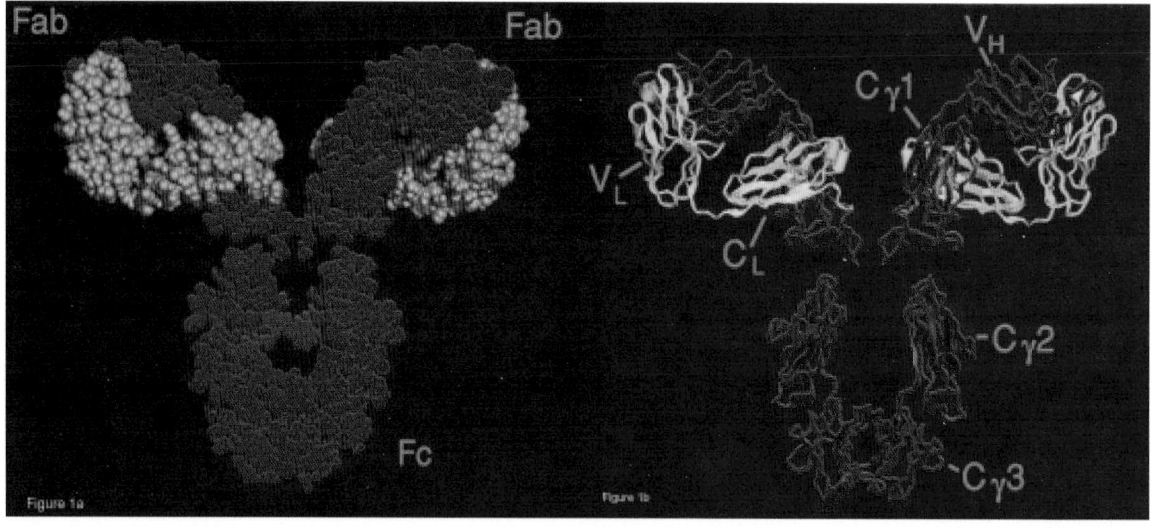

(a)   **(b)**

Fig. 3.1 An immunoglobulin (Ig) molecule. (**a**) Model of human IgG1 composed of two heavy chains (red) and two light chains (yellow). (**b**) Graphic representation of IgG1 in which secondary structure of a carbon backbone is shown. The CH2 domains are thought to be of primary importance in determining Fc effector functions such as complement activation and FcR binding. (Images courtesy of Dr Mike Clark, University of Cambridge, Department of Pathology; further images available at www.path.cam.ac.uk/mrc7/mikeimages.html.)

Table 3.1 Human immunoglobulin (Ig) Isotypes

	IgM	IgG	IgA	IgD	IgE
Heavy chain	μ	γ	α	δ	ε
Molecular weight (kDa)	970	146	160	184	188
Polymeric form	Pentameric	Monomeric	Dimeric	Monomeric	Monomeric
Total Ig in adults (%)	8	73	18	< 1	< 0.5
Principal site	Blood	Blood secretions	Mucosal	Blood	Blood
Placental transfer	No	Yes	No	No	No
Complement activation	+++	+++	+	–	–
Classical (C) Alternative (A)	C	C	A	–	–
Cellular binding/ activation	Macrophages/ phagocytes	–	Macrophages/ phagocytes	–	Mast cells/ basophils

Table 3.2 B-cell and antibody function

	Antibody isotype
B-cell function	
Antigen presentation to T-cells	–
Antibody production	–
Antibody effector function	
Activation of NK cells (ADCC)	IgG
Facilitation of phagocytosis (opsonization)	IgG/IgA
Activation of complement	IgM/IgA/IgG

ADCC, Antibody-dependent cell-mediated cytotoxity; Ig, immunoglobulin; NK, natural killer.

1.2 B-cell development

The purpose of B-cell development is to produce cells with a diverse range of receptor specificities capable of responding to foreign, but not self, antigen. The genes encoding antibodies are grouped in three clusters: the *IGH* cluster encoding the heavy chain, the *IGK* cluster encoding the κ light chain and the *IGL* cluster encoding the λ light chain. Within each heavy-chain cluster there are a number of each of the four gene segments, *V*, *D*, *J* and *C*. The light chain gene has *V*, *J* and *C* segments only. The different *V*, (*D*), *J* and *C* segments are then recombined to form a unique heavy or light chain. This process produces a B-cell repertoire of up to 10^8 different antibody specificities.[1,2,5]

B-cells develop from pluripotent stem cells in the bone marrow. The first member of the committed B-cell lineage is the pro-B-cell, in which there is significant heavy-chain rearrangement. This results in the expression of intact μ chain in combination with a surrogate light chain (composed of λ5 and VpreB) to form the pre-B-cell receptor complex, marking the large pre-B-cell. It is thought that the surrogate light chain, by associating with the heavy chain, identifies those heavy chains that are functional. Pre-B-cells with unfavourable heavy-chain structures die by apoptosis. Those cells with suitable heavy-chain rearrangements subsequently divide, giving rise to small pre-B-cells in which successful light-chain gene *VJ* gene rearrangement allows the assembly of surface IgM molecules in the immature B-cell. These immature B-cells are subject to selection for self-reactivity (see section 2) and undergo further differentiation to become mature B-cells, expressing both IgM and IgD (Fig. 3.2).[6,7] Thus, B-cell development is an orderly sequence of proliferation, immunoglobulin gene

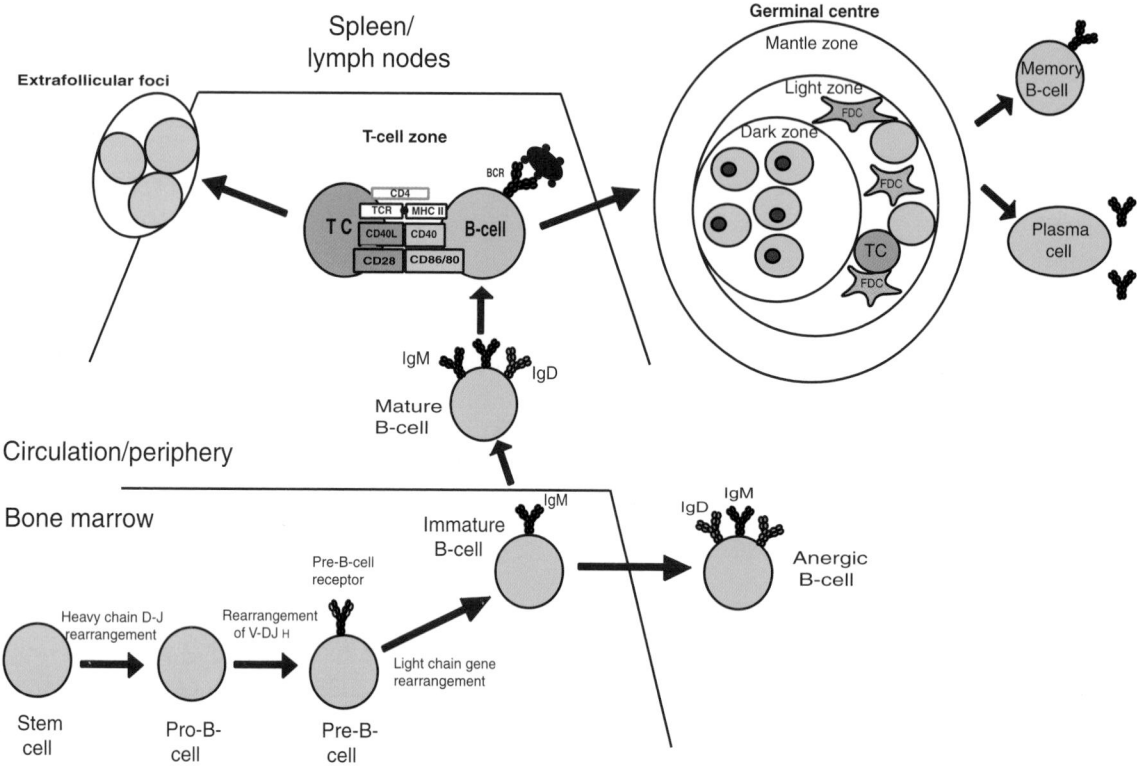

Fig. 3.2 B-cell development and tolerance. Differentiation and expansion of B-cell precursors are accompanied by sequential rearrangement of immunoglobulin (Ig) *V* genes. B-cells failing to make a normal pre-B- or B-cell receptor die at the pre-B- and immature B-cell stages, respectively. Those binding self-antigen are eliminated, anergized or undergo receptor editing. B-cells interacting with antigen and a cognate T-cell form foci of plasmablasts or germinal centres. Germinal centres are the source of high-affinity plasma and memory cells.

rearrangement, with selection of cells possessing productive rearrangements, and death of unselected or autoreactive cells.

A subset of B-cells, termed B-1-cells, arise early in ontogeny, populate the pleural and peritoneal cavities and are usually characterized by the expression of CD5. B1-cells are autonomously self-renewing and produce low-affinity, polyreactive antibodies which undergo little somatic hypermutation. It has been suggested that B1-cells are not subject to the same tolerogenic checkpoints as conventional B-cells (see section 2) and may be responsible for the production of some autoantibodies.[8]

1.3   B-cell response to antigen

Antigens that elicit an antibody response can be divided into two groups on the basis of their need for T-cell assistance. Antigens that require B- and T-cell collaboration in order to generate an antibody response, and thus fail to produce a response in athymic mice, are known as T-dependent (TD) antigens. The second group of antigens can stimulate antibody production in athymic mice, in the absence of conventional T-cell help, and are termed T-independent (TI) antigens.

1.3.1 TD antigens

Upon antigen recognition, adaptive immune responses are generated in the spleen, lymph nodes and mucosa-associated lymphoid tissue, known collectively as secondary lymphoid tissue (Fig. 3.2). Mature B-cells may circulate though lymphoid organs in order to increase the likelihood of antigen encounter. Encountered protein antigen is bound to the B-cell receptor (BCR; surface immunoglobulin) where it is internalized, processed and returned to the cell surface bound to major histocompatibility complex (MHC) class II molecules. On entering lymphoid tissue, these B-cells engage antigen-specific T-cells in the T-cell zone. The peptide/MHC complex is recognized by specific CD4+ T-cells, triggering the production of a variety of cytokines [in particular interleukin (IL)-4] and interaction between surface molecules, e.g. CD40 ligand (CD40L) on T-cells and CD40 on B-cells.[9,10] This interaction prompts some B-cells to proliferate in extrafollicular foci, rapidly producing large quantities of low-affinity antibody before undergoing apoptosis.[11] Other B-cells migrate to primary follicles where they form germinal centres. Here they proliferate and undergo somatic hypermutation, allowing single nucleotide exchanges to be introduced into the rearranged V-region genes. These cells then undergo a selection process in which those B-cells with low-affinity antibody–antigen interactions are eliminated by apoptosis. High-affinity antigen-specific B-cells eventually predominate, differentiating into memory B-cells and plasma cells.[12,13]

1.3.2 TI antigens

Thymus-independent antigens fall into two classes. High concentrations of TI-1 antigens, e.g. bacterial lipopolysaccharides, can induce polyclonal B-cell activation and proliferation, regardless of antigen specificity of the B-cells involved. At lower concentrations, only antigen-specific B-cells are activated. TI-2 antigens, e.g. dextrans and pneumococcal polysaccharides, do not act as polyclonal stimulators and can only activate mature B-cells. TI-1 antigens are generally inefficient inducers of isotype switching, germinal centre and memory B-cell formation. However, they do provide a prompt response to encapsulated pyogenic bacteria.[14]

2. B-CELL TOLERANCE AND ITS BREAKDOWN

The adaptive immune response provides an efficient defence against infection but if turned against self can cause severe tissue damage, a concept which Ehrlich[15] termed *horror autotoxicus*. Individuals do not usually mount a sustained immune response against self, since autoreactive cells are eliminated thus rendering the individual 'tolerant' to self, a theory proposed by Burnet[16] and confirmed by Medawar and Brent.[17] Autoreactive cells may be eliminated by clonal deletion, rendered anergic or self-antigens may be prevented from encountering the immune system, resulting in immune ignorance. However, in some circumstances, these measures of self-protection breakdown, resulting in autoimmune disease. There are a number of 'checkpoints' at which autoreactive B-cells are eliminated or silenced, thus ensuring B-cell tolerance. Mechanisms which might underlie B-cell tolerance both during B-cell development (central tolerance) and following antigen encounter in the periphery (peripheral tolerance) will be outlined in the following sections.

2.1 Central tolerance

In the bone marrow, immature B-cells (at the stage of light-gene rearrangement) encountering antigen capable of cross-linking their BCR are either eliminated (clonal deletion), become unresponsive and short-lived (anergic), or undergo revision of their BCR to eliminate self-reactivity (receptor editing). High-affinity interactions with membrane-bound antigen results in deletion, whereas lower affinity interactions and encounter with soluble antigen allows editing or anergy (the latter is characterized by expression of IgD and downregulation of IgM). Immature cells that do not encounter antigen mature normally and migrate from the bone marrow to the peripheral lymphoid tissue (Fig. 3.2).[18–20]

2.2 Peripheral tolerance

There are a number of processes maintain tolerance in the periphery (see Fig. 3.2).

- *T-cell tolerance.* In many cases B-cells fail to undergo TD activation due to the absence of appropriate T-cell help. T-cell tolerance can thus, by depriving the B-cell of help, impose tolerance on the B-cell repertoire. This may well be the most important mechanism in preventing TD B-cell autoreactivity.[18,21,22]

  It is also possible that autoreactive B-cells presenting antigen to CD4+ T-cells can be eliminated by delivery of a death signal from Fas ligand (FasL) on T-cells (see section 2.3.1). Naïve B-cells binding antigen become activated, resistant to apoptosis and capable of clonal expansion, whereas self-reactive B-cells, 'desensitized' by chronic binding of autoantigen, downregulate CD86/80 and remain sensitive to apoptosis. They may thus be eliminated in the T-cell zone.[18]

- *Deletion in germinal centres.* Once in germinal centres, unwanted autoreactive B-cell clones may be produced as a result of somatic hypermutation. Those binding foreign antigen immobilized on follicular dendritic cells are selected for survival, whereas those binding soluble antigen undergo apoptosis, perhaps providing a mechanism for the deletion of autoreactive germinal-centre B-cells.[23,24]

- *Antigen sequestration.* Some self-antigens are sequestered inside cells or within native protein folds, or exist in sites of immunological privilege (e.g. the eye), and are thus hidden from B-cells. Tolerance to them is therefore never developed in normal circumstances, as they are not exposed to the immune system, a state termed 'immunological ignorance'.[1]

- *Negative regulators of B-cell function.* B-cell activity is kept in check by a number of negative regulatory molecules, e.g. CD22, CD32 (FcγRIIb), CD72 and PIR-B (see section 2.3.3).

2.3 Breakdown of tolerance

The mechanism by which B-cells escape control measures and begin to produce pathological autoantibodies is complex and incompletely understood. A number of factors may contribute to the breakdown of tolerance, some of which will be considered in more detail.

2.3.1 Defects in apoptosis

Apoptosis is crucial for the removal of autoreactive B-cells, both centrally and peripherally. Abnormalities in a number of apoptotic pathways have been linked with the development of autoimmunity. Two of these will be discussed here.

CD95 (Fas) is a member of the nerve growth factor/tumor necrosis factor (TNF) receptor superfamily and can initiate a signal transduction cascade leading to apoptosis. It is expressed at high levels in activated lymphocytes and acts as a major pathway for the peripheral deletion of antigen-primed lymphocytes.[25] Humans with Fas mutations develop an autoimmune lymphoproliferative syndrome (ALPS), which is characterized by massive lymphadenopathy and autoimmune disease.[26] Mice homozygous for the *lpr* or *gdl* mutation (leading to nonfunctional Fas or FasL proteins, respectively) have increased numbers of B- and T-cells (the latter are CD4-CD8-B220+) and autoantibodies, and develop lymphadenopathy and immune complex-mediated glomerulonephritis.[27, 28]

The proto-oncogene *bcl-2* was originally identified as the result of its chromosomal translocation in follicular lymphoma[29] and encodes a 24 kDa membrane-associated protein which protects cells from apoptosis.[30] Transgenic overexpression of Bcl-2 in B-cells prevents apoptosis, blocks peripheral self-tolerance and can predispose to autoantibody production and immune-mediated glomerulonephritis.[31] Thus, breakdown of pathways of programmed cell death may well lead to the survival of autoreactive cells and to autoimmune disease.

2.3.2 Altered antigen processing and presentation

- *Exposure of sequestered antigen.* Tissue damage and inflammation may expose previously concealed autoantigens or induce presentation of certain cryptic self-antigens, as seen in sympathetic orchitis or ophthalmia. Other processes contributing to the recognition of previously hidden self-antigen include the binding of a foreign antigen to a self-protein, the alteration of protein structure due to somatic mutation, or abnormal protein degradation.[1]

- *The inflammatory response.* In addition to releasing previously concealed antigen, inflammation also focuses activated immunologically relevant cells on the newly exposed self-antigen. Complement deposition may make self-antigen more antigenic, e.g. C3d attached to antigen recruits the CD19/CD21 complex, lowering the threshold for B-cell activation and perhaps allowing tolerance to be broken.[32,33]
- *Molecular mimicry.* A variety of infections have been associated with autoantibody production or autoimmune disease (e.g. coxsackie virus and autoimmune myocarditis). It has therefore been proposed that autoantibody production might begin as a monospecific response to an epitope shared by a microbial antigen and a self-antigen. This autoantigen may then be processed and presented by B-cells, thus priming autoreactive T-cells.[34] Using a transgenic mouse model it has recently been shown that challenge with a self-mimicking foreign antigen can release B-cells from peripheral tolerance independent of T-cell help.[35]

2.3.3 Alteration of B-cell activation thresholds

A number of lines of evidence suggest that B-cell hyperactivity can contribute to the development of autoimmunity. Upon antigen binding to the BCR, B-cell activation thresholds are determined by the net effects of positive and negative regulatory molecules.[36] If the balance between these inputs is disturbed then autoimmunity can result.

FcγRII (CD32) is an inhibitor of cellular activation which is expressed on B-cells, macrophages and other cells of the myeloid lineage. FcγRIIb can also generate a pro-apoptotic signal and may well have a role in maintaining peripheral tolerance.[37] FcγRIIb deficient mice have elevated immunoglobulin titres, hyperactive B-cells, are susceptible to inducible autoimmune disease and, on certain genetic backgrounds, develop spontaneous SLE[38,39](see section 5.1).

CD22 is a B-cell-specific negative regulator.[33] CD22-deficient mice show B-cell hyperresponsiveness which correlates with the development

of autoantibodies directed against double-stranded DNA.[40] Mice deficient in other molecules involved in the inhibitory pathway, such as Lyn and SHP-1, also display B-cell hyperresponsiveness and autoimmune disease.[33,41] Thus, defective negative regulation of B-cell activation can lead to B-cell hyperactivity and autoimmunity.

CD19 is a cell-surface glycoprotein expressed exclusively on B-cells, in a complex with CD21 (complement receptor 2), CD81 and Leu 13.[33] CD19 modulates the proliferation and activation signals delivered to the B-cell by immunoglobulin. Coligation of the CD19/CD21/CD81 complex to the BCR results in a massive decrease in the activation threshold of B-cells stimulated through surface IgM.[42] Overexpression of human CD19 in mice leads to elevated levels of immunoglobulin and hyperactive B-cells.[43,44] Transgenic mice which express a model autoantigen, soluble hen egg lysosyme (sHEL), and high-affinity HEL-specific antigen receptors are functionally anergic and do not produce autoantibodies. However, overexpression of CD19 in these mice results in the breakdown of peripheral tolerance and the production of anti-HEL antibodies.[45] In addition, upregulation of CD19 has been noted in patients with systemic sclerosis.[46] Thus, by lowering the activation threshold on B-cells, CD19 overexpression may contribute to the breakdown of tolerance and the development of autoimmune disease.

3. B-CELLS, AUTOANTIBODY AND DISEASE

Autoantibodies have been found in association with a number of diseases (Table 3.3). In some of these it is clear that these antibodies are directly pathogenic, inducing disease without recourse to inflammation. In others, the antibodies form immune complexes (IC) that become deposited in tissues causing inflammation, subsequent tissue damage and thus disease. The third broad group comprises diseases associated with autoantibodies but in which no definitive link has been made between the antibodies and the pathogenesis of disease. In some of these there is some evidence for

Table 3.3 Autoantibodies and disease

Disease	Antigen (Ref)
Autoimmune diseases caused by directly pathogenic autoantibodies	
Graves's disease	Thyroid-stimulating hormone receptor (44)
Myasthenia gravis	Acetylcholine receptor (45)
Cold autoimmune haemolytic anaemia	I antigen (red blood cell surface antigen)
Thrombocytopenic purpura	GpIIb/IIIa fibrinogen receptor on platelets (50)
Lambert–Eaton syndrome	Presynaptic calcium channel
Anti-phospholipid syndrome	Phospholipid (55)
Pemphigus vulgaris	Desmoglein 3 (Fig. 4.4a)
Diseases associated with immune complex (IC) mediated inflammation	
Cryoglobulinaemia	IgG
Goodpasture's disease	α3 Chain of type IV collagen in glomerular basement membrane (Fig. 4.4b) (70)
Systemic lupus erythematosus	See Table 4.4 and Fig. 4.4 c and d
Diseases with autoantibodies of unknown significance	
Atherosclerosis	Oxidized LDL, cardiolipin, β2-glycoprotein-I, HSP-60/65 (100–102)
Autoimmune chronic active hepatitis	Smooth muscle, anti-LKM antibody
Coeliac disease	α-gliadin, endomysium, reticulin
Congenital heart block/subacute cutaneous lupus erythematosus	Ro/SSA (cytoplasmic protein-RNA complex) (50)
CREST syndrome	Centromeres (50)
Diabetes mellitus	Insulin, islet cell, glutamic acid decarboxylase, tyrosine phosphatase antibodies (90–92)
Guillain-Barré syndrome	GM1
Microscopic polyangiitis	pANCA (Fig. 4.4f)
Miller–Fisher syndrome	Gq1b
Multiple sclerosis	MOG, MBP (97,98)
Autoimmune myositis	Histydyl-tRNA synthetase (Jo-1) (50)
Pernicious anaemia	Parietal cell, intrinsic factor
Primary biliary cirrhosis	Mitochondrial (M2 antibody)
Rheumatoid arthritis	IgG (83)
Sjogren's syndrome	Ro/SSA, La/SSB (cytoplasmic protein-RNA complex) (50)
Systemic sclerosis	DNA topoisomerase (50)
Wegener's granulomatosis	Neutrophil proteinase-3 (Fig. 4.4e) (75)

ANCA, Anti-neutrophil cytoplasmic antibody; GP, glycoprotein; HSP, heat-shock protein; Ig, immunoglobulin; LDL, low-density lipoprotein; LKM, liver kidney microsomal; MBP, myelin basic protein; MOG, myelin oligodendrocyte; tRNA, transfer RNA.

antibody-mediated pathogenesis, which may strengthen over time. In others the presence of autoantibody might well indicate that B-cells are playing an important role, perhaps via antigen presentation, but the antibodies themselves are not pathogenic. Finally, in some diseases, autoantibodies may be an epiphenomenon, their presence reflecting inflammation and tissue damage alone. Even in this situation their detection could still be of diagnostic or prognostic use. Each of these three groups of diseases will be discussed in turn and illustrated by selected examples.

4. DISEASES WITH DIRECTLY PATHOGENIC AUTOANTIBODY

There are a number of diseases in which the autoantibody produced is thought to be directly pathogenic independent of inflammation. Two examples are Graves's disease and myasthenia gravis.

4.1 Graves's disease

In Graves's disease, autoantibody directed against the thyroid-stimulating hormone receptor persistently binds and stimulates the excessive production of thyroxine, resulting in thyrotoxicosis. The pathogenic action of the autoantibody has been demonstrated in animal models, e.g. serum taken from a patient with Graves's disease injected into a healthy rat produces thyroid activation. In addition, these autoantibodies can cross the placenta, leading to hyperthyroidism in the neonate.[47]

4.2 Myasthenia gravis

Patients with myasthenia gravis develop muscle weakness (particularly of the extraocular and respiratory muscles) due to a failure of signal transmission at the neuromuscular junction. The disease is characterized by autoantibodies directed against the α chain of the nicotinic acetylcholine receptor found on the postsynaptic membrane. Binding of the autoantibody causes complement-mediated lysis of the membrane and acceleration of the normal degradative processes of the receptor, thus preventing signal transmission.[48] Transfer of human IgG obtained from myasthenics to mice reproduces the precise electrophysiological features of myasthenia gravis.[49] As is the case in Graves's disease, transplacental transfer of the IgG autoantibody can cause disease in neonates.[50] Removal of the antibody by plasmapheresis is an effective treatment for severe disease.[51]

5. DISEASES ASSOCIATED WITH IMMUNE COMPLEX (IC)-MEDIATED INFLAMMATION

The interaction of autoantibody and antigen leads to the formation of IC. If there is an excess of antigen, then soluble IC are formed. These may circulate and become deposited in tissues and initiate inflammation by activating complement or phagocytic cells. Alternatively, antibodies may bind to fixed antigen, with *in situ* IC formation. The inflammatory response to these IC subsequently leads to local tissue damage. In some diseases, such as Goodpasture's disease, the specificity of the autoantibody limits the sites affected by inflammatory processes. In others, e.g. SLE, antibodies are raised against numerous autoantigens (see Table 3.4), including some ubiquitous cellular antigens, and the IC formation and deposition is therefore more widespread and variable.

5.1 SLE

SLE is a multisystem autoimmune disease characterized by autoantibody production, IC deposition and complement activation. Clinical manifestations range from dermatological lesions and immune cytopenias to necrotizing glomerulonephritis.[52]

It useful to describe what is understood of the pathogenesis in two phases (Fig. 3.3). In the first, self-tolerance is broken and autoimmunity results. Self- or cross-reactive antigens are presented by professional antigen-presenting cells (APCs), such as macrophages, dendritic cells and B-cells to autoreactive CD4+ T-cells. These T-cells then activate B-cells and autoantibodies are produced. The second phase involves inflammation due to IC deposition, and the recruitment and activation of macrophages,

Table 3.4 Autoantibodies in systemic lupus erythematosus (SLE)[50]

Antigen	Prevalence in SLE (%)
Single-stranded DNA	70–90
Ubiquitin (DNA/chromatin-binding protein)	60–80
Double-stranded DNA	50–70
Histones	60–80
Lymphocyte (including CD24, TCR, CD4, IL–2R)	30–50
SSA/Ro (cytoplasmic antigen)	30–40
Ku (DNA-binding protein, involved in repair complex)	30–40
U1 RNP (nuclear RNA–associated protein)	30–40
Sm (soluble nuclear RNA protein)	20–30
Phospholipid	20–30
Red cell (causing haemolytic anaemia)	20–30
Proliferating cell nuclear antigen	<5
SSB/La (cytoplasmic antigen)	15–25
Platelet (causing immune thombocytopenic purpura)	10–25
Ribosomal P0, P1, P2	10–20
Mitotic-spindle-associated proteins (NuMA-1)	<5
Vimentin (extracellular matrix component)	Unknown
Heat-shock proteins (cytoplasmic antigen)	Unknown

IL, Interleukin; TCR, T-cell receptor.

CD8+ cytotoxic T-lymphocytes and granulocytes. Inflammation exposes further autoantigen to the immune system, which may amplify the disease process.

5.1.1 Antibodies and IC-mediated inflammation in SLE

The exact role played by autoantibodies in the pathogenesis of SLE is incompletely defined. Many older patients have detectable antinuclear antibodies (ANA) and anti-double-stranded (ds) DNA antibodies but never develop disease. Others develop SLE in the absence of detectable circulating autoantibodies. Nonetheless the association of ANA with SLE is remarkably strong. Certain ANA are relatively specific for the diagnosis of SLE. Anti-dsDNA antibodies are found in 70% of patients with

SLE and have a 95% specificity for the diagnosis. Anti-Sm antibodies are found in up to 25% of SLE patients' sera and are virtually pathognomonic of SLE.[53]

As discussed previously, the presence of autoantibodies does not necessarily imply a direct role in disease processes. However, IC deposition is a consistent histopathological feature in affected tissues in SLE. For example, in both major types of glomerulonephritis associated with SLE there is prominent IC deposition. In membranous glomerulonephritis (Fig. 3.4c), subepithelial deposits are seen, whereas in diffuse proliferative lupus nephritis more widespread deposition, including sub-endothelial (with so-called 'full-house' immunofluorescence for IgG, IgM, C1q and C3) is seen (Fig. 3.4d).

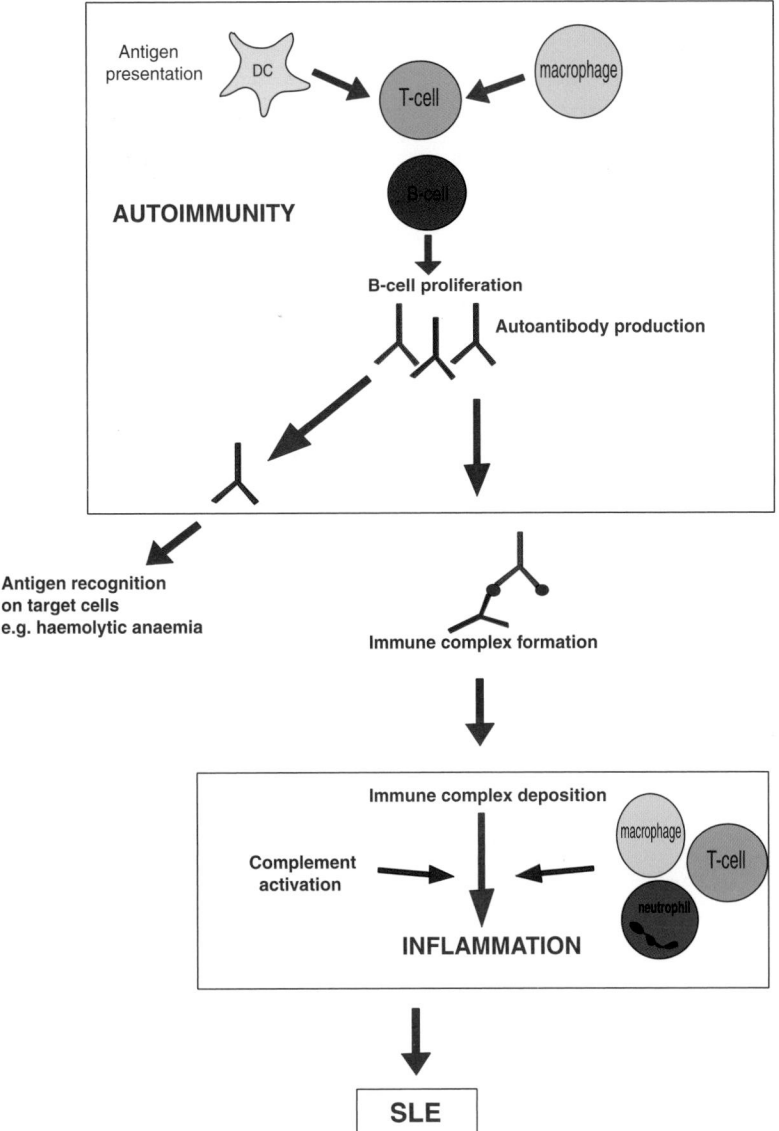

Fig. 4.3 The pathogenesis of systemic lupus erythematosus (SLE). Two-stage process in which autoimmunity and inflammation lead to disease.

In animal models of SLE, anti-DNA antibodies have been shown to cause, at least indirectly, some pathological features, particularly renal manifestations. Infusion of anti-DNA antibodies obtained from lupus-prone mouse strains such as MRL, into normal mice prompts the development of a proliferative glomerulonephritis.[51] Intraperitoneal administration of a monoclonal anti-DNA antibody-secreting hybridoma into control mice can also induce glomerulonephritis, proteinuria and a dermal vasculitis.[54] In addition, mouse and human anti-DNA IgG applied to the isolated perfused rat kidney binds avidly to glomeruli and is associated with proteinuria and a reduction in inulin clearance.[55]

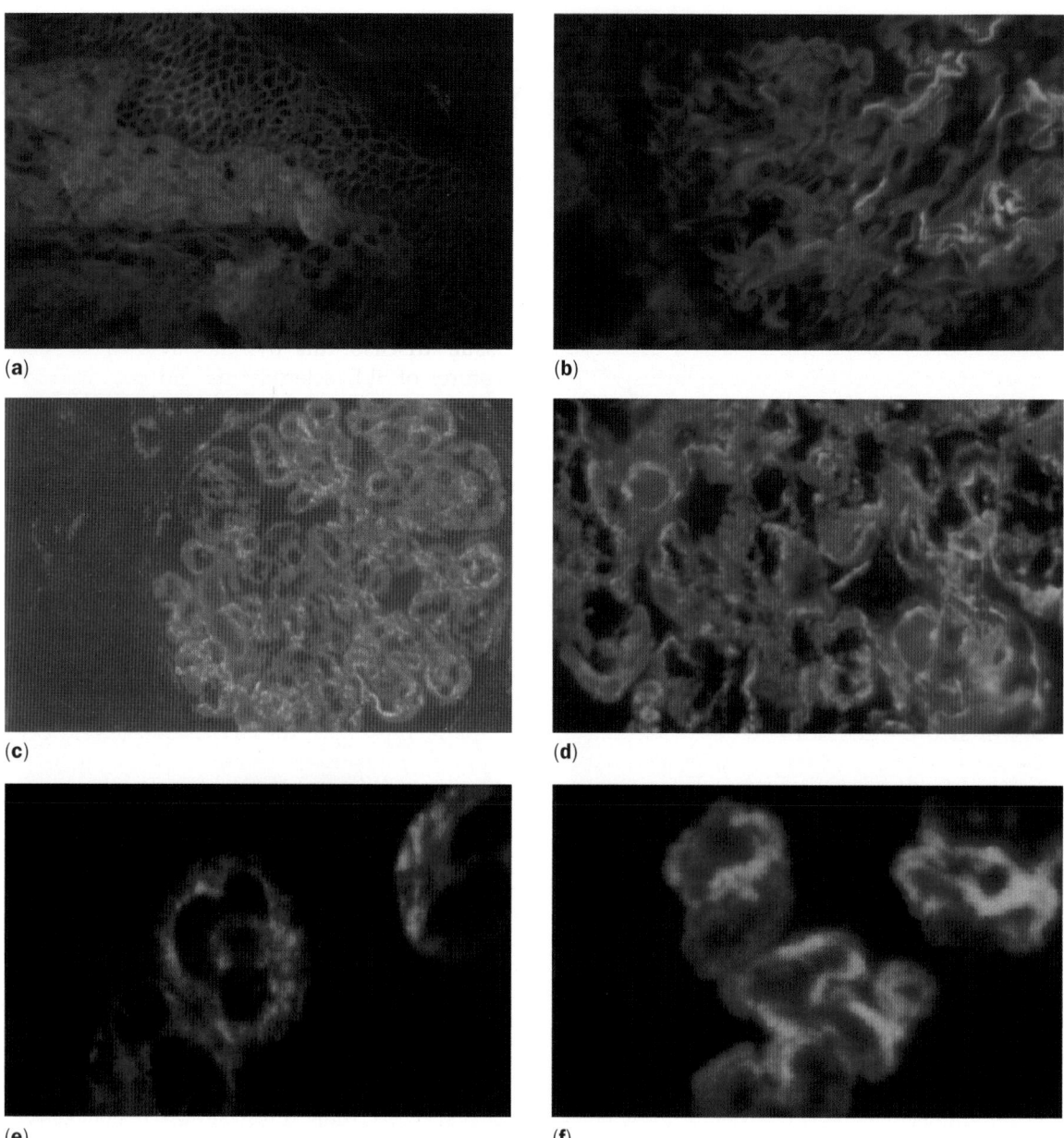

Fig. 3.4 (**a**) *Pemphigus.* Antibody deposition between epidermal cells leading to subsequent disruption and blistering. [Immunofluorescence for immunoglobulin (Ig) G, courtesy of Dr E Rytina, Department of Histopathology, Addenbrookes Hospital, Cambridge.] (**b**) *Goodpasture's disease* – Anti-GBM (glomerular basement membrane) antibody binding to the basement membrane of a glomerulus in a patient with Goodpasture's disease. (Immunofluorescence for IgG, courtesy of Dr S Thiru, Department of Pathology, Addenbrookes Hospital, Cambridge.) (**c**) Subendothelial immune complex deposition in *membranous glomerulonephritis* associated with systemic lupus erythematosus (SLE). (Immunofluorescence for IgG). (**d**) Widespread immune complex (IC) deposition in *diffuse proliferative lupus nephritis.* (Immunofluorescence for IgG). (**e**) auto-neutrophil cytoplasmic antibody (ANCA) staining pattern associated with proteinase-3 in *Wegener's granulomatosis.* (**f**) pANCA staining pattern due to myeloperoxidase in *microscopic polyangitis.* [(e) and (f) show immunofluorescence of serum IgG binding to fixed neutrophils, and were kindly provided by Dr D Jayne, Department of Nephrology, Addenbrookes Hospital, Cambridge.]

Even in animal models, however, the presence of antibody does not necessarily lead to disease. B6.NZMc1 congenic mice develop IgG ANA in the absence of nephritis.[56] One of the mechanisms coupling cytotoxic antibodies/IC and effector cells are FcγR. Deletion of activatory FcγR protects mice from antibody-mediated spontaneous or induced autoimmune disease without altering expression of autoantibodies, as demonstrated in the FcRγ-deficient NZB/NZW F1 mice which develop autoantibodies, and also have significant IC deposition but do not develop glomerulonephritis.[57] Loss of negative regulatory molecules, such as CD22, leads to the development of high-affinity autoantibodies against DNA, cardiolipin and myeloperoxidase but not to disease,[40] suggesting that additional factors are required for disease causation. Thus, it seems that autoantibodies in SLE are necessary but not sufficient to cause disease.

5.1.2 Directly pathogenic antibodies
Some antibodies directly cause specific disease manifestations. Autoimmune haemolytic anaemia is an initial feature in 5% of patients with SLE and occurs in up to one third of patients with SLE. Autoantibodies (usually IgG) bind to red cell membrane components, causing autoagglutination of erythrocytes within the splenic pulp and subsequent removal by phagocytes (warm autoimmune haemolytic anaemia).[53] Similarly, autoantibody-mediated thrombocytopenia, neutropenia and lymphopenia may occur in SLE.

5.1.3 Antibodies associated with particular clinical features
Anti-phospholipid antibodies, which recognize a variety of phospholipids including cardiolipin, phosphatidylserine and β_2-glycoprotein I (β_2-GPI), are strongly associated with recurrent episodes of arterial and venous thrombosis, spontaneous fetal loss, and thrombocytopenia. This triad, termed antiphospholipid syndrome, is seen in the presence of antiphospholipid antibodies in patients with and without SLE. A number of pathogenic mechanisms have been proposed for this association. Anti-β_2-GPI

antibodies are thought to interfere with the β_2-GPI inhibition of factor Xa production by activated platelets. In addition, autoantibody binding to β_2-GPI on the endothelial cell surface induces the expression of a number of adhesion molecules, e.g. VCAM-1 (vascular cell adhesion molecule-1) and E-selectin, thus enhancing monocyte adhesion to endothelial cells.[58] Other clinical syndrome–autoantibody associations include that of neonatal heart block in mothers with anti-Ro antibodies and mixed connective tissue disease (an overlap syndrome with features of SLE, scleroderma and polymyositis) with anti-nRNP antibodies.[53]

5.1.4 Autoantibodies in SLE – TD or TI
There is good evidence to suggest that autoantibody production in SLE occurs by both TD and TI mechanisms. TD is suggested by the predominance of IgG2a ANA in MRL mice and by the observation that lower levels of autoantibodies occur in MRL and NZB/W mice treated with anti-CD4 antibodies. In addition, analysis of autoantibody V regions shows a high degree of somatic mutation, indicative of autoantigen-driven TD B-cell activation.[59]

In contrast, low-affinity, polyreactive single-stranded (ss) DNA autoantibodies, bearing germline V-region sequences, have also been identified in SLE. It is thought these antibodies may be produced by B1 cells in a TI fashion.[60]

5.1.5 B-cell hyperactivity
B-cell activation thresholds following antigen binding to the BCR are determined by the net effects of positive and negative regulatory molecules.[36] If the balance between these inputs is disturbed then autoimmunity can result. CD32 (FcγRIIb) is a single-chain transmembrane glycoprotein expressed on B-cells, macrophages, neutrophils and other cells of the myeloid lineage. FcγRIIb binds IgG with low affinity via its extracellular domain and mediates its inhibitory activity through its immunoreceptor tyrosine-based inhibitory motif (ITIM).[37] FcγRIIb-deficient mice are susceptible to collagen-induced arthritis,[38] IC-induced alveolitis[61] and, on certain genetic backgrounds, develop SLE.[39] In addition, defects in FcγRIIb also seem to be

important in polygenic mouse models of SLE. A deletion in the promoter region of the FcγRII gene, which is associated with a reduction in its surface expression, has been found in all strains prone to spontaneous SLE, including the NZB, MRL and BXSB strains, and this defect has been associated with macrophage hyperactivity[62] and autoantibody production.[63]

CD22 is a B-cell-specific negative regulator that acts to dampen signals generated through the BCR via its ITIM.[33] CD22-deficient mice show increased B-cell hyperresponsiveness that correlates with the development of autoantibodies directed against dsDNA.[40] Mice deficient in other molecules downstream in the inhibitory pathway, such as Lyn and SHP-1, also display B-cell hyperresponsiveness and autoimmune disease.[41]

Patients with SLE have been noted to have spontaneously active polyclonal antibody-forming cells in their peripheral blood that demonstrate an exaggerated intracellular calcium response to BCR stimulation, similar to that seen in mice with defective negative regulatory pathways.[64]

5.1.6 B-cell as an antigen-presenting cell
Antigen presentation by B-cells may also be important in the pathogenesis of SLE. J_HD-MRL/*lpr* mice (a B-cell deficient version of the lupus-prone MRL/*lpr* mouse) fail to develop nephritis and dermatitis, emphasizing the importance of B-cells in disease.[65] However, mIgM.MRL/*lpr* transgenic mice that have B-cells but are unable to secrete antibody, develop substantial nephritis and vasculitis, suggesting pathogenic B-cell activity independent of antibody production.[66] It may be that, in this model, B-cell autoantigen presentation plays a more important role than the production of autoantibody in the development of lupus.

5.1.7 Role of cytokines
The TNF superfamily is involved in the regulation of cell proliferation, differentiation and apoptosis. Most of these are membrane proteins and contain a 150 amino-acid-conserved domain which can be proteolytically cleaved, releasing a soluble, functional form.[67] B-lymphocyte stimulator (BLyS; also known as

BAFF or TALL-1) is a member of the TNF superfamily and stimulates B-cell proliferation. BLyS-transgenic mice develop B-cell hyperplasia and hyperactivity, anti-DNA antibodies and circulating IC which become deposited in glomeruli.[68] In murine models of lupus (MRL and NZB/NZW F1), increased levels of BLyS have been noted, which correlate with the severity of glomerulonephritis.[69] In addition, soluble BLyS activates B-cells *in vitro* and is elevated in patients with SLE compared with controls.[70]

B-lymphocyte chemokine (BLC; also known as BCA-1/CXCL13) is a potent B-cell chemo-attractant expressed predominantly by follicular dendritic cells in secondary lymphoid tissues and is thought to play a role in attracting naïve B-cells to form germinal centres. It has recently been reported that the expression of BLC is markedly increased in the thymus and kidneys of lupus-prone (NZB×NZW) F1 mice. Interestingly, BLC shows preferential chemotactic activity for B1-cells (thought by some to be responsible for autoantibody production), and in the (NZB×NZW) F1 mice the B1/B2 cell ratio in the thymus was markedly increased in favour of B1-cells. These observations raise the possibility that high expression of BLC by dendritic cells in target organs may play a role in the breakdown of tolerance.[71]

5.1.8 Role of complement
Although not obviously related to autoantibody production, nonetheless, the role of complement in SLE is worthy of comment. The complement system is known to be important in facilitating the disposal of IC by the mononuclear phagocytic system. IC that fix complement are transported in the blood [bound to erythrocytes via complement receptor 1 (CR1)] to the spleen and liver where they are disposed of by phagocytic cells. Interestingly, hereditary complement deficiencies (particularly early complement components, such as C1q, C2 and C4) predispose to the development of SLE, presumably due to the accumulation of IC.[53] This is supported by the observation that C1q-deficient mice have a significantly reduced splenic uptake of IC compared with controls and develop SLE.[72]

5.2 Goodpasture's disease

The classical clinical features of Goodpasture's disease are that of a proliferative glomerulo-nephritis and pulmonary haemorrhage. Autoantibodies are formed against the carboxy-terminal, non-collagenous domain of the α_3 chain of type IV collagen.[73] Type IV collagen is only found in basement membrane. Antibodies bind to the basement membranes of renal glomeruli (Fig. 3.4b) and pulmonary alveoli and, by activating complement and phagocytes, initiate inflammation producing the clinical features observed. There is usually a correlation between the autoantibody titre and severity of renal disease.[74] In addition, antibody eluted from the kidneys of patients with Goodpasture's disease can bind to the glomerular basement membrane of squirrel monkeys *in vivo* and cause pathological glomerular changes.[75] The proposed pathogenic role of antibody in Goodpasture's disease provides the rationale for the use of plasma exchange in treatment.[76] Interestingly, lung haemorrhage is a variable feature of Goodpasture's disease and shows a very poor correlation with antibody titre. Although the Goodpasture's antigen is present in pulmonary basement membrane, it is usually shielded from direct contact with circulating antibody and lymphocytes by a non-fenestrated vascular endothelium. If this barrier is disturbed, e.g. by infection or smoking, then pulmonary haemorrhage may occur.[77]

6. DISEASES IN WHICH B-CELLS PLAY AN UNCERTAIN ROLE

The third group of diseases are those associated with autoantibodies but in which no definitive link has been made between the antibodies and the pathogenesis of disease. In some, the presence of autoantibody may indicate that B-cells are playing an important role, either through antibody production or antigen presentation. In others, autoimmunity might be due to a breakdown in T-cell tolerance, with autoantibody production resulting from this but not in itself causing disease. Finally, autoantibody production may be an epiphenomenon, occurring merely as a result of tissue damage.

6.1 Wegener's granulomatosis

Wegener's granulomatosis is a small-vessel vasculitis predominantly affecting upper and lower respiratory tracts and kidneys. It is characterized by the presence of anti-neutrophil cytoplasmic antibody (cANCA), an autoantibody usually directed against proteinase-3, a serine protease found in the azurophilic granules of neutrophils (Fig. 3.4e). The antibody is thought to bind near the catalytic domain of the molecule and interfere with its inactivation by α_1-antitrypsin.[78]

Direct evidence for the pathogenicity of cANCA is lacking in particular, ANCA transferred to healthy animals does not induce disease. However, considerable circumstantial evidence implicates autoantibodies in pathogenesis. Histopathological studies have shown that in ANCA-associated glomerulonephritis, the earliest changes affect the vascular endothelium and are associated with the presence of numerous neutrophils within affected vessels. In addition, numbers of neutrophils seem to correspond to the extent of renal function loss. *In vitro*, ANCA can activate neutrophils to produce reactive oxygen species and release lytic enzymes and proinflammatory cytokines. However, these neutrophils require priming with proinflammatory cytokines such as TNF-α before they can be activated in this way. This priming results in surface expression of proteinase-3, making the antigen available for interaction with cANCA.[79] ANCA-associated activation appears to occur by interaction of the antibody with FcγRIIa and FcγRIII, and also requires integrin-mediated adhesion. Finally, when primed, neutrophils and endothelial cells are incubated *in vitro* with ANCA, endothelial cell damage results. In the clinical setting, in patients with ANCA-positive vasculitis, the neutrophil-activating capacity of ANCA-positive IgG fractions correlate better with disease activity than levels of ANCA alone.[80] Together, these observations support, but do not yet prove, a pathogenic role for ANCA in Wegener's granulomatosis via neutrophil activation.

6.2 Rheumatoid arthritis (RA)

RA is a chronic, debilitating disorder characterized by synovial inflammation. This inflammation results in hyperplasia of synoviocytes, infiltration of mononuclear cells, neoangiogenesis, pannus formation and joint destruction. These effector-phase processes are relatively well delineated but the upstream initiating events remain unclear.

The classical model of RA proposes that it is T-cells within joints that recognize autoantigen presented to them and produce the inflammatory cytokines that initiate a predominantly type 1 helper T-cell (Th1) response within the synovium.[81] This is supported by the observed association of certain MHC class II haplotypes with RA, the presence of T-cells in synovial tissue and evidence from animal models of RA in which T-cell clones can provoke disease in normal mice.[82]

The K/BxN transgenic mouse model of inflammatory arthritis has led to an alternative model of rheumatoid pathogenesis. K/BxN mice express a transgenic T-cell receptor (TCR) that recognizes glucose-6-phosphate isomerase (GPI), an ubiquitous self-antigen.[83] TCR engagement with antigen provokes the differentiation and proliferation of B-cells to produce anti-GPI antibodies. Injection of these antibodies into healthy animals produces arthritis in the absence of lymphocytes within the joint. This model of RA suggests that the initial T-cell–antigen encounter may occur outside of the joint, that the autoantigen involved may not be joint specific and that T-cells can then induce B-cells to produce pathogenic autoantibodies.[84]

An aggressive arthritis, similar to RA, can be induced in susceptible mice by immunization with collagen. B-cell-deficient mice do not develop this collagen-induced arthritis[85] and thus B-cells seem to play a key role in its pathogenesis.

6.2.1 Rheumatoid factor

Approximately 80% of patients with RA develop circulating antibodies to IgG (rheumatoid factor). The relevance of rheumatoid factor to pathogenesis is not clear-cut, since it is absent in a proportion of cases and is also found in other instances of chronic immune stimulation.[86] Rheumatoid factor exists in the circulation as oligomers and dimers. The IgG dimers are of a sufficiently small size to pass out of the circulation and access tissue macrophages. Studies have shown that there are high levels of expression of the IgG receptor FcγRIIIa (an activatory receptor) in macrophages found in tissues affected by RA. The binding of IgG to FcγRIIIa may then induce the release of both TNF-α and oxygen radical species, providing a possible mechanism for a pathogenic role of rheumatoid factor in RA.[87,88]

6.2.2 Synovial germinal centres

The immune response is normally restricted to the secondary lymphoid organs (see section 1). However, in patients with RA, large perivascular, cellular aggregates with an organized follicular structure have been noted in the synovium.[89] Most cells in these aggregates are B-cells, some of which have a germinal centre phenotype and have somatically mutated *V* genes.[90] However, at present the significance of these synovial germinal centres is unclear.

6.2.3 B-cell depletion – a treatment for RA?

Recent evidence suggests that B-cell depletion in patients with RA may alleviate disease. CD20 is found exclusively on B-cells, and humanized anti-CD20 monoclonal antibody has been used previously in the treatment of B-cell lymphoma. In this group of patients it was coincidentally noted to be very effective in treating RA.[91] Further trials using anti-CD20 antibody in rheumatoid patients without lymphoma have supported the suggestion that B-cell depletion can induce disease remission.[92]

In summary, although RA has traditionally been considered to be a T-cell-mediated disease, there is increasing evidence to suggest that B-cells and antibody play an important role.

6.3 Diabetes mellitus (DM)

Type 1 (insulin-dependent) DM (IDDM) is caused by immune destruction of the insulin-secreting B-cells in the islets of Langerhans within the pancreas. A number of autoantibodies have been identified in IDDM patients, including anti-islet cell, anti-insulin, anti-glutamic acid decarboxylase (GAD), and anti-tyrosine phosphatase IA2 antibodies.[93] Anti-islet cell autoantibodies can be detected in early infancy and their presence in first-degree relatives of patients with IDDM is strongly predictive for the development of disease.[94] In addition, the presence of multiple autoantibodies makes progression to IDDM more likely.[95] Whether these autoantibodies are involved in disease pathogenesis, or reflect anti-islet T-cell immunity, has not yet been resolved.

The murine model of IDDM, the non-obese diabetic (NOD) mouse, also develops diabetes spontaneously due to islet cell destruction.[96] Transgenic NOD mice (NOD.$Ig\mu^{null}$) deficient in B-lymphocytes fail to develop disease,[97] and immunoglobulin infusions from NOD mice fail to restore disease. However, disease susceptibility in the NOD.$Ig\mu^{null}$ mice can be restored by B-lymphocytes transferred from NOD mice.[98] Thus, B-cells may well act to process and present antigen to autoreactive T-cells in diabetes.

6.4 Multiple sclerosis (MS)

MS is a chronic inflammatory demyelinating disorder of unknown cause that affects the central nervous system (CNS). The principal pathological features in brain and spinal cord are focal areas of demyelinating plaques surrounded by an inflammatory infiltrate consisting of B-cells, T-cells and macrophages.[99]

Experimental autoimmune encephalitis (EAE) (an animal model of MS) can be induced in genetically susceptible animals by immunization with numerous CNS, derived antigens, including myelin basic protein (MBP). T-cells reactive to MBP taken from an animal with EAE can transfer disease to a healthy recipient.[100] This model seems to implicate the importance of a T-cell-driven Th1 immune process in the pathogenesis of MS.

Some circumstantial evidence collected from histological and molecular studies suggest a substantive role for antibody in plaque development. MS is characterized by elevated IgG levels in the cerebrospinal fluid (CSF), identified isoelectrically as oligoclonal bands. Correspondingly large quantities of IgG mRNA have been isolated from brain plaques compared with normal brain. B-cells also appear to be more abundant in acute lesions in which there is ongoing demyelination than in older, inactive lesions. In addition, IgG deposited around the borders of actively demyelinating plaques has been shown to correlate with the presence of activated complement fragments. Sequence analysis of complementarity-determining regions of the antibodies found in the CSF of MS patients reveals a predominance of the variable heavy chain-4 in which there was extensive somatic mutation. These results suggest antigen-driven TD B-cell selection. Extensive efforts to identify the antigen specificity of the CSF antibodies in MS have yielded multiple candidates, including myelin-associated protein, MBP, myelin oligodendrocyte glycoprotein, heat-shock protein-60 (HSP-60) and human transaldolase, but some of these antibodies can be found in normal individuals as well as those with MS. EAE can be elicited by a number of autoantigens, but myelin oligodendrocyte glycoprotein in particular produces demyelinating plaques almost identical to those seen in MS. In addition, autoantibodies to myelin oligodendrocyte glycoprotein can enhance the clinical severity of EAE.[101] More recently, high-affinity anti-DNA antibodies have been isolated from the CSF of patients with MS,[102] and these antibodies bind efficiently to the surface of neuronal cells and oligodendrocytes. Studies investigating whether these autoantibodies can initiate or exacerbate demyelinating disease *in vivo* are awaited.

6.5 Atherosclerosis

The development of atheroscerotic plaques is increasingly recognized as an inflammatory process. Atherosclerotic lesions contain large quantities of IgG and several autoantibodies have been described in association with atheroma (see Table 3.3), including those directed against HSP-60/65 and oxidized low-density lipoprotein (LDL). HSP are a group of proteins with high interspecies homology. They are not expressed constitutively but may be induced by stress. Animal models provide evidence for the association between an immune response against HSP-65 and atherosclerosis. Rabbits immunized with HSP-65 develop atherosclerotic lesions. Patients with atherosclerosis have elevated levels of anti-HSP-65 antibodies compared with controls. It has been suggested that 'stressed' arterial endothelial cells may express HSP, which invoke an inflammatory and autoimmune response that initiates or aggravates atherosclerosis.[103,104]

Antibodies to oxidized LDL have also been linked to atherosclerosis, although the association appears to be more complex. Anti-oxidized LDL antibodies are increased in patients with early-onset peripheral vascular disease and angiographically verified coronary artery disease. In addition, elevated levels of these antibodies are predictive for disease progression and mortality from myocardial infarction. Conversely, long-term follow-up of a group of IDDM patients showed that those who remained free of coronary artery disease had lower levels of anti-oxidized LDL antibodies. In animal models, immunization with oxidized LDL resulted in suppression of early atherosclerosis. It is therefore possible that in healthy subjects, oxidized LDL antibodies may have a role in clearing LDL from the circulation. However, in advanced atherosclerosis an elevated humoral response to oxidized LDL may have a different significance.[104,105]

Although it is clear that some autoantibodies are associated with atherosclerosis, their significance is unclear. However, long-term follow-up of autoantibody levels may eventually define them as useful predictors or markers of disease.

7. CONCLUSIONS

There are many diseases associated with autoantibodies. In some, the antibody is directly pathogenic and in others they appear to cause disease via IC-mediated inflammation. However, in many, the role of the B-cell and autoantibody is poorly defined.

Knowledge about the role of individual components of the immune system in disease pathogenesis is vital if effective treatments are to be established. The use of plasma exchange to remove causative antibodies in Goodpasture's disease and myasthenia gravis illustrates the effectiveness of rational therapies founded on understanding the basic pathogenic processes involved. As evidence emerges implicating B-cells in disease, specific B-cell immunosuppression may provide targeted treatment in appropriate patients. Finally, autoantibodies have been an essential diagnostic tool for decades and indeed form part of the diagnostic criteria for SLE. It may be that in some diseases, such as IDDM, the early identification of auto-antibodies before irreversible tissue damage will allow pre-emptive treatment prior to disease progression. It is therefore imperative that the precise mechanisms involved in the pathogenesis of autoimmune diseases, and in particular the role of B-cells, continue to be unravelled by both basic science and clinical observation.

REFERENCES

Scientific papers

1. Janeway CA, Travers P, Walport M, Capra JD. *Immunobiology – The Immune System in Health and Disease*. London: Elsevier Science Ltd, 1999.
2. Edelman GM. Antibody structure and molecular immunology. *Science* 1973; **180**: 830–40.
3. Ravetch JV, Kinet J. Fc receptors. *Annu Rev Immunol* 1993; **9**: 457–92.
4. Tomlinson S. Complement defence mechanisms. *Curr Opin Immunol* 1993; **5**: 83–9.
5. Tonegawa S. Somatic generation of antibody diversity. *Nature* 1983; **302**: 575–81.
6. Melchers F, Rolink A. B cell development and biology. In: Paul WE, ed. *Fundamental Immunology*, 4th edn. Philadelphia: Lippincott-Raven Publishers, 1999.
7. Hardy RR, Hayakawa K. B cell development pathways. *Annu Rev Immunol* 2001; **19**: 595–621.
8. Fagarason S, Watanabe N, Honjo T. Generation, expansion, migration and activation of mouse B1 cells. *Immunol Rev* 2000; **176**: 205–15.
9. Parker DC. T cell dependent B cell activation. *Annu Rev Immunol* 1993; **11**: 331–40.
10. Foy TM, Aruffo A, Bajorath J et al. Immune regulation by CD40 and its ligand GP39. *Annu Rev Immunol* 1996; **14**: 591–617.
11. Tarlinton D, Smith KGC. Apoptosis and the B cell response to antigen. *Int Rev Immunol* 1997; **15**: 53–71.

12. Smith KGC, Light A, Nossal GJV, Tarlinton DM. The extent of affinity maturation differs between the memory and antibody-forming cell compartments in the primary immune response. *Eur Molec Biol Org J* 1997; **16**: 2996–3006.
13. Tarlinton D, Smith KGC. Dissecting affinity maturation: a model explaining selection of antibody forming cells and memory B cells in the germinal centre. *Immunol Today* 2000; **21**: 436–41.
14. Fagarasan S, Honjo T. T independent immune response: new aspects of B cell biology. *Science* 2000; **290**: 89–92.
15. Ehrlich P, Morgenroth J. Zytotoxine als antikorper. *Berl Klin Wochenschr* 1901; **38**: 251–60.
16. Burnet FM, Fenner F. *The Production of Antibodies.* Monographs of the Walter and Elisa Hall Institute, Melbourne. Melbourne: Macmillan, 1949.
17. Billingham RE, Brent L, Medawer PB. Actively acquired tolerance of foreign cells. *Nature* 1953; **172**: 603–6.
18. Goodnow CC. Balancing immunity and tolerance: deleting and tuning lymphocyte repertoires. *Proc Natl Acad Sci USA* 1996; **93**: 2264–71.
19. Pike BL, Boyd AW, Nossal GJV. Clonal anergy: the universally anergic B lymphocyte. *Proc Natl Acad Sci USA* 1982; **79**: 2013–17.
20. Casellas R, Shih TAY, Kleinewietfeld M et al. Contribution of receptor editing to the antibody repertoire. *Science* 2001; **291**: 1541–44.
21. Gu H, Tarlinton D, Muller W et al. Most peripheral B cells are ligand selected. *J Exp Med* 1991; **173**: 1357–71.
22. Fulcher DA, Basten A. B cell activation versus tolerance – the central role of immunoglobulin receptor engagement and T cell help. *Int Rev Immunol* 1997; **15**: 33–52.
23. Pulendran B, Kannourakis G, Nouri S et al. Soluble antigen can cause enhanced apoptosis of germinal centre B cells. *Nature* 1995; **375**: 331–4.
24. Shokat KM, Goodnow CC. Antigen-induced B cell death and elimination during germinal centre immune responses. *Nature* 1995; **375**: 334–8.
25. Nagata S. Apoptosis by death factor. *Cell* 1997; **88**: 355–65.
26. Fisher GH, Rosenberg FJ, Straus SE et al. Dominant interfering Fas gene mutations impair apoptosis in a human autoimmune lymphoproliferative syndrome. *Cell* 1995; **81**: 935–46.
27. Bossu P, Singer GG, Andreas P et al. Mature CD4+ lymphocytes from MRL/lpr mice are resistant to receptor-mediated tolerance and apoptosis. *J Immunol* 1993; **151**: 7233–9.
28. Russell JH, Wang R. Autoimmune *gld* mutation uncouples suicide and cytokine/proliferation pathways in T cells. *Eur J Immunol* 1993; **23**: 2379–82.
29. Tsujimoto Y, Cossman J, Jaffe E, Croce CM. Involvement of the bcl-2 gene in human follicular lymphoma. *Science* 1985; **228**: 1440–3.
30. Vaux DL, Cory S, Adams JM. Bcl-2 gene promotes haemopoetic cell survival and cooperates with c-myc to immortalise pre-B cells. *Nature* 1988; **335**: 440–2.
31. Strasser A, Whittingham S, Vaux DL et al. Enforced Bcl-2 expression in B lymphoid cells prolongs antibody responses and elicits autoimmune disease. *Proc Natl Acad Sci USA* 1991; **88**: 8661–5.
32. Dempsey PW, Fearon DT. Complement: instructing the acquired immune system through the CD21/CD19 complex. *Res Immunol* 1996; **147**: 71–5.
33. Smith KGC, Fearon DT. Receptor modulators of B cell receptor signalling – CD19/CD22. *Curr Top Microbiol Immunol* 2000; **245**: 195–212.
34. Von Herrath MG, Oldstone MB. Virus-induced autoimmune disease. *Curr Opin Immunol* 1996; **8**: 878–85.
35. Kouskoff V, Lacaud G, Nemazee D. T cell-independent rescue of B lymphocytes from peripheral immune tolerance. *Science* 2000; **287**: 2501–3.
36. Ravetch JV. Fc receptors. *Curr Opin Immunol* 1997; **9**: 121–5.
37. Ravetch JV, Lanier LL. Inhibitory immune receptors. *Science* 2000; **290**: 84–9.
38. Bolland S, Ravetch JV. Spontaneous autoimmune disease in FcγRIIB-deficient mice results from strain-specific epistasis. *Immunity* 2000; **13**: 277–85.
39. Yuasa T, Kubo S, Yoshino T et al. Deletion of Fcγ receptor IIB renders H-2^b mice susceptible to collagen-induced arthritis. *J Exp Med* 1999; **189**: 187–94.
40. O'Keefe TL, Williams GT, Batista FD, Neuberger MS. Deficiency in CD22, a B cell specific inhibitory receptor, is sufficient to predispose to the development of high affinity autoantibodies. *J Exp Med* 1999; **189**: 1307–13.
41. Hibbs ML, Tarlinton DM, Armes J et al. Multiple defects in the immune system of Lyn-deficient mice, culminate in autoimmune disease. *Cell* 1995; **83**: 301–311.
42. Carter RH, Fearon DT. CD19: lowering the threshold for antigen receptor stimulation by B lymphocytes. *Science* 1992; **256**: 105–7.
43. Rickert RC, Rajewski K, Roes J. Impairment of T cell dependent B cell responses and B1

cell development in CD19 deficient mice. *Nature* 1995; **376**: 352–5.

44. Sato S, Ono N, Steeber DA et al. CD19 regulates B lymphocyte signalling thresholds for the development of B1 lineage cells. *J Immunol* 1996; **156**: 4371–8.

45. Inaoki M, Sato S, Weintraub BC et al. CD19-regulated signalling thresholds control peripheral tolerance and autoimmunity and antibody production in B lymphocytes. *J Exp Med* 1997; **186**: 1923–31.

46. Sato S, Hasegawa M, Fujimoto M et al. Quantitative genetic variation in CD19 expression correlates with autoimmunity. *J Immunol* 2000; **165**: 6635–43.

47. Bottazzo GF, Doniach D. Autoimmune thyroid disease. *Annu Rev Med* 1986; **37**: 353–9.

48. Newsom-Davis J, Vincent A. Antibody-mediated neurological disease. *Curr Opin Neurobiol* 1991; **1**: 430–5.

49. Toyka KV, Brachman DB, Pestronk A, Kao I. Myasthenia gravis: passive transfer from man to mouse. *Science* 1975; **190**: 397–9.

50. Vernet der Garabedian B, Lacokova M, Eymard B et al. Association of neonatal myasthenia gravis with antibodies against the fetal acetylcholine receptor. *J Clin Invest* 1994; **94**: 555–9.

51. Newsom-Davis J, Pinching AJ, Vincent A, Wilson SG. Function of circulating antibody to acetylcholine receptors in myasthenia gravis: investigation by plasma exchange. *Neurology* 1978; **28**: 266–72.

52. Tan EM, Cohen AS, Freis JF et al. The 1982 revised criteria for the classification of SLE. *Arthritis Rheum* 1982; **25**: 1271–7.

53. Lahita RG. *Systemic Lupus Erythematosus*, 3rd edn. London: Academic Press, 1999.

54. Vlahakos DV, Foster MH, Adams S et al. Anti-DNA antibodies form immune deposits at distinct glomerular and vascular sites. *Kidney Int* 1992; **41**: 1690–700.

55. Raz E, Brezis M, Rosenmann E, Eliat D. Anti-DNA antibodies bind directly to renal antigens and induce kidney dysfunction in the isolated perfused rat kidney. *J Immunol* 1989; **142**: 3076–83.

56. Morel L, Mohan C, Yu Y et al. Functional dissection of systemic lupus erythematosus using congenic mouse strains. *J Immunol* 1997; **158**: 6019–28.

57. Clynes R, Dumitru C, Ravetch JC. Uncoupling of immune complex formation and kidney damage in autoimmune glomerulonephritis. *Science* 1998; **279**: 1052–4.

58. Myones BL, McCurdy D. The anti-phospholipid syndrome: immunologic and clinical aspects. Clinical spectrum and treatment. *J Rheumatol* 2000; **27**: 20–8.

59. Craft J, Peng S, Fujii T et al. Autoreactive T cells in murine lupus: origins and roles in autoantibody production. *Immunol Res* 1999; **19**: 245–57.

60. Suzuki N, Sakane T, Engelman EG. Anti-DNA antibody production by CD5+ and CD5- B cells of patients with SLE. *J Clin Invest* 1990; **85**: 238-45.

61. Clynes R, Maizes JS, Guinamard R et al. Modulation of complex-induced inflammation in vivo by the coordinate expression of activatory and inhibitory Fc receptors. *J Exp Med* 1999; **189**: 179–85.

62. Jiang Y, Hirose S, Abe M et al. Polymorphisms in IgG Fc receptor IIB regulatory regions asociated with autoimmune susceptibility. *Immunogenetics* 2000; **51**: 429–35.

63. Pritchard NR, Cutler AJ, Uribe S et al. Autoimmune-prone mice share a promoter haplotype associated with reduced expression and function of the Fc receptor FcγRII. *Curr Biol* 2000; **10**: 227–30.

64. Liossis SN, Kovacs B, Dinnis G et al. B cells from patients with SLE display abnormal antigen receptor-mediated signal transduction events. *J Clin Invest* 1996; **98**: 2549–57.

65. Chan OTM, Madaio MP, Shlomchik MJ. The central and multiple roles of B cells in lupus pathogenesis. *Immunol Rev* 1999; **169**: 107–21.

66. Chan O, Shlomchik MJ. A new role for B cells in systemic autoimmunity: B cells promote spontaneous T cell activation in MRL-lpr/lpr mice. *J Immunol* 1998; **160**: 51–9.

67. Smith CA, Farrh T, Goodwin RG. The TNF superfamily of cellular and viral proteins: activation, costimulation and death. *Cell* 1994; **76**: 959–62.

68. Mackay F, Woodcock SA, Lawton P et al. Mice transgenic for BAFF develop lymphocytic disorders along with autoimmune manifestations. *J Exp Med* 1999; **190**: 1697–710.

69. Gross JA, Johnston J, Mudri S et al. TACI and BCMA are receptors for a TNF homologue implicated in B cell autoimmune disease. *Nature* 2000; **404**: 995–8.

70. Zhang J, Roschke V, Baker KP et al. Cutting edge: a role for B cell lymphocyte stimulator in systemic lupus erythematosus. *J Immunol* 2001; **166**: 6–10.

71. Ishikawa S, Sato T, Abe M et al. Aberrant high expression of B lymphocyte chemokine

(BLC/CXCL13) by C11b+ and CD11c+ dendritic cells in murine lupus and preferential chemotaxis of B1 cells towards BLC. *J Exp Med* 2001; **193**: 1393–402.

72. Nash JT, Taylor PR, Botto M et al. Immune complex processing in C1q deficient mice. *Clin Exp Immunol* 2001; **123**: 196–202.

73. Turner N, Mason PJ, Brown R et al. Molecular cloning of the human Goodpasture's antigen demonstrates it to be the α3 chain of type IV collagen. *J Clin Invest* 1992; **89**: 592–601.

74. Savage COS, Pusey CD, Bowman C et al. Anti-glomerular basement membrane antibody mediated disease in the British Isles 1980–4. *Br Med J* 1986; **292**: 301–4.

75. Lerner RA, Glassock KJ, Dixon FJ. The role of antiglomerular basement membrane antibody in the pathogenesis of human glomerulonephritis. *J Exp Med* 1967; **129**: 989–1004.

76. Lockwood CM, Rees AJ, Pearson M et al. Immunosuppression and plasma exchange in the treatment of Goodpasture's Syndrome. *Lancet* 1976; **i**: 711–15.

77. Donaghy M, Rees AJ. Cigarette smoking and lung haemorrhage in glomerulonephritis caused by autoantibodies to glomerular basement membrane. *Lancet* 1983; **ii**: 1390–3.

78. van De Weil A, Dolman KM, van der Meer-Gerritsen CH et al. Interference of Wegener's Granulomatosis autoantibodies with neutrophil protease-3 activity. *Clin Exp Immunol* 1992; **90**: 409–14.

79. Hewins P, Tervaert JWC, Savage COS et al. Is Wegener's granulomatosis an autoimmune disease? *Curr Opin Rheumatol* 2000; **12**: 3–10.

80. Harper L, Savage COS. Pathogenesis of ANCA-associated systemic vasculitis. *J Pathol* 2000; **190**: 349–59.

81. Feldman M, Brennan FM, Maini RN. Rheumatoid arthritis. *Cell* 1996; **85**: 307–10.

82. Fox DA. The role of the T cell in the pathogenesis of rheumatoid arthritis: new perspectives. *Arthritis Rheum* 1997; **40**: 598–609.

83. Ji H, Korganow AS, Mangialaio S et al. Different modes of pathogenesis in T cell-dependent autoimmunity: clues from two transgenic systems. *Immunol Rev* 1999; **169**: 139–46.

84. Matsumoto I, Staub A, Benoist C, Mathis D. Arthritis provoked by linked T and B call recognition of a glycolytic enzyme. *Science* 1999; **286**: 1732–5.

85. Svensson L, Jirholt J, Holmdahl R, Jansson L. B cell deficient mice do not develop type II colla-gen-induced arthritis. *Clin Exp Immunol* 1998; **111**: 521–6.

86. Carson DA. Rheumatoid factor. In: *Textbook of Rheumatology*. Philadelphia: WB Saunders, 1993.

87. Bhatia A, Blades S, Cambridge G, Edwards JCW. Differential distribution of FcγRIIIa in normal human tissues and co-localisation with DAP and fibrillin-1: implication for immunological microenvironments. *Immunology* 1998; **94**: 65–8.

88. Abrahams VM, Cambridge G, Edwards JCW. FcγRIIIa mediates TNFα secretion by human monocytes/macrophges. *Br J Rheumatol* 1998; **37**: 90.

89. Kim HJ, Krenn V, Steinhauser G et al. Plasma cell development in synovial germinal centres in patients with rheumatoid and reactive arthritis. *J Immunol* 1999; **162**: 3053–62.

90. Kim HJ, Berek C. B cells in rheumatoid arthritis. *Arthritis Res* 2000; **2**: 126–31.

91. Protheroe A, Edwards JC, Simmons A et al. Remission of inflammatory arthropathy in association with anti-CD20 therapy for Hodgkin's lymphoma. *Rheumatology* 1999; **38**: 1150–2.

92. Edwards JC, Cambridge G. Sustained improvement in rheumatoid arthritis following a protocol designed to deplete B lymphocytes. *Rheumatology* 2001; **40**: 205–11.

93. Riley WJ, Atkinson MA, Schatz DA, Maclaren NK. Comparison of islet cell autoantibodies in pre-diabetes and recommendations for screening. *J Autoimmun* 1990; **3**: 47–51.

94. Riley WJ, Maclaren NK, Krischer J et al. A prospective study of the development of diabetes in relatives of patients with insulin dependent diabetes. *N Engl J Med* 1990; **323**: 1167–72.

95. Verge CF, Gianani R, Kawasaki E et al. Prediction of type I diabetes in first degree relatives using a combination of insulin, GAD, ICA512bdc/IA-2 autoantibodies. *Diabetes* 1996; **45**: 926–33.

96. Delovitch TL, Singh B. The non-obese diabetic mouse as a model of autoimmune diabetes: immune dysregulation gets the NOD. *Immunity* 1997; **7**: 727–33.

97. Serreze DV, Chapman HD, Varnum MS et al. B lymphocytes are essential for the initiation of T cell mediated autoimmune diabetes: analysis of a new 'speed congenic' stock of NOD.*Igμ^null* mice. *J Exp Med* 1996; **184**: 2049–55.

98. Serreze DV, Fleming SA, Chapman HD et al. B lymphocytes are critical antigen presenting cells for the initiation of T cell-mediated autoimmune diabetes in non-obese diabetic mice. *J Immunol* 1998; **161**: 3912–18.

99. Trapp BD, Peterson J, Ransohoff RM et al. Axonal transection in multiple sclerosis. *N Engl J Med* 1998; **338**: 278–85.

100. Zamvil SS, Mitchell DJ, Moore AC et al. T-cell epitope of the autoantigen myelin basic protein that induced encephalomyelitis. *Nature* 1986; **324**: 258–60.

101. Archelos JJ, Storch MK, Hartung HP. The role of B cells and autoantibodies in multiple sclerosis. *Ann Neurol* 2000; **47**: 694–70.

102. Williamson AR, Burgoon MP, Owens GP et al. Anti-DNA antibodies are a major component of the intrathecal B cell response in multiple sclerosis. *PNAS* 2001; **98**: 1793–8.

103. Xu Q, Willeit J, Marosi M et al. Association of serum antibodies to heat shock protein 65 with carotid atherosclerosis. *Lancet* 1993; **341**: 255–9.

104. Schoenfeld Y, Sherer Y, George J, Harats D. Autoantibodies associated with atherosclerosis. *Ann Med* 2000; 32S1: 37–40.

105. Salonen JT, Yla-Herttuala S, Moutsatsos G et al. Autoantibodies against oxidised LDL and progression of carotid atherosclerosis, *Lancet* 1992; **339**: 883–7.

4

Complement, Fc receptors and immune complexes

Kevin A Davies

Objectives • Overview • Physiology and pathology of immune complexes • Immune complex processing – soluble and particulate complexes compared • Role of the complement system in immune complex-mediated autoimmune disease • Fcγ receptors – new insights into structure and function • References

OBJECTIVES

(1) To review the physiology and pathophysiology of immune complex (IC) formation and clearance.

(2) To review how abnormalities – genetic or acquired – in the complement system and Fcγ receptors can alter IC handling and contribute to autoimmunity and infections.

OVERVIEW

There are a number of important similarities between the receptors for immunoglobulin (Ig) (described as Fcγ receptors or FcγR) and the complement system. Both biological systems constitute key links between humoral and cellular aspects of the immune cascade, and both play an important role in the processes by which opsonized material, both endogenous and of foreign origin, are identified and processed by the immune system. Detailed discussion of both FcγR and complement biology would be beyond the scope of this chapter, so the focus will be on the role of complement and FcγR in the processing of

immune complexes (IC). Complexes, of course, have a potential to interact with either the complement or the FcγR systems; the former as a consequence of activation of the complement system and the resultant opsonization with complement proteins, and the latter as a consequence of direct interaction of the Fc portion of Ig with the cellular receptors themselves.

Complement is a major multicomponent part of the human host defence system. The system comprises a number of proteins that are partitioned between the plasma and the membranes of cells in the tissues and in the blood. As a consequence of activation by pathogens – bacterial, parasitic or viral – the complement system generates fragments and complexes of its constituent proteins that can mediate inflammatory reactions, direct killing of pathogenic organisms, and the clearance of foreign cells, molecules and IC. The three main mechanisms by which complement is activated are illustrated in Figure 4.1. Many of these key functions are mediated through the activation and attraction of phagocytic cells, mast cells, platelets or the endothelium. The activation of cells can

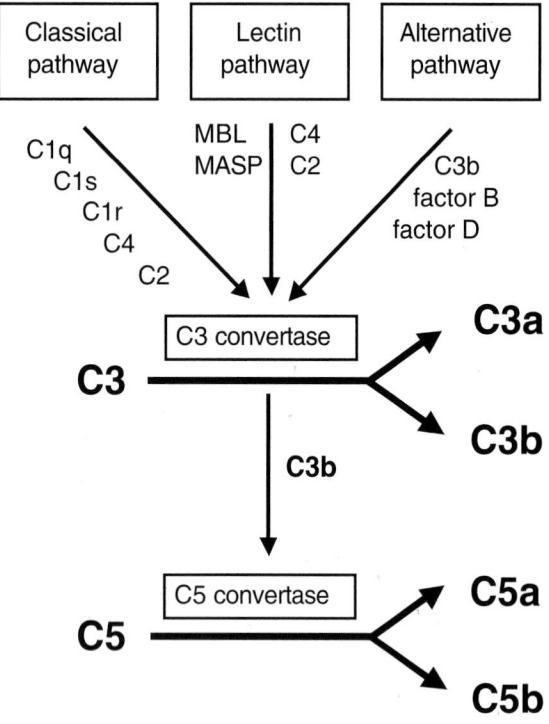

Fig. 4.1 Simplified diagram illustrating the three main pathways of complement activation. (MBL, mannose-binding protein.)

either be mediated by the direct insertion of protein complexes into the cell membrane or by the binding of complement proteins, or fragments thereof, to specific cellular receptors. Complement also plays a role in the regulation of adaptive immune responses and there is increasing interest in this area. However, this will not be considered in this chapter, but suffice it to say that the engagement of complement receptors on B-cells has a role in optimizing antibody responses to T-cell-dependent antigens.

FcγR are a diverse group of molecules dispersed on the cell surface of leucocytes, and the molecules are often found in inhibitory and stimulatory pairings. The activation of stimulatory FcγR can lead to a number of biological consequences, including antibody-dependent cell-mediated cytotoxicity, phagocytosis and the stimulation of the cell to release a range of inflammatory mediators such as proteases, reactive oxidant species and a variety of

cytokines. A number of insights have recently been gained from the study of cellular interactions *in vitro* and from the study of murine models genetically engineered to be deficient in stimulatory FcγR. Such studies have demonstrated that stimulatory FcγR can trigger the Arthus reaction, and have a role to play in mediating auto-immune cytopenias, arthritis and glomerulonephritis. Stimulatory FcγR have also been shown to play a critical role in initiating type 3 and type 2 hypersensitivity reactions. Inhibitory FcγR have an important role to play in altering the threshold for cellular activation by IC and other stimuli, and these receptors can also interfere with stimulatory signals. As will be discussed in detail later, they therefore have a key role in the regulation of the effector functions in the immune system. A number of insights have also been gained from the study of knockout mice deficient in inhibitory FcγR, demonstrating, for example, that these animals have enhanced antibody responses and have a tendency towards developing an enhanced inflammatory response in the context of antibody-induced hypersensitivity. Understanding of the genetics and structure of this family of molecules has advanced greatly in recent years, and in the second part of the chapter some of the new insights gained from a variety of murine and human experimental models into the structure and function of these molecules will be considered. We shall focus briefly on signal transduction mechanisms, and the factors which influence the cellular expression and function of the molecules in humans, as well as reviewing the importance of some newly described polymorphic variants of FcγR II and III in both infectious and autoimmune disease.

1. PHYSIOLOGY AND PATHOLOGY OF IMMUNE COMPLEXES

1.1 Normal physiology

Immune complexes (IC) comprise any combination of antibody with antigen. The composition of IC is highly variable. In addition to antigen and antibody there may be complement proteins associated with IC, covalently bound in the case of C3 and C4, or non-covalently in the case of

C1q. The biological and physicochemical properties of an IC vary according to the antibody isotype and according to the antigen, which may be soluble or particulate, such as bacteria or cells.

IC formation is a physiological consequence of an adaptive humoral immune response. Binding of antibody to antigen is designed to promote removal of foreign antigens, the stimulation of an appropriate adaptive immune response and the development of specific immunological memory by the focusing of complexes to 'professional' antigen-presenting cells within the immune system.

1.2 Pathophysiology

IC are also a very important cause of pathological tissue damage. This occurs in two situations. The first of these is when antigen persists as a consequence of ineffective clearance by formation of IC. This may occur in various circumstances, e.g. when the antigen is an autoantigen which cannot be removed from the body and, in the case of persistent infection, where the immune response does not effectively control the infection and there is persistent production of antigens from the infectious agent. The second circumstance in which IC cause tissue injury is when the physiological clearance mechanisms are overwhelmed by formation of a large amount of IC, e.g. in serum sickness. Failure to eliminate potentially harmful IC may result in their persistence, either in the circulation or in the tissues, with potentially phlogistic effects. Alternatively, failure of effective antigen presentation in IC to 'professional' antigen-presenting cells (e.g. in the spleen) may result in an abnormal immune response, consequences of which may be the failure of antigen clearance or the development of persistent autoimmunity. These mechanisms are discussed in detail below.

2. IMMUNE COMPLEX (IC) PROCESSING – SOLUBLE AND PARTICULATE COMPLEXES COMPARED

Both Fc receptors (FcγR) and complement play critical roles in the processing of IC. Incorporation of complement proteins into IC modifies the lattice structure (see below).

Covalently incorporated cleavage products of components C3 and C4 can then influence the fate of IC by serving as ligands; firstly, for receptors on cells which transport IC through the body and, secondly, for receptors on cells within the reticuloendothelial system which take up and process the complexes. Cellular uptake of IC results in the catabolism of foreign antigen and presentation to T- and B-lymphocytes leading to a specific immune response to that antigen. IC may be classified into those that contain soluble antigens, such as proteins, and those containing particulate antigens, such as cells and bacteria. The clearance mechanisms are not the same for soluble and particulate IC, and the different processes involved are reviewed below.

2.1 Soluble IC

2.1.1 Role of complement in the modification of IC structure

The incorporation of proteins of the complement system into IC is a key element in the way in which complement mediates IC processing, and was first recognized during the 1940s with the finding that immune precipitates contained more nitrogen when they formed in normal compared with heat-treated serum.[1] It was subsequently demonstrated that the presence of complement reduced the rate of immune precipitation, a phenomenon rediscovered 20 years later by investigators developing radio-immunoassays, who observed that complement interfered with the precipitation reaction.[2,3] It was later discovered that complement not only inhibits the formation of immune precipitates but can also solubilize immune precipitates that have already formed.[4] Inhibition of immune precipitation is primarily mediated through activation of the classical pathway of complement.[5,6] Solubilization of immune precipitates, on the other hand, is mediated by the alternative pathway.[4] The capacity of complement to inhibit immune precipitation has been studied in several *in vitro* model systems. For example, it was demonstrated that complexes formed between bovine serum albumin (BSA) and rabbit anti-BSA at 37°C were kept soluble more easily when formed in antibody excess. During the first minutes of the reaction, IC were kept soluble by classical pathway components alone but in the later stages the alternative pathway was essential.[6] Binding of C3 fragments is necessary for maintaining IC solubility. C3 and C4 binding is covalent and, in the case of ovalbumin/rabbit anti-ovalbumin IC studied *in vitro*, has been shown to involve amide bonds between C3b and the immunoglobulin (Ig) G heavy chain.[7]

How do complement proteins facilitate the modification of IC solubility? Two possible explanations have been adduced. The first is that the incorporation of complement proteins into the lattice reduces the valency of antibody for antigen by occupying sites of interaction between antibody and antigen (reviewed by Lachman and Walport[8]). The second possibility is that complement incorporation interferes with non-covalent Fc–Fc interactions that promote the rapid aggregation of IC.[9]

A number of properties of the antibody component of an IC determines the efficiency of inhibition of immune precipitation. For example, only antibody isotypes that activate the classical pathway will induce complement-mediated inhibition of immune precipitation. Thus, inhibition of immune precipitation occurs with IgG and IgM complexes but not with IgA complexes.[10] The ability of an IC to activate the classical pathway of complement does not precisely parallel its ability to incorporate C3b into the lattice. This is of some clinical relevance as, for example, complexes of monoclonal IgM rheumatoid factor and IgG, found in patients with mixed essential cryoglobulinaemia, deplete complement rapidly but do not effectively incorporate C3 into the complex.[11] The formation of immune precipitates can activate the alternative pathway of complement. Solubilization of immune precipitates is associated with covalent binding of C3b to antigen and antibody molecules. A fraction of antibody may be released from the complex during solubilization though the mechanism whereby bound C3b interferes with primary antigen–antibody bonds is unclear. This solubilization reaction is relatively inefficient, requiring a considerable amount of complement activation (approximately one molecule of

C3b needs to bind per antibody molecule to induce solubilization[12]). Since <10% of activated C3 binds to an immune aggregate, it follows that large quantities of complement are consumed during solubilization, which may result in deposition of the membrane attack complex and release of potentially proinflammatory complement split products and anaphylatoxins into the tissues. The degree of complement activation required for solubilization can be generated only by alternative pathway amplification; insoluble immune aggregates appear to form 'protected' surfaces to which factor H has little access, thereby providing sites where amplification of complement activation is favoured.[13] All the proteins of the alternative pathway, including properdin, are required. Activation of the classical pathway alone is neither necessary nor sufficient to solubilize immune precipitates, although partial solubilization by classical pathway activation has been demonstrated *in vitro* using immune precipitates.[14,15] To summarize, there are two important differences between the processes of inhibition of IC precipitation and solubilization of precipitates. Firstly, the capacity of the complement system to inhibit immune precipitation is 10 times greater than its capacity for solubilization, probably reflecting the ease of prevention of Fc–Fc interactions and lattice enlargement, compared with disruption of a lattice that is already formed. Secondly, the reactions differ in their capacity to induce inflammation, as inhibition of immune precipitation generates smaller amounts of the anaphylatoxins C3a and C5a than does solubilization.[16]

2.1.2 Complement receptor type 1 (CR1) and IC transport

IC that enter the circulation, or are formed within it, may have to travel some distance around the body before reaching one of the organs of the fixed mononuclear phagocytic system. There is evidence that most IC travel through the circulation bound to receptors on the surface of circulating cells (erythrocytes in primates) rather than free in plasma. When IC arrive in the organs of the fixed mononuclear phagocytic system, they are transferred from the carrier cell to fixed macrophages. This binding of IC to receptors on carrier cells was first described for complement-coated microorganisms over 80 years ago. Pneumococci were injected intravenously into immune rabbits and the clustering of bacteria around platelets in blood taken by cardiac puncture was observed.[17] Rieckenberg[18] found that the serum of rats that had recovered from infection with *Trypanosoma brucei* caused platelets to adhere to *T brucei in vitro*. It was subsequently found in humans and other primates that red blood cells, rather than platelets, were the main cell in blood to which opsonized trypanosomes would bind in this 'immune adherence' reaction.[19] The role of complement in mediating these binding reactions was initially suggested by Russian scientists in the 1920s, who observed that heat-inactivated serum would not mediate binding.[20] It was then shown specifically that erythrocyte adherence reactions could be abolished by heat treatment of sera or by dilute ammonia (which facilitates inactivation of C4[21–23]). The observation that treatment of serum with cobra venom factor prevented adherence reactions showed an essential role for C'3.[23] Many of these early observations were mainly published in minor European and British journals and were overlooked between the late 1930s and early 1950s. No mention is made of any of the work on complement-dependent adherence reactions described above in two major reviews on the complement system published at this time.[24,25]

It was Nelson,[26] in 1953, who rediscovered adherence reactions between human erythrocytes and specifically opsonized treponemes and pneumococci.[26] He confirmed the complement-dependent nature of these reactions and first coined the term immune adherence. The modern era of studies on this phenomenon followed the isolation by Fearon[27] of the molecule responsible for the adherence reactions of human erythrocytes, the C3b/iC3b receptor (CR1, CD35). This receptor bound large IC and was shown to play a role in the transport of soluble IC *in vivo* in primates.[28] CR1 is a receptor for C3b and iC3b, and has a number of different biological activities. These include: (1) the uptake by phagocytic cells of C3b- and iC3b-coated IC and particles; (2) the activation of B-cells by antigen in the form of complement-coated IC; (3) acting as a cofactor for factor-I-mediated cleavage of C3b to iC3b and then C3dg; and (4) serving as the key transport molecule for IC, both soluble and particulate. It is the last of these functions that is of critical importance in understanding the role of IC processing in autoimmunity and our discussion will focus on this area. The sites of CR1 expression vary substantially between different species. In humans and other primates, the majority of CR1 in the circulation is located in a clustered form on erythrocytes. The number of CR1 molecules per red cell is very low, varying between 50 and approximately 1000 receptors per cell in humans.[29,30] This compares with 5000 to 50,000 receptors per neutrophil (PMN) (numbers vary depending on the state of cellular activation).[31] Red cells, however, play an important role in the binding and transport of C3b- and iC3b-coated IC and particles through the circulation for two reasons. The first is the vast numerical majority of red cells in the blood compared with other cell types (approximately 1000 erythrocytes for every PMN). The second is the spatial organization of CR1 on the cell surface, which on red cells is clustered.[32] This facilitates very high avidity interactions with ligand, in comparison to PMN and lymphocytes, on which the receptor is expressed as cell-surface monomers. In other species a hybrid molecule sharing the activities shown by human CR1 and CR2 is expressed on leucocytes and platelets.[33]

In the light of the key role that CR1 plays in the binding and transport of IC, there has been a great deal of interest in polymorphisms of the molecule in autoimmune disease. There are two types of genetic polymorphism of CR1, each of which may show functional variation in respect to the transport of IC. The first is a structural polymorphism. Four alleles of CR1 have been characterized with molecular weights of ~ 210 kDa [F' (or C) allotype], ~ 250 kDa [F (or A) allotype], ~ 290 kDa [S (or B) allotype] and ~ 330 kDa. This variation of ~ 40 kDa between allelic variants is due to variable internal repetition of the long homologous repeats forming the structural core of the receptor. The ~ 210 kDa [F' (or C)] allotype has reduced binding affinity for C3b dimers, corresponding to the absence of one long homologous repeat containing a C3b binding site.[34] This uncommon variant appears to have an increased prevalence amongst patients with systemic lupus erythematosus (SLE),[35] though is very uncommon even in this population. The potential contributory role of abnormalities in CR1 function in the pathophysiology of autoimmune disease is discussed in detail in section 3.2.1.

CR1 also exhibits a numerical polymorphism of expression on red cells in the normal population, numbers varying between 50 and 500 CR1/erythrocyte. This numerical variation of CR1 expression on erythrocytes was first identified following the discovery of normal subjects whose erythrocytes failed to show immune adherence and was subsequently shown to be an inherited trait.[36] Studies have confirmed the numerical polymorphism by direct enumeration of the receptor using radioligand binding assays.[37]

2.1.3 How do IC interact with other circulating cells?

PMN have both complement and FcγR. On resting PMN, the number of CR1/cell is approximately 10-fold higher than on erythrocytes,[33] raising the possibility that PMN might have a role to play in IC binding and transport. However, the kinetics of the interaction between PMN CR1 and IC are quite different to the kinetics of erythrocyte CR1–IC binding.[38] IC that are not opsonized react only very slowly with PMN and pre-coating the complexes with C3b accelerates the reaction only marginally. Only CR1 appears to be involved in this inefficient binding, since it is inhibited by a monoclonal anti-CR1 antibody. In spite of the greater numbers per cell, PMN do not bind C3b-coated IC better than erythrocytes, a discrepancy largely explained by electron microscopic studies which showed that CR1 are not clustered on PMN. Activation of PMN with C5a, interleukin (IL)-8 and FMLP (formyl methionyl leucyl phenylalanine) does not modify this distribution, in spite of stimulating a 5–10-fold increase in the total number of CR1 expressed on the PMN surface.[39] These observations suggest that, in primates at least, CR1-dependent binding of IC to circulating

leucocytes is not of major importance in IC processing. In fact, one of the primary roles of erythrocyte CR1 may be in preventing potentially harmful interactions between IC, leucocytes and vascular endothelium, by maintaining the complexes within the central stream of the vessel. This hypothesis is supported by *in vitro* observations that erythrocyte CR1 can protect cultured human umbilical vascular endothelial cells from IC/PMN-mediated injury.[40]

2.1.4 Soluble IC processing: in vivo *studies*

The main site of clearance of IC is the fixed mononuclear phagocytic system. In the majority of species, including primates, rodents and lagomorphs, the liver and spleen are the primary sites in the circulation in which tissue macrophages are located.[41] Pulmonary intravascular macrophages are also found in pigs, cows, sheep, goats and cats, and these have been shown to be important both in the clearance of particles[42] and soluble IC.[43] Important findings that have emerged from the study of the mechanisms of IC processing include: (1) identification of the sites of processing of IC; (2) the finding that the nature of the antigen in the complex may influence clearance kinetics; (3) observations that IC uptake by the mononuclear phagocytic system is saturable; and (4) characterization of receptors on circulating cells which act as transport receptors for IC in the circulation. For example, in rodents and lagomorphs, as in humans, soluble IC, injected intravenously, were predominantly removed in the liver and spleen,[44–47] but the complexes were not transported in the circulation bound to erythrocytes, which in these species do not bear CR1. Platelets in these species carry C3b receptors and in one study, rapid *in vivo* binding of IC to platelets was observed following intravenous injection.[44]

The antigen component, as well as the antibody, of an IC has a role in determining the mode and kinetics of its clearance. Evidence in support of this came from studies of the clearance in mice of IC containing as antigen either orosomucoid or caeruloplasmin or their desialylated derivatives.[48] The asialo-orosomucoid-containing complexes were cleared 20-fold more rapidly than those containing the sialylated molecule, and blocking studies showed that the rapid clearance phase was mediated by a hepatocyte carbohydrate receptor. The importance of receptors (e.g. the recently described family of 'scavenger' receptors), other than those designed to bind complement proteins or Ig, in the clearance of IC in humans remains to be elucidated.

IC clearance mechanisms have been shown to be saturable in rabbits injected with escalating doses of soluble IC. After saturation of hepatic uptake, spillover of IC into other organs was observed.[46] It remains unclear the extent to which this mechanism may operate in human disease.

The first *in vivo* demonstration of the physiologic importance of erythrocyte R1 in IC clearance was in a series of studies performed in baboons.[49–51] Radiolabelled IC comprising BSA/anti-BSA were initially employed, and shown to localize mainly in the liver.[52] In de-complemented animals, the IC did not bind to red cells and were cleared more rapidly, depositing in other organs including the kidney. IgA-containing complexes, which fixed complement poorly, failed to bind to baboon erythrocyte CR1, were cleared rapidly and localized in other organs.[51]

A number of model IC have been employed to explore the *in vivo* processing of exogenously administered soluble IC in humans. The three main models which have been employed are heat-aggregated IgG, tetanus toxoid (TT):anti-TT and hepatitis B surface Ag (HBsAg):anti-HBsAg IC. Radiolabelled heat-aggregated IgG injected intravenously into normal subjects was shown by scintigraphy to be cleared mainly in the liver and spleen.[53] The roles of complement and CR1 in soluble IC clearance mechanisms in humans were first studied *in vivo* using ^{125}I-labelled TT:anti-TT complexes.[54] IC bound to erythrocyte CR1 receptors in a complement-dependent manner and the CR1 number correlated with the level of uptake. In subjects with low CR1 numbers and hypocomplementaemia there was a very rapid initial disappearance of IC. A second phase of clearance was more or less monoexponential, and the observed elimination rate correlated inversely with CR1 numbers and the binding of IC to red cells. Important differences were seen between normal control subjects and patients with SLE, and these are discussed in more detail below.

Extensive *in vivo* studies of soluble IC clearance have also been performed using a different model – ^{123}I-labelled HBsAg:anti-HBsAg IC. The fate of these complexes was monitored by blood sampling and external scanning to define the sites and kinetics of processing in normal subjects, patients with SLE and a single patient with homozygous C2-deficiency.[55,56] In normal subjects, complexes were cleared in the liver and spleen. The majority of the injected complexes bound rapidly to red cells. In all subjects there was a very close correlation between *in vivo* binding to red cells and CR1 number. Results of studies using this model in SLE patients are discussed further below (section 3.2.3).

A major criticism of all of the studies of IC processing described above is that they all involve the exogenous administration of large IC prepared *in vitro*, in the absence of complement, and may not therefore be representative of potentially pathogenic IC that may form *in vivo*. Similar results have, however, been obtained from studies performed with IC that form *in vivo*, both in an animal model and in humans. For example, the successive infusion of human anti-double-stranded (ds) DNA antibodies and dsDNA into monkeys and rabbits led to rapid formation of IC that bound to red cell CR1.[57] The formation and fate of IC formed *in vivo* in patients receiving radio-immunotherapy has also been studied.[58] The successive administration of a radiolabelled mouse antitumour antibody and a human anti-mouse antibody was shown to result in the formation of IC comprising the two antibody species. Rapid clearance of complexes was observed with significant binding of the complexed material to red cell CR1. Systemic complement activation and a 30% fall in erythrocyte CR1 numbers were observed. Clearance took place primarily in the liver.

2.2 Particulate complexes

2.2.1 Clearance of an autoantigen – red blood cells

Autoimmune haemolysis and pathological platelet destruction within the fixed macrophage system are important clinical features of lupus. The site of clearance of particulate IC depends on the class of antibody bound to the antigen. Studies of autoimmune haemolytic anaemia, which constitutes an important clinical example of a persistent IC disease involving a particulate autoantigen, namely erythrocytes, demonstrate this well. Cold agglutinin disease is mediated by IgM anti-I antibodies, which stimulate efficient classical pathway activation and fixation of C4 and C3 to erythrocytes. The role of anti-I and complement in mediating cell lysis was first studied in a rabbit model.[59] IgM cold agglutinin was injected into C3-depleted and C6-deficient rabbits. The latter developed thrombocytopenia, neutropenia and a fall in haemoglobin and PCV, with only minimal haemoglobinaemia, but a rapid decrease in plasma C3 levels. Circulating red cells could be readily agglutinated with anti-C3 antibodies and *in vivo* immune adherence of platelets to red cells occurred. In the C3-depleted animals, injection of the anti-I IgM produced no significant haematological changes. It has also been possible to model the fate of erythrocytes in cold agglutinin disease in non-human primates using radiolabelled cells coated with an IgM cold agglutinin.[60] The main site of red cell uptake was the liver and transient retention of cells in this organ occurred, thought to be mediated by reversible binding to complement receptors. In patients with cold agglutinin disease, circulating red cells are characterized by morphologic change to a microspherocytic form, associated with the presence of several thousand C3dg molecules bound per cell.

On the other hand, in IgG-mediated warm haemolytic anaemia, uptake of erythrocytes occurs predominantly in the spleen by Fc-dependent pathways. ^{51}Cr-labelled incompatible red cells, transfused into recipients with non-complement fixing antibodies, were removed from the circulation monoexponentially with a half-time of 18–20 minutes.[61] Splenic uptake exhibited similar kinetics. No uptake was detectable elsewhere, notably in the liver. As the spleen exclusively removed cells, and this organ receives only a relatively small fraction of the cardiac output, it was reasoned that the splenic extraction efficiency was very high. It was subsequently shown that the site of sensitized red cell destruction was dependent on the degree of antibody coating, with more heavily coated cells being destroyed predominantly by the liver.[62]

Radiolabelled erythrocytes, coated with antibody (IgG), have been extensively studied as a probe of mononuclear phagocytic function in various diseases.[63] In humans and other species, these cells are cleared primarily in the spleen. The mechanisms by which this probe exhibits primarily splenic clearance, while soluble IC (see above) and cells coated with IgM and C3 localize predominantly in the liver, are poorly understood. Tissue macrophages in the liver and spleen bear both FcR and CR (CR1, CR3 and CR4),[64] while follicular dendritic cells within the spleen and lymph nodes also bear the C3dg receptor CR2. The FcγR on monocytes/macrophages primarily involved in interactions with IC or Ig aggregates are the relatively low-affinity receptors FcγRII and FcγRIII.[65,66] The biology, structure and function of these molecules are reviewed in section 4. There is evidence from *in vitro* experiments, performed using magnetic anti-IgG probes, that the potential 'availability' of IgG on red cells to interact with fixed cellular receptors may be different depending on whether the immunoglobulin is distributed at multiple sites on the red cell surface, adjacent to the cell membrane, or presented in IC bound to clustered CR1, away from the erythrocyte cell membrane.[67] In the latter case, it has been postulated that IgG may be 'safely' stripped from the cells as a consequence of interaction with fixed macrophages, with little associated damage to the red cell. In the instance of the antibody-coated erythrocytes used to study the function of the fixed macrophage system in the type of *in vivo* study discussed above, multiple more intimate contacts with receptors on fixed macrophages may result in cellular destruction, especially in the spleen (reviewed in Peters[68]).

It has also been suggested that the anatomy of the splenic circulation favours the uptake of particulate rather than soluble IC. The haematocrit in the spleen is relatively high compared with that in major arteries and veins.[69] The converse applies in the sinusoids of the liver that have a low haematocrit in comparison with major blood vessels. This reflects observations that hepatic sinusoidal macrophages are very efficient at clearing soluble IC from plasma and the splenic macrophages play an important role in handling IgG-coated erythrocytes. After splenectomy, the peripheral blood contains abnormal red cells bearing denatured haemoglobin, known as Heinz bodies, and nuclear remnants, known as Howell-Jolly bodies, clearly illustrating the physiologic role of the spleen in the processing of abnormal red blood cells.[70]

2.2.2 Bacterial and endotoxin clearance

Mortality and morbidity due to infection are major problems in patients with SLE. Many factors have been implicated, including the use of corticosteroids and immunosuppressive drugs. However, lupus patients with hypocomplementaemia and low red cell CR1 numbers may also be susceptible to both Gram-positive and Gram-negative infections, due to defective clearance of bacteria and endotoxin. *In vivo* bacterial clearance has not been studied experimentally in humans but has been evaluated in a variety of animal models. A number of important interspecies differences have been observed and care is required in extrapolating observations in animal models to the human situation. Variations in the site of clearance may have a major influence on the pathophysiologic consequences of bacteraemia. For example, pigs are extremely susceptible to the development of adult respiratory distress syndrome (ARDS).[71] Equivalent doses (on a weight basis) of *Pseudomonas aeruginosa* administered in parallel to pigs and dogs were well tolerated by the latter but were associated with acute pulmonary failure in pigs, in which there was selective lung uptake of the organisms. Complement – but not PMN – depletion abrogated the development of ARDS. These findings suggest that the susceptibility of pigs to ARDS may be specifically related to the pulmonary vascular location of the mononuclear phagocytic system and the local release of inflammatory mediators. The role of natural antibody and complement in the clearance of endotoxin from the circulation remains unclear. Recently reported experiments in mice rendered C3 or C4 deficient by gene

targeting, have demonstrated defective lipopolysaccharide (LPS) clearance in the complement-deficient animals, and enhanced mortality.[72] RAG–/– mice, which are unable to produce Ig also exhibit defective LPS processing.[73] However, attempts in humans to enhance LPS clearance, and to reduce mortality in septic shock, by the administration of exogenous IgM anti-lipid A antibodies, have proved largely unsuccessful (reviewed in Lynn and Cohen[74]), even though the reagents used have been shown *in vitro* to complex with LPS, fix complement and mediate binding to erythrocyte CR1.[75,76]

3. THE ROLE OF THE COMPLEMENT SYSTEM IN IMMUNE-COMPLEX (IC)-MEDIATED AUTOIMMUNE DISEASE

Complement plays both beneficial and deleterious roles in autoimmune disease. There is a large evidence base showing that complement causes inflammatory injury to tissues in patients and experimental animals in which IC form in the circulation or locally in tissues. However, it is also clear that either inherited or acquired deficiencies of classical pathway complement proteins, in humans, are associated with increased susceptibility to the development of IC disease typical of SLE.

3.1 Complement deficiency and lupus

3.1.1 Clinical observations

Inherited homozygous deficiency of C1q, C1r, C1s, C4 or C2 has each been strongly associated with the development of SLE. There is a hierarchy of severity and susceptibility to SLE according to the position of the missing protein in the pathway of classical pathway complement activation. More than 90% of patients with homozygous C1q deficiency develop SLE, typically at an early age.[77] Disease is characterized by severe rashes with a significant proportion of patients developing glomerulonephritis and/or cerebral lupus. A wide range of autoantibodies to extractable nuclear antigens, including anti-Ro, anti-Sm and anti-RNP, are found in these patients, although anti-dsDNA antibodies are much less common. Approximately one third of patients with C2 deficiency develop SLE[78] and the autoantibody profile tends to be restricted to the presence of anti-Ro antibodies. The severity of disease is similar to that seen in lupus patients without homozygous complement deficiency. C3 deficiency, on the other hand, is usually not associated with the development of full-blown SLE and typically presents with recurrent pyogenic infections.[79] Up to one third of C3-deficient patients develop a prominent rash in association with pyogenic infections, which in one case was associated with a dense neutrophilic cutaneous infiltrate.[80] Lupus-associated autoantibodies are only exceptionally identified in patients with C3 deficiency, although about one quarter of C3-deficient patients develop a mesangiocapillary glomeru-lonephritis. Deficiency of two of the alternative pathway control proteins, factor I and factor H, are each associated with severe secondary C3 deficiency, due to failure of regulation of the alternative pathway and amplification loop of C3 cleavage.[81] These patients show a similar phenotype to C3 deficiency and typically suffer from recurrent pyogenic infections, with only occasional development of glomerulonephritis without significant autoantibody formation.

Numerous studies have shown associations between specific gene products of the major histocompatibility complex (MHC) and the development of SLE and other autoimmune diseases. Because of the phenomenon of linkage disequilibrium, it is frequently extremely difficult to dissect which associations between MHC gene products and specific diseases are primary and which are due to other linked genes in the MHC. All four complement genes (C4A, C4B, C2 and factor B) located in the class III region of the MHC exhibit extensive genetic polymorphism, which in the case of C4A and C4B includes frequent null alleles which do not encode the production of a protein product. The observation that homozygous complement deficiency was associated with lupus raised the possibility that null alleles of C4 might show an association with the disease. This was found to be the case[82,83] and the results of early studies have been confirmed in a number of different ethnic populations,[84] strengthening the likelihood that the C4 null allele is the relevant gene.

However, the association between C4A null alleles and SLE is not confirmed by all studies and remains controversial.[85]

An increased prevalence of alleles of mannose-binding lectin (MBL), associated with reduced serum levels of the protein amongst two populations of patients with SLE, has recently been reported.[86] The significance of these results is not certain and the role of MBL in the pathophysiology of IC-mediated auto-immune disease remains to be defined.

There is an increased prevalence of both antinuclear antibodies and the development of both SLE and a range of other autoimmune disorders (including glomerulonephritis, Sjögren's syndrome, inflammatory bowel disease and thyroiditis)[87,88] in patients with hereditary angioedema due to heterozygous C1-inhibitor deficiency. These patients show prolonged reduction in C4 and C2 levels due to partially unregulated activity of C1r and C1s, and disordered regulation of both cell-mediated and humoral immunity has been described.[89] Similarly, patients with prolonged acquired C3 deficiency due to the presence of the autoantibody (C3 nephritic factor) may develop SLE many years after presentation with partial lipodystrophy or mesangiocapillary glomerulo-nephritis with dense deposits.[90] These associations of acquired complement deficiency and IC-mediated autoimmune disease strongly support the hypothesis that complement has a key role to play in the pathophysiology of these conditions. However, the possibility remains that the associations of complement deficiency with SLE are due to an ascertainment artefact, as a consequence of the fact that complement levels are mainly measured in patients with diseases associated with complement activation. This would mean that any examples of complement deficiency detected would inevitably be associated with those conditions. However, extensive surveys performed in normal populations have shown that inherited homozygous complement deficiency in healthy individuals is extremely rare.[91,92]

Further evidence for the role of complement and IC in autoimmunity comes from a number of animal models of complement deficiency that have been described. For example, dogs from a colony with C3 deficiency develop a very similar pattern of glomerulonephritis to that seen in C3-deficient humans.[93] A strain of pigs in Norway develop a severe mesangiocapillary glomerulonephritis of early onset and these animals have been shown to have hereditary factor H deficiency.[94] Mice with targeted deletions of C4,[95] C3,[72] C1q,[79] factor B[96] and the *Cr2* locus[97] have recently been developed. Our own data show that C1q-deficient mice develop antinuclear antibodies and a significant proportion of the animals die with crescentic glomerulonephritis.[98]

3.1.2 Possible mechanisms

A number of physiologic activities of the complement system may explain the clinical associations of hypocomplementaemia and autoimmune disease discussed above. One of the most important of these is the role of complement in the processing of IC. Defective IC processing and clearance may result in the inefficient clearance of IC by the fixed mononuclear phagocytic system with deposition of IC in many tissues. This in turn causes inflammation, the release of autoantigens and stimulation of an autoimmune response. Direct evidence for the abnormal processing of IC in hypocomplementaemic patients is discussed in detail later.

Two other roles of the complement system may also be relevant in the pathophysiology of lupus. Complement has an important role in host defence against infection and in antigen processing and presentation in germinal centres. Detailed discussion of these areas is beyond the scope of the present chapter, which relates primarily to the role of IC, complement and FcγR in autoimmunty. However, it is worth considering the possibility that the classical pathway of complement normally provides defence against an infectious agent that induces SLE. Complement proteins are known to play an important role in host defence against pyogenic infections. However, it seems unlikely that this is a major factor in the induction of SLE as other abnormalities of host defence associated with recurrent pyogenic disease are not associated with development of the disease.

There is evidence for a role of complement in host defence against C-type retroviruses[99,100] and it remains an unproven possibility that SLE is an autoimmune response following infection by an unidentified virus of this type.

3.2 Do primary or secondary defects exist in IC clearance and processing mechanisms?

3.2.1 Defects in CR1

CR1 has a key role in the clearance of soluble and particulate IC in humans, as discussed above. The number of receptors per red cell of CR1 varies widely between individuals, and the level of expression is under genetic control at the CR1 locus.[30,36] The molecular mechanism of this is not clear, but a restriction fragment length polymorphism within the CR1 gene is correlated with high or low expression of CR1 on red cells.[101,102] It has been demonstrated that patients with SLE express reduced numbers of receptors per cell compared with healthy individuals.[37] This raised the possibility that low expression of CR1 might constitute a disease susceptibility gene for the development of SLE. However, a number of studies showed that low expression of CR1 in SLE and in certain other conditions associated with complement activation on erythrocytes or in the fluid phase, is very likely to be due to acquired mechanisms. These mechanisms may be related to partial cleavage of CR1 during IC transfer from red cells to cells of the fixed mononuclear phagocytic system in the liver and spleen.[37]

3.2.2 FcγR function

The nomenclature and structure of specific FcγR are discussed in section 4. In this section we review the evidence, mainly from *in vivo* studies, that functional defects in FcγR function may occur in autoimmune diseases such as SLE. It has long been mooted that defects in mononuclear phagocytic function predispose to the development of SLE by impairment of IC clearance. This hypothesis originally stemmed from experimental studies of the clearance of colloidal carbon particles in animals,[41] which showed that uptake by the mononuclear phagocytic system was saturable. IC injected into rabbits also showed saturable uptake in the liver, followed by spillover into other organs.[46] However, in spite of these experimental data in animals, there is no firm evidence that saturation of soluble IC clearance mechanisms occurs in human disease.

A number of different methods have been used to study whether there is indeed impaired processing of IC in SLE by the mononuclear phagocytic system. Studies of the clearance of IgG-coated erythrocytes by the spleen showed delayed uptake in SLE, and correlations were found between clearance rate, disease activity, and levels of circulating IC in patients with lupus.[103,104] However, as discussed above, IgG-coated erythrocytes may not be an appropriate surrogate measure for Fc- and complement-dependent clearance mechanisms of soluble IC. The clearance of soluble IC in a C2-deficient patient with SLE was totally corrected by complement repletion, largely excluding a primary defect in mononuclear phagocytic function as the explanation for defective IC clearance in that patient.[56]

Mononuclear cell phagocytic function in SLE may also be addressed by studying genetic variation in FcγR and complement receptors. Support for the idea that FcγR function is abnormal in SLE has come from recent studies of a functionally important polymorphism of the Fc receptor FCγRIIa. An allotypic variant of FcγRIIa, FcγRIIa-HR (FcγRIIa-R131), has been shown *in vitro* to reduce the capacity of phagocytic cells to bind and internalize IgG-containing IC and IgG-opsonized erythrocytes.[105] This receptor mainly binds IgG2. A number of groups have addressed the question of whether there is an overrepresentation of this allotypic variant in patients with SLE, either by genotype analysis or by determination of receptor phenotype on peripheral blood leucocytes by FACS analysis using specific monoclonal antibodies. An excess of FcγRIIa-R131 homozygotes was found in African-American patients with lupus nephritis[106] and in Dutch patients with SLE.[107] However, we were unable to confirm this finding in groups of Caucasian, Afro-Caribbean or Chinese patients with lupus.[108] Further studies are needed to test whether this polymorphic variant of FcγRIIa is a disease susceptibility

gene for SLE or, more specifically, for lupus nephritis. This area is reviewed in more detail in section 4.2.

3.2.3 Processing of IC in patients with abnormal CR1 and complement function

The *in vivo* clearance of soluble IC in human disease has been studied using all of the three models described earlier in section 2.1.4, i.e. IgG aggregates (AIgG), TT complexes and anti-HBsAg:HBsAg complexes. Important differences in the clearance of radiolabelled aggregated γ-globulin were seen between normal subjects and patients with SLE.[109] The mean half-time for initial clearance of AIgG was shorter in patients than in controls, and binding of AIgG to erythrocytes was significantly lower in patients compared with normal subjects. Liver/spleen uptake ratios were also significantly higher in patients than in controls, attributable to reduced splenic uptake of AIgG. Accelerated clearance of AIgG was also observed in two C3-deficient patients studied using the same model complexes.[110] Similar observations were made in patients with SLE and hypocomplementaemia in studies that employed ^{125}I-labelled TT:anti-TT complexes as probes of the pathways of IC processing.[54] The most striking finding was the enhanced rapid initial clearance of complexes in patients with lupus and low complement levels, most marked in a patient with C1q deficiency.

The explanation for these results, notably for the rapid initial clearance of IC in hypocomplementaemic patients, came from our own studies using ^{123}I-labelled HBsAg:anti-HBsAg IC. As in normal individuals, the liver and spleen were the main sites of complex uptake. However, the initial clearance of IC from blood was more rapid in patients with SLE than in normal controls due to more rapid uptake in the liver. In SLE patients, however, there was significant release of complexes from the liver after 30–40 minutes, which was not seen in normal subjects. Binding of IC to erythrocytes was greatly reduced in the patients as a consequence of hypocomplementaemia and reduced CR1 numbers. As discussed above, in a C2-deficient patient studied before and after therapy with

FFP, there was no uptake of IC in the spleen prior to therapy, but both the kinetics and sites of complex clearance reverted to normal after normalization of classical pathway complement activity.[56]

To summarize, the main findings of these studies of *in vivo* IC processing in SLE patients are as follows:

- More rapid initial clearance of complexes from the circulation takes place in patients than controls, followed by release of IC back into the circulation.
- The splenic uptake of IC is reduced in patients. It is possible that the impaired uptake of complexes in the spleen in SLE may be related to the mode of delivery of IC to the fixed mononuclear phagocytic system.
- Reduced binding to red cell CR1 was observed in all three models in SLE patients, with a resultant increase in the numbers of complexes delivered to the fixed macrophage system in the fluid phase. As discussed previously, the anatomy of the spleen favours the uptake of particles.[68] The haematocrit in the splenic vasculature is relatively high compared with major blood vessels, and splenic macrophages play a key role in the processing of IgG-coated erythrocytes (discussed in section 2.2). It might therefore be expected that IC bound to red cell CR1 would be selectively processed in the spleen, while complexes presented in the fluid phase would localize to the liver.

The explanation for the observed release of IC back into the circulation from the liver is unclear. One possibility is that it is only complexes which are able to interact efficiently with both complement and FcγR on fixed macrophages, with subsequent internalization and processing, that are retained efficiently within the liver and spleen. IC bearing relatively little C3b, which are delivered in the fluid phase, may bind rapidly to the relatively low-affinity Fcγ-R (II and III), but ligation of these receptors alone may be insufficient to trigger efficient internalization of the complexes.

3.3 Role of IC and complement in causing inflammation

3.3.1 Background
IC induce tissue injury primarily by activation of the complement system. Three main mechanisms are involved.

- Complement proteins attached, covalently (C3 and C4) or non-covalently (C1q), to IC may ligate receptors on leucocytes and lymphocytes, triggering these cells to express effector activities.
- Formation of the membrane-attack complex may cause direct cellular damage or, at sublytic levels, stimulate local cell activation.
- Complement activation may cause anaphylatoxin generation.

The architecture of the affected tissues is an important factor in determining the nature of IC-mediated inflammatory tissue injury. A good example of this is in glomerular renal inflammation, where the glomerular basement membrane is a barrier to the exit of leucocytes from glomerular capillaries. Tissue injury in membranous glomerulonephritis, in which IC form in the subepithelium, is induced by the complement membrane-attack complex in the absence of inflammatory leucocytes.[111] On the other hand, when IC form, or are deposited, in the subendothelium, as in SLE or Goodpasture's disease, then tissue injury is induced by a combination of leucocytes and complement.[112]

The study of animals with gene-targeted deletions of complement and FcγR has greatly facilitated further exploration of the triggering mechanisms of inflammation by IC. One such model system that has been widely used is the reverse passive Arthus reaction. In this model, antibody is injected into the skin, or introduced into the lungs, of an animal that has been injected intravenously with antigen. In skin, the reverse passive Arthus reaction is dependent on both Fc- and complement-mediated pathways.[113–115] Complement depletion alone did not significantly reduce the inflammatory response. Deficiency of FcγRIII diminished the response to a variable degree, which correlated inversely with the level of haemolytic complement expressed in individual animals.[114] Complete abolition of the response was only seen in FcγRIII-deficient animals following depletion of complement with cobra venom factor. These observations are similar to those made some years ago in C5-deficient and cobra-venom-factor-treated mice which showed that, at low concentrations of antibody, complement-dependent inflammatory pathways dominated, whereas, at high concentrations, complement-independent pathways played a more critical role.[115] The results of studies of the reverse passive Arthus reaction in the lung are similar to those in the skin. In this model, however, complement depletion, or deficiency of C5, seem to block the inflammatory response more effectively than in the skin.[116] A role for the anaphylatoxin, C5a, and/or the membrane-attack complex, may be inferred from the observation that C5 deficiency has some protective effect against the Arthus reaction in the lung,[114] as in the skin.

Several lines of evidence support an important role for mast cells in triggering tissue injury in response to IC in the Arthus reaction. Studies performed in a strain of mice lacking mast cells due to deficiency of stem cell factor, c-kit, showed a markedly reduced reverse passive Arthus reaction.[117] Reconstitution studies have been performed in these animals with mast cells derived from animals deficient or sufficient in the FcR γ-chain.[118] The Arthus response was only effectively restored to normal in mice reconstituted with mast cells bearing FcγRIII, showing that IC, in this model, trigger mast cells to release their mediators and cause inflammation by ligation of this FcγR.

Intrapulmonary IC formation has also been studied in mice with gene-targeted deletions of either the NK-1R substance-P receptor or the C5a receptor.[119] The induction of the inflammatory response following intrapulmonary IC formation was abrogated in NK-1R–/–mice and was also absent in C5aR–/– mice. These observations suggest an additional role for the tachykinin, substance P, in IC-mediated inflammation. Substance P, found in C-type nerve fibres, is also found in macrophages and mast cells, as is NK-1R.

3.3.2 In situ *IC formation and the deposition of complexes from the circulation*

The relative importance of *in situ* IC formation, and the deposition of IC from the circulation, in causing inflammation, has long been the subject of debate. In solution, when antigen meets antibody at equivalence or in antibody excess, rapid precipitation occurs. This reaction requires intact IgG molecules, as distinct from $F(ab')_2$ fragments, suggesting that Fc–Fc interactions are important in promoting precipitation.[120] Large complexes also promote the aggregation of small complexes on their surface.[9] Such interactions bring the reacting molecules into close proximity and this is followed by formation of an 'infinite lattice' of alternating antigen–antibody bonds, resulting in the precipitation of an insoluble IC. Such a lattice can also build up on an antigen or antibody located within tissues, either as an intrinsic component or 'planted' from the circulation. *In situ* formation of IC in this way has been demonstrated in experimental glomerulonephritis, in which planted antigen (or antibody) exposed successively to further antibody and antigen leads to the development of large, microscopically visible, deposits.[121]

Continuous overproduction of antibody, often antigen driven, is a major factor in the pathophysiology of autoimmune diseases such as SLE and in infections such as bacterial endocarditis, in which IC are thought to play an important role. In these diseases, IC are formed in large antibody excess and are likely to be large, complement-activating aggregates. Immobilization of these IC in tissues, either from *in situ* formation or deposition from the blood stream, causes inflammation and organ injury. The complement system has a role in limiting such injury by inhibiting the formation of large IC, as discussed above, and promoting their safe disposal by the mononuclear phagocytic system.

3.3.3 Role of autoantibodies to complement components in amplifying IC-mediated tissue damage

A number of autoantibodies to complement components may have a role in amplifying the phlogistic effects of IC. The two best characterized examples are C3 nephritic factor (C3 NeF) and antibodies to the collagenous part of the C1q molecule [anti-C1q(CLR) – collagen-like region].

C3 NeF is an IgG autoantibody directed against neo-antigenic determinants on the alternative pathway C3 convertase, C3bBb. C3 NeF stabilizes the enzyme, causing dysregulated complement activation, leading to a severe secondary deficiency of C3.[122] C3 NeF is associated clinically with partial lipodystrophy and type II membranoproliferative glomerulonephritis, in which electron-dense deposits occur in the glomerulus. These deposits do not generally contain Ig, though C3 is usually demonstrable. The mechanism of the association of C3 NeF with glomerulonephritis is not understood. One hypothesis is that C3 NeF causes secondary C3 deficiency which, in turn, is responsible for the development of nephritis. This hypothesis is supported by observations that homozygous C3 deficiency is associated in some humans and in dogs with development of mesangiocapillary glomerulonephritis, though not with the typical electron-dense deposits that define type II mesangiocapillary glomerulonephritis. The mechanism of the association of C3 deficiency with glomerulonephritis also remains uncertain. Attempts to induce renal injury in experimental animals rendered hypocomplementaemic by non-immune mechanisms have been generally unsuccessful,[123,124] and nephritis in the context of NeF may coexist with normal complement levels.[122]

A second possible explanation for the association of C3 NeF with glomerulonephritis is that C3 NeF can activate complement locally in the kidney. This explanation could also account for the association of factor H and I deficiencies with glomerulonephritis, in which C3, locally synthesized in the kidney, may undergo unregulated activation and cause local tissue injury. In support of this hypothesis are *in vitro* experiments showing that heat-killed kidney cells may activate complement and bind a NeF-stabilized C3 convertase.[125] There is also a report of a patient with mesangiocapillary glomerulonephritis, hypocomplementaemia and systemic candidiasis. The glomerular deposits in this patient contained both C3 and *Candida albicans*, a known alternative pathway activator.[126]

It is becoming clear that antibodies to C1q are important in some types of autoimmune disease. The pathogenic role of these anti-C1q(CLR), IgG autoantibodies to neo-epitopes on the collagenous part of the C1q molecule is, however, poorly understood. The antibodies exhibit a number of specific clinical associations, notably with SLE and hypocomplementaemic urticarial vasculitis syndrome,[127,128] and are strongly associated with classical pathway complement activation, causing very low levels of C3, C4 and C1q. It is possible that they may augment activation of the complement system by IC in tissues. This idea is supported by recent observations that anti-C1q antibodies, purified from two patients with SLE, deposited in mouse glomeruli in the presence of human C1q.[129]

A range of other autoantibodies to complement neo-antigens has also been described. For example, IgG autoantibodies that stabilize the classical pathway convertase, C4b2a, have been reported in a patient with post-streptococcal glomerulonephritis and in some patients with SLE.[130,131]

4. Fcγ RECEPTORS (FcγR) – NEW INSIGHTS INTO STRUCTURE AND FUNCTION

4.1 Genetics and structure

A detailed description of the genetics of this complex family of molecules is beyond the scope of this chapter. A diagram illustrating the main structural characteristics of the different groups of FcγR is shown in Figure 4.2. We shall consider the inhibitory and stimulatory groups of receptors separately.

4.1.1 Inhibitory FcγR
The inhibitory FcγR (FcγRIIb) comprise single-chain, low-affinity receptors. These molecules have extracellular domains that are highly homologous to the similar activating molecules and they have cytoplasmic domains that contain immunoreceptor tyrosine-based inhibitory motifs (ITIM).[132] FcγRIIb are widely expressed on haematopoietic cells – FcγRIIb2 on cells of myeloid origin and FcγRIIb1 on B-cells.

Neither of these molecules can trigger cellular activation. These receptors are encoded by a single gene on chromosome 1q 23–24 and the two different isoforms are generated by alternative splicing. There is an insertion of 19 amino acids in FcγRIIb1.

Negative regulation of cellular activation occurs when both isoforms of FcγRIIb co-aggregate with ITIM-bearing receptors. The intracytoplasmic insertion in FcγRIIb1 inhibits internalization of exogenous molecules. FcγRIIb2 has a role in the endocytosis of multivalent antigens by both antigen-presenting cells and phagocytes. The function of this group of molecules is highly dependent on the co-aggregation of FcγRIIb and ITIM-expressing receptors in the presence of a multivalent ligand.[133] It has been demonstrated that the co-aggregation of FcγRIIb with IgG-opsonized particles, and also of FcγRIIa, will inhibit phagocytosis. Proliferation of B-cells may also be inhibited by FcγRIIb co-ligation to B-cell receptors (BCR) by IC.

4.1.2 Stimulatory FcγR

FcγR in this group are a multichain structure, comprising an α subunit which is ligand binding and which confers affinity and ligand specificity. The molecules also have subunits with immunoreceptor tyrosine-based activating motifs (ITAM) in the cytoplasmic domains and it is this part of the molecule that plays a key role in the triggering of cellular activation (see below).

The α-chains of FcγR are mainly found on myeloid cells. These subunits are transmembrane molecules, and there are variations in their affinity for IgG and also variations in the capacity of the different variants for binding different IgG subclasses. The capacity of this group of molecules to bind IgG subclasses is also influenced by allelic variations in the ligand-binding region of the molecules. These allelic variants also have an important effect in the way in which phagocytic cells respond to antigenic stimuli that are opsonized by IgG.[105,106,134]

There are two main multichain FcγR isoforms – FcγRI (a receptor for IgG of high affinity, binding the monomeric form of the molecule) and FcγRIIIa (a receptor which binds only multivalent Ig with intermediate/low affinity). The transducing molecules for these two receptors comprise homodimeric γ-chains. Additionally, homodimers of ζ-chains, or γ-ζ

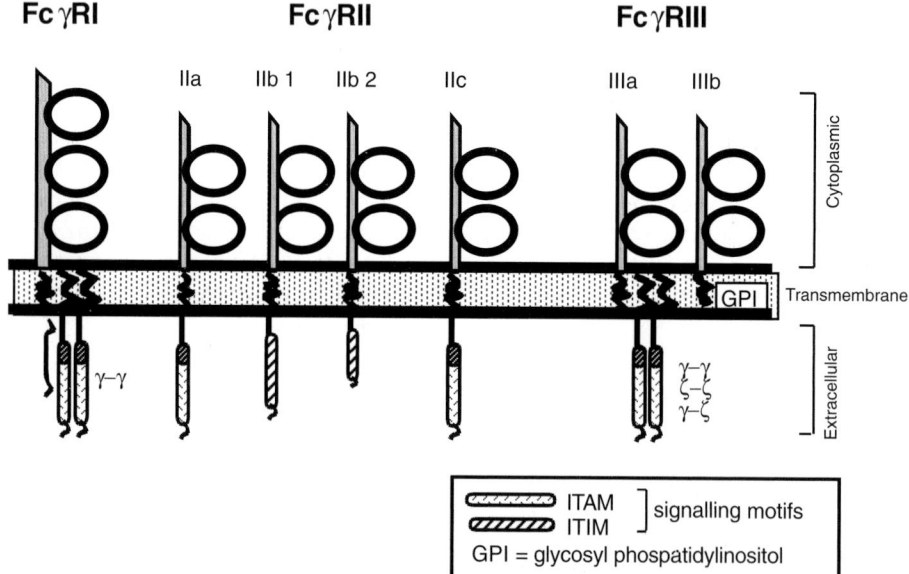

Fig. 4.2 Fc-receptors: diagrammatic representation of the structure of the three main types of gamma receptor. ITAM, immunoreceptor tyrosine-based activating motifs; ITIM, immunoreceptor tyrosine-based inhibitory motifs.

heterodimers, have the capacity to transduce signals through FcγRIIIa in natural killer (NK) cells in humans.[135]

In humans, three further types of stimulatory FcγR exist – FcγRIIa, FcγRIIc and FcγRIIIb. The two former molecules are low-affinity, single-chain receptors that bear an ITAM-containing cytoplasmic domain, while FcγRIIIb has neither an ITAM nor a transmembrane domain, but is a glucose-6-phosphate isomerase (GPI)-linked molecule. It is generally the case that it is the cell type expressing the activating FcγR that determines the type of response that follows the interaction of a ligand and the FcγR. For example, on dendritic cells, FcγR which bear ITAM have a role in the transport of IC into the cell, and in antigen processing and presentation. FcγRIIa on platelets induce degranulation and aggregation. The same receptor on polymorphonuclear leucocytes can trigger a respiratory burst. On mast cells, ligation of stimulatory FcγR can trigger the production of a range of inflammatory mediators, including key cytokines such as tumour necrosis factor (TNF)-α.[136]

4.2 FcγR polymorphisms and disease

A detailed discussion of this evolving and complex area is beyond the scope of this chapter and the reader should consult one of the recent comprehensive reviews.[137,138] FcγRIIa, expressed on monocytes, platelets and PMN, is encoded by two co-dominantly expressed alleles (H and R131) that bear either a histidine or an arginine at amino acid position 131. The two variants differ in their capacity to bind Ig. The H131 variant binds IgG2 very efficiently, while R131 is a low binder. FcγRIIIa (expressed on NK cells and monocytes) similarly has two co-dominantly expressed allelic variants (F176 and V176), differing in one amino acid (phenylalanine or valine). Homozygosity for V176 results in more avid binding of IgG1 and IgG3 than is the case for F176 homozygotes. Two common allelic variants of the PMN receptor FcγRIIIb have also been described (NA1 and NA2), differing by five nucleotides. At the protein level, a substitution of four amino acids

in one of the extracellular domains of the molecule results, but IgG binding is not affected.[139–142] There is some evidence, however, that FcγRIIIb NA1/NA1 homozygous PMN have enhanced phagocytic responses compared with NA2/NA2 cells, as a result of greater degranulation and oxidative burst responses in the former.[141–143] Allelic variants of FcγRIIa, FcγRIIIa and of the PMN receptor FcγRIIIb have been implicated in the pathogenesis of autoimmune disease and in influencing susceptibility to certain infections. These are considered in turn.

4.2.1 FcγR polymorphisms and autoimmunity

It has been suggested by many authors that FcγR genetic variants, which encode receptors with an impaired capacity to ligate IgG in IC, are likely to be susceptibility genes for SLE. This contention is partly supported by association studies in some populations which suggest that FcγRIIa-R131 and FcγRIIIa-F176 are enriched in patients with the disease.[106,144–147] More recent evidence from genome scanning performed in African-American patients with SLE has also linked the FcγR gene cluster on chromosome 1q with lupus.[148] However, this area remains controversial and associations between SLE and low-binding alleles has not been demonstrated in all populations studied.[105,108,149,150] Current evidence would support an association between SLE and the FcγRIIa-R131 allele in African-American patients, while in Caucasians, the link with the FcγRIIIa-F176 variant appears more convincing. More specific associations with lupus nephritis, anti-C1q autoantibodies and the FcγRIIa-R131 variant have been described independently by this group[151] and Salmon's[152] suggesting that these genes may play a role in dictating severity of disease, rather than acting as simple susceptibility factors.

FcγR allelic variants have also been studied in anti-neutrophil cytoplasmic antibody (ANCA)-positive vasculitis (Wegener's granulomatosis) and in rheumatoid arthritis. In the latter, an increased frequency of FcγRIIIa-F176 homozygosity has been observed.[153] In Wegener's, the situation remains unresolved, but there is some evidence that a high-binding variant of FcγRIIIb on PMN may predispose to more severe disease, possibly as a consequence of facilitation of the binding of pathogenic ANCA to PMN.

4.2.2 FcγR polymorphisms and susceptibility to infection

IgG2-mediated humoral immune responses are critical in host defence against many encapsulated bacterial pathogens, e.g. *Streptococcus pneumoniae*, *Haemophilus influenzae*, and *Neisseria meningitidis*. FcγRIIa-R131 has been shown to predispose to severe pnemococcal infection in patients with lupus, and to fulminant meningococcal sepsis and recurrent respiratory tract infection in children.[154] The recent observation that C-reactive protein binds to FcγRIIa suggest that this receptor may have a key role in defence against organisms in this group, particularly pneumococci.

It has been proposed that the differences in the capacity of the V-176 and F-176 variants of FcγRIIIa to bind IgG may have an effect on 'immune' surveillance mediated by the humoral immune system. This contention is supported by the observation that there is a decreased frequency of Kaposi's sarcoma in HIV-infected individuals homozygous for the F176 allele.[155] In chronic granulomatous disease, there is a well-described association between the forma-

tion of granulomas in the genitourinary and gastrointestinal tracts and FcγRIIIb genotypes.[156]

In certain clinical situations, the coexistence of genetically determined abnormalities in the immune system may have an additive role in increasing susceptibility to infection. An excellent example exists with respect to the complement and FcγR systems. There is increased susceptibility to *N meningitidis* in patients with deficiency of terminal complement components 6 or 8, who are also homozygotes for FcγRIIa-R131 and FcγRIIIb-NA2.[157]

4.3 Fc gamma receptor-mediated Ic

As discussed above, there is clear evidence that complement and its receptors are involved in Ic clearance, and that abnormalities in these mechanisms exist in SLE. Much of this evidence comes from *in vivo* studies using complement-fixing HbsAg : anti-HbsAg immune complexes in humans.[55] More recently, we have performed similar studies in man employing similar complexes, the size of which was modified to facilitate their clearance primarily by Fc-mediated mechanisms.[158] In this model, a number of fundamental differences were observed compared with larger complement-fixing complexes of the same species. We found that complexes were cleared mainly in the liver,

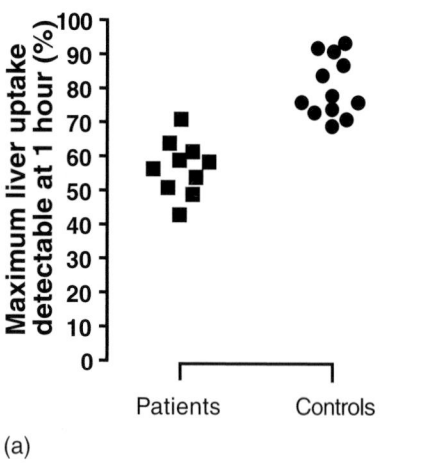

(a)

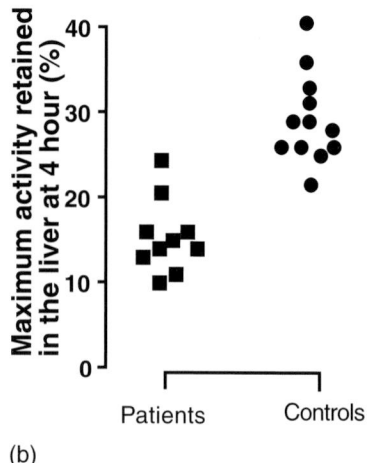

(b)

Fig. 4.3 Impaired retention of experimental soluble immune complexes in the liver is seen in SLE (from ref. 158 with permission).

confirming our previous observations that IC uptake in the spleen is a complement-dependent phenomenon. Perhaps the most interesting observations were in patients with SLE, in whom there was a failure effectively to retain IC in the liver, after their initial uptake (Figure 4.3). This obviously raises the possibility that there is indeed abnormal Fc receptor function in this condition, and may in part provide the link between the Fc-receptor polymorphisms discussed above, and severe SLE characterized by IC-mediated renal damage.

5. CONCLUDING REMARKS

There is clearly a number of functional similarities between the complement system and the FC-receptor network. Both have key roles to play in linking the innate and adaptive immune systems; both have a role in the clearance of immune complexes and particulate antigens, and both groups of molecules are involved in processes with both pro- and anti-inflammatory biological consequences. In addition, genetically-determined deficiencies (in the case of complement), and structural variations in the case of Fc-receptors in particular, may predispose to infectious or auto-immune diseases, or influence their severity. There is no doubt that both systems are at present only relatively poorly understood, and it is likely that further research in this area will in due course result in the development of new therapeutic strategies in a wide range of infectious, inflammatory and auto-immune conditions.

REFERENCES

Scientific papers

1. Heidelberger M. Quantitative chemical studies on complement or alexin. I A method. *J Exp Med* 1941; **73**: 691–4.
2. Morgan CR, Sorenson RL, Lazarow A. Further studies of an inhibitor of the two antibody immunoassay system. *Diabetes* 1964; **13**: 579–84.
3. Utiger RD, Daughaday WH. Studies on human growth hormone. I. A radioimmunoassay for human growth hormone. *J Clin Invest* 1962; **41**: 254–61.
4. Miller GW, Nussenzweig V. A new complement function: solubilization of antigen–antibody aggregates. *Proc Natl Acad Sci USA* 1975; **72**: 418–22.
5. Schifferli JA, Morris SM, Dash A, Peters DK. Complement-mediated solubilization in patients with systemic lupus erythematosus, nephritis or vasculitis. *Clin Exp Immunol* 1981; **46**: 557–64.
6. Schifferli JA, Bartolotti SR, Peters DK. Inhibition of immune precipitation by complement. *Clin Exp Immunol* 1980; **42**: 387–94.
7. Hong K, Takata Y, Sayama K et al. Inhibition of immune precipitation by complement. *J Immunol* 1984; **133**: 1464–70.
8. Lachmann PJ, Walport MJ. Deficiency of the effector mechanisms of the immune response and autoimmunity. In: Whelan J, ed. *Autoimmunity and Autoimmune Disease, Ciba Foundation Symposium #129*. Chichester: Wiley Ltd, 1987.
9. Moller NP, Steengaard J. Fc mediated immune precipitation. I. A new role of the Fc portion of IgG. *Immunology* 1983; **38**: 631–40.
10. Johnson A, Harkin S, Steward MW, Whaley K. The effects of immunoglobulin isotype and antibody affinity on complement-mediated inhibition of immune precipitation and solubilization. *Molec Immunol* 1987; **24**: 1211–17.
11. Ng YC, Peters DK, Walport MJ. Monoclonal rheumatoid factor-IgG IC. Poor fixation of opsonic C4 and C3 despite efficient complement activation. *Arthritis Rheum* 1987; **31**: 99–107.
12. Takahashi M, Tack BF, Nussenzweig V. Requirements for the solubilization of immune aggregates by complement: assembly of a factor B-dependent C3-convertase on the IC. *J Exp Med* 1977; **145**: 86–100.
13. Fries LF, Gaither TA, Hammer CH, Frank MM. C3b covalently bound to IgG demonstrates a reduced rate of inactivation by factors H and I. *J Exp Med* 1984; **160**: 1640–55.
14. Spath PJ, Pascual M, Meyer Hanni L et al. Solubilization of immune precipitates by complement in the absence of properdin or factor D. *FEBS Lett* 1988; **234**: 131–4.
15. Volanakis JE. Complement-induced solubilization of C-reactive protein–pneumococcal C-polysaccharide precipitates: evidence for covalent binding of complement proteins to C-reactive protein and to pneumococcal C-polysaccharide. *J Immunol* 1982; **128**: 2745–50.
16. Schifferli JA, Steiger G, Paccaud JP. Complement mediated inhibition of immune precipitation and solubilization generate different concentrations

of complement anaphylatoxins (C4a, C3a, C5a). *Clin Exp Immunol* 1986; **64**: 407–14.

17. Bull CG. The agglutination of bacteria *in vivo*. *J Exp Med* 1915; **22**: 484–91.

18. Rieckenberg H. Eine neue immuninitasreaktion bei experimentaller trypanosomen-infection: die blutpattchen-probe. *Immunitatsforsch* 1917; **26**: 53–64.

19. Duke HL, Wallace JM. 'Red-cell adhesion' in trypanosomiasis of man and animals. *Parasitology* 1930; **22**: 414–56.

20. Kritschewsky IL, Tscherikower RS. Uber anti-korper, die micro-organismen mit blutpattchen beladen (thrombozytobarinen). *Zeitschrift fur immunitatsforsch* 1925; **42**: 131–49.

21. Gordon J, Whitehead HR, Wormall A. The action of ammonia on complement. The fourth component. *Biochem J* 1926; **20**: 1028–35.

22. Wallace JM, Wormall A. Red cell adhesion in trypanosomiasis of man and other animals. II Some experiments on the mechanism of the reaction. *Parasitology* 1931; **23**: 346–59.

23. Brown HC, Broom JC. Studies in trypanosomiasis. II. Observations on the red cell adhesion test. *Trans R Soc Trop Med Hyg* 1938; **32**: 209–22.

24. Osborne TWB. *Complement or Alexin*. London: Oxford University Press, 1937.

25. Ecker EE, Pillemer L. Complement. *Ann NY Acad Sci* 1942; **43**: 63–83.

26. Nelson Jr, RA. The immune adherence phenomenon: an immunologically specific reaction between micro-organisms and erythrocytes leading to enhanced phagocytosis. *Science* 1953; **118**: 733–7.

27. Fearon DT. Identification of the membrane glycoprotein that is the C3b receptor of the human erythrocyte, polymorphonuclear leukocyte, B lymphocyte, and monocyte. *J Exp Med* 1980; **152**: 20–30.

28. Hebert LA, Cosio FG. The erythrocyte–IC–glomerulonephritis connection in man. *Kidney Int* 1987; **31**: 877–85.

29. Walport MJ, Ross GD, Mackworth-Young C et al. Family studies of erythrocyte complement receptor type 1 levels: reduced levels in patients with SLE are acquired, not inherited. *Clin Exp Immunol* 1985; **59**: 547–54.

30. Wilson JG, Wong WW, Schur PH, Fearon DT. Mode of inheritance of decreased C3b receptors on erythrocytes of patients with systemic lupus erythematosus. *N Engl J Med* 1982; **307**: 981–6.

31. Fearon DT, Collins LA. Increased expression of C3b receptors on polymorphonuclear leukocytes induced by chemotactic factors and by purification procedures. *J Immunol* 1983; **130**: 370–5.

32. Paccaud J-P, Carpentier J-L, Schifferli JA. Direct evidence for the clustered nature of complement receptors type 1 on the erythrocyte membrane. *J Immunol* 1988; **141**: 3889–94.

33. Fearon DT. Cellular receptors for fragments of the third component of complement. *Immunol Today* 1984; **5**: 105–10.

34. Wong WW. Structural and functional correlation of the human complement receptor type 1. *J Invest Dermatol* 1990; **94**: 64S–67S.

35. Van Dyne S, Holers VM, Lublin DM, Atkinson JP. The polymorphism of the C3b/C4b receptor in the normal population and in patients with systemic lupus erythematosus. *Clin Exp Immunol* 1987; **68**: 570–9.

36. Klopstock A, Schartz J, Bleiberg Y et al. Hereditary nature of the behaviour of erythrocytes in immune adherence – haemagglutination phenomenon. *Vox Sang* 1965; **10**: 177–87.

37. Walport MJ, Lachmann PJ. Erythrocyte complement receptor type 1, IC and the rheumatic diseases. *Arthritis Rheum* 1987; **31**: 153–8.

38. Paccaud JP, Carpentier JL, Schifferli JA. Difference in the clustering of complement receptor type 1 (CR1) on polymorphonuclear leukocytes and erythrocytes: effect on immune adherence. *Eur J Immunol* 1990; **20**: 283–9.

39. Paccaud JP, Schifferli JA, Baggiolini M. NAP-1/IL-8 induces up-regulation of CR1 receptors in human neutrophil leukocytes. *Biochem Biophys Res Commun* 1990; **166**: 187–92.

40. Beynon HLC, Davies KA, Haskard DO, Walport MJ. Erythrocyte complement receptor type 1 and interactions between IC, neutrophils and endothelium. *J Immunol* 1994; **153**: 3160–7.

41. Biozzi G, Benacerraf B, Halpern BN. Quantitative study of the granulopectic activity of the reticuloendothelial system II. *BJ Exp Path* 1953; **34**: 441–57.

42. Niehaus GD, Shumacker PR, Saba TM. Reticuloendothelial clearance of blood-borne particulates: relevance to experimental lung microembolization and vascular injury. *Ann Surg* 1980; **191**: 479–87.

43. Davies KA, Chapman PT, Norsworthy PJ et al. Clearance pathways of IC in the pig. Insight into the adaptive nature of antigen clearance in humans. *J Immunol* 1995; **155**: 5760–8.

44. Taylor RP, Kujala G, Wilson K et al. In vivo and in vitro studies of the binding of antibody/dsDNA IC to rabbit and guinea pig platelets. *J Immunol* 1985; **134**: 2550–8.

45. Edberg JC, Kujala GA, Taylor RP. Rapid immune adherence reactivity of nascent, soluble

antibody/DNA IC in the circulation. *J Immunol* 1987; **139**: 1240–4.

46. Haakenstad AO, Mannik M. Saturation of the reticuloendothelial system with soluble IC. *J Immunol* 1974; **112**: 1939–48.

47. Finbloom DS, Plotz PH. Studies of reticuloendothelial function in the mouse with model IC: II. Serum clearance, tissue uptake and reticuloendothelial saturation in NZB/W mice. *J Immunol* 1979; **123**: 1600–3.

48. Finbloom DS, Magilavy DB, Harford JB et al. Influence of antigen on IC behavior in mice. *J Clin Invest* 1981; **68**: 214–24.

49. Cornacoff JB, Hebert LA, Smead WL et al. Primate erythrocyte–IC clearing mechanism. *J Clin Invest* 1983; **71**: 236–47.

50. Waxman FJ, Hebert LA, Cornacoff JB et al. Complement depletion accelerates the clearance of IC from the circulation of primates. *J Clin Invest* 1984; **74**: 1329–40.

51. Waxman FJ, Hebert LA, Cosio FG et al. Differential binding of immunoglobulin A and immunoglobulin G1 IC to primate erythrocytes *in vivo*: immunoglobulin A IC bind less well to erythrocytes and are preferentially deposited in glomeruli. *J Clin Invest* 1986; **77**: 82–9.

52. Cornacoff JB, Hebert LA, Birmingham DJ, Waxman FJ. Factors influencing the binding of large IC primate erythrocyte CR1 receptor. *Clin Immunol Immunopathol* 1984; **30**: 255–64.

53. Lobatto S, Daha MR, Voetman AA et al. Clearance of soluble aggregates of immunoglobulin G in healthy volunteers and chimpanzees. *Clin Exp Immunol* 1987; **68**: 133.

54. Schifferli JA, Ng YC, Estreicher J, Walport MJ. The clearance of tetanus toxoid/anti-tetanus toxoid IC from the circulation of humans. Complement- and erythrocyte complement receptor 1-dependent mechanisms. *J Immunol* 1988; **140**: 899–904.

55. Davies KA, Peters AM, Beynon HLC, Walport MJ. IC processing in patients with systemic lupus erythematosus – *in vivo* imaging and clearance studies. *J Clin Invest* 1992; **90**: 2075–83.

56. Davies KA, Erlendsson K, Beynon HLC et al. Splenic uptake of IC in man is complement-dependent. *J Immunol* 1993; **151**: 3866–73.

57. Edberg JC, Kujala GA, Taylor RP. Rapid immune adherence reactivity of nascent, soluble antibody/DNA IC in the circulation. *J Immunol* 1987; **139**: 1240.

58. Davies KA, Hird V, Stewart S et al. A study of *in vivo* IC formation and clearance in man. *J Immunol* 1990; **144**: 4613–20.

59. Brown DL, Lachmann PJ, Dacie JV. The *in vivo* behavior of complement-coated red cells: studies in C6-deficient, C3-depleted, and normal rabbits. *Clin Exp Immunol* 1970; **7**: 401–22.

60. Atkinson JP, Frank MM. Studies on the *in vivo* effects of antibody. Interaction of IgM antibody and complement in the immune clearance and destruction of erythrocytes in man. *J Clin Invest* 1974; **54**: 339–48.

61. Hughes-Jones NC, Mollison PL, Mollison PN. Removal of incompatible red cells by the spleen. *Br J Haematol* 1957; **3**: 125–33.

62. Mollison PL, Crome P, Hughes-Jones NC, Rochna E. Rate of removal from the circulation of red cells sensitised with different amounts of antibody. *Br J Haematol* 1965; **11**: 461–70.

63. Frank MM, Lawley TJ, Hamburger MI, Brown EJ. Immunoglobulin G Fc receptor-mediated clearance in autoimmune diseases. *Ann Intern Med* 1983; **98**: 206–18.

64. Smedsrod B, Pertoft H, Eggertsen G, Sundstrom C. Functional and morphological characterization of cultures of Kupffer cells and liver endothelial cells prepared by means of density separation in Percoll, and selective substrate adherence. *Cell Tiss Res* 1985; **241**: 639–49.

65. Ross GD, Newman SL. Regulation of macrophage functions by complement, complement receptors, and IgG-Fc receptors. In: Bellanti JA, Herscowitz HB, eds. *The Reticuloendothelial System, A Comprehensive Treatise*, Vol. 6. New York: Plenum Publishing, 1984.

66. Unkeless JC, Fleit H, Mellman IS. Structural aspects and heterogeneity of immunoglobulin Fc receptors. *Adv Immunol* 1981; **31**: 247–70.

67. Reist CJ, Wright JD, Labuguen RH, Taylor RP. Human IgG in IC bound to human erythrocyte CR1 is recognized differently than human IgG bound to an erythrocyte surface antigen. *J Immunol Methods* 1993; **163**: 199–208.

68. Peters AM. Splenic blood flow and blood cell kinetics. *Clin Haematol* 1983; **12**: 421–47.

69. Weiss L. The spleen. In: Weiss L, ed. *Cell and Tissue Biology*, 2nd edn. Baltimore: Urban and Schwarzenberg, 1988.

70. Robertson DA, Bullen AW, Hall R, Losowsky MS. Blood film appearances in the hyposplenism of coeliac disease. *Br J Clin Pract* 1983; **37**: 19–22.

71. Crocker SH, Eddy DO, Obenauf RN et al. Bacteremia: host specific lung clearance and pulmonary failure. *J Trauma* 1981; **21**: 215–20.

72. Wessels MR, Butko P, Ma M et al. Studies of group B streptococcal infection in mice deficient in complement component C3 or C4 demonstrate

an essential role for complement in both innate and acquired immunity. *Proc Natl Acad Sci USA* 1995; **92**: 11490–4.

73. Reid R, Prodeus AP, Khan W, Carroll MC. Natural antibody and complement are critical for endotoxin clearance from the circulation. *Molec Immunol* 1996; **33**: 78 (abstract).

74. Lynn WA, Cohen J. Adjunctive therapy for septic shock: a review of experimental approaches. *Clin Infect Dis* 1995; **20**: 143–58.

75. Seelen MA, Athanassiou P, Lynn WA et al. The anti-lipid A monoclonal antibody E5 binds to rough gram-negative bacteria, fixes C3, and facilitates binding of bacterial IC to both erythrocytes and monocytes. *Immunology* 1995; **84**: 653–61.

76. Tonoli M, Davies KA, Norsworthy PJ et al. The anti-lipid antibody HA-1A binds to rough Gram-negative bacteria, fixes complement and facilitates binding to erythrocyte CR1(CD35). *Clin Exp Immunol* 1993; **92**: 232–8.

77. Bowness P, Davies KA, Norsworthy PJ et al. Hereditary C1q deficiency and systemic lupus erythematosus. *Q J Med* 1994; **87**: 455–64.

78. Ruddy S. Component deficiencies 3. The second component. *Prog Allergy* 1986; **39**: 250–67.

79. Botto M, Fong KY, So AK et al. Homozygous hereditary C3 deficiency due to a partial gene deletion. *Proc Natl Acad Sci USA* 1992; **89**: 4957–61.

80. Botto M, Walport MJ. Hereditary deficiency of C3 in animals and humans. *Int Rev Immunol* 1993; **10**: 37–50.

81. Vyse TJ, Spath PJ, Davies KA et al. Hereditary complement factor I deficiency. *Q J Med* 1994; **87**: 385–401.

82. Fielder AH, Walport MJ, Batchelor JR et al. Family study of the major histocompatibility complex in patients with systemic lupus erythematosus: importance of null alleles of C4A and C4B in determining disease susceptibility. *Br Med J Clin Res* 1983; **286**: 425–8.

83. Christiansen FT, Dawkins RL, Uko G et al. Complement allotyping in SLE: association with C4A null. *Aust NZ J Med* 1983; **13**: 483–8.

84. Howard PF, Hochberg MC, Bias WB et al. Relationship between C4 null genes, HLA-D region antigens, and genetic susceptibility to systemic lupus erythematosus in Caucasian and black Americans. *Am J Med* 1986; **81**: 187–93.

85. Hartung K, Baur MP, Coldewey R et al. Major histocompatibility complex haplotypes and complement C4 alleles in systemic lupus erythematosus. Results of a multicenter study. *J Clin Invest* 1992; **90**: 1346–51.

86. Davies EJ, Snowden N, Hillarby MC et al. Mannose-binding protein gene polymorphism in systemic lupus erythematosus. *Arthritis Rheum* 1995; **38**: 110–14.

87. Donaldson VH, Hess EV, McAdams AJ. Lupus-erythematosus-like disease in three unrelated women with hereditary angioneurotic edema [letter]. *Ann Intern Med* 1977; **86**: 312–13.

88. Brickman CM, Tsokos GC, Balow JE et al. Immunoregulatory disorders associated with hereditary angioedema. I. Clinical manifestations of autoimmune disease. *J Allergy Clin Immunol* 1986; **77**: 749–57.

89. Brickman CM, Tsokos GC, Chused TM et al. Immunoregulatory disorders associated with hereditary angioedema. II. Serologic and cellular abnormalities. *J Allergy Clin Immunol* 1986; **77**: 758–67.

90. Walport MJ, Davies KA, Botto M et al. C3 nephritic factor and SLE. *Q J Med* 1994; **87**: 609–15.

91. Inai S, Akagaki Y, Moriyama T et al. Inherited deficiencies of the late-acting complement components other than C9 found among healthy blood donors. *Int Arch Allergy Appl Immunol* 1989; **90**: 274–9.

92. Hassig A, Borel JF, Ammann P et al. Essentielle hypokomplementamie. *Pathol Microbiol* 1964; **27**: 542.

93. Cork CL, Morris JM, Olson JL et al. Membranoproliferative glomerulonephritis in dogs with a genetically determined deficiency of the third component of complement. *Clin Immunol Immunopathol* 1991; **60**: 455–70.

94. Hogasen K, Jansen JH, Mollnes TE et al. Hereditary porcine membranoproliferative glomerulonephritis type II is caused by factor H deficiency. *J Clin Invest* 1995; **95**: 1054–61.

95. Fischer MB, Ma M, Goerg S et al. Regulation of the B cell response to T-dependent antigens by classical pathway complement. *J Immunol* 1996; **157**: 549–56.

96. Matsumoto M, Fukada W, Goellner J et al. Abrogation of the alternative complement pathway by targeted deletion of murine factor B. *Proc Natl Acad Sci USA* 1997; **94**: 8720–5.

97. Ahearn JM, Fischer MB, Croix D et al. Disruption of the Cr2 locus results in a reduction in B-1a cells and in an impaired B cell response to T-dependent antigen. *Immunity* 1996; **4**: 251–62.

98. Botto M, Dell'Agnola C, Bygrave AE et al. Homozygous C1q deficiency causes glomerulonephritis associated with multiple apoptotic bodies. *Nature Genet* 1998; **19**: 56–9.

99. Takeuchi Y, Cosset FL, Lachmann PJ et al. Type C retrovirus inactivation by human complement is determined by both the viral genome and the producer cell. *J Virol* 1994; **68**: 8001–7.

100. Rother RP, Fodor WL, Springhorn JP et al. A novel mechanism of retrovirus inactivation in human serum mediated by anti-alpha-galactosyl natural antibody. *J Exp Med* 1995; **182**: 1345–55.

101. Cornillet P, Philbert F, Kazatchkine MD, Cohen JH. Genomic determination of the CR1 (CD35) density polymorphism on erythrocytes using polymerase chain reaction amplification and HindIII restriction enzyme digestion. *J Immunol Methods* 1991; **136**: 193–7.

102. Moldenhauer F, David J, Fielder AHL et al. Inherited deficiency of erythrocyte complement receptor type 1 does not cause susceptibility to systemic lupus erythematosus. *Arthritis Rheum* 1987; **30**: 961–6.

103. Frank MM, Hamburger MI, Lawley TJ et al. Defective reticuloendothelial system Fc-receptor function in systemic lupus erythematosus. *N Engl J Med* 1979; **300**: 518–23.

104. Hamburger MI, Lawley TJ, Kimberly RP et al. A serial study of splenic reticuloendothelial sysyem Fc-receptor function in systemic lupus erythematosus. *Arthritis Rheum* 1982; **25**: 48.

105. Salmon JE, Brogle NL, Edberg JC, Kimberly RP. Allelic polymorphisms of human Fcγ receptor IIA and Fcγ receptor IIIB; independent mechanisms for differences in human phagocyte function. *J Clin Invest* 1992; **89**: 1274–81.

106. Salmon JE, Millard S, Schachter LA et al. Fcγ RIIA alleles are heritable risk factors for lupus nephritis in African Americans. *J Clin Invest* 1996; **97**: 1348–54.

107. Duits AJ, Bootsma H, Derksen RHWM et al. Skewed distribution of IgG Fcγ receptor IIa is associated with renal disease in systemic lupus erythematosus patients. *Arthritis Rheum* 1995; **39**: 1832–6.

108. Botto M, Theodoridis E, Thompson EM et al. Fcγ RIIa polymorphism in systemic lupus erythematosus (SLE): no association with disease. *Clin Exp Immunol* 1996; **104**: 264–8.

109. Halma C, Breedveld FC, Daha MR et al. Elimination of soluble 123I-labeled aggregates of IgG in patients with systemic lupus erythematosus. Effect of serum IgG and numbers of erythrocyte complement receptor type 1. *Arthritis Rheum* 1991; **34**: 442–52.

110. Halma C, Daha MR, Camps JA et al. Deficiency of complement component C3 is associated with accelerated removal of soluble 123I-labelled aggregates of IgG from the circulation. *Clin Exp Immunol* 1992; **90**: 394–400.

111. Cochrane CJ. Mediation of immunologic glomerular injury. *Transplant Proc* 1969; **1**: 949–56.

112. Henson PM, Cochrane CG. The effects of complement depletion on experimental tissue injury. *Ann NY Acad Sci* 1975; **256**: 426–40.

113. Sylvestre DL, Ravetch JV. Fc receptors initiate the Arthus reaction: redefining the inflammatory cascade. *Science* 1994; **265**: 1095–8.

114. Hazenbos WLW, Gessner JE, Hofhuis FMA et al. Impaired IgG dependent anaphylaxis and Arthus reaction in Fcγ RIII (CD16) deficient mice. *Immunity* 1996; **5**: 181–8.

115. Ben-Efraim S, Cinader B. The role of complement in the passive cutaneous reaction of mice. *J Exp Med* 1964; **120**: 925–42.

116. Larsen GL, Mitchell BC, Henson PM. The pulmonary response of C5 sufficient and deficient mice to IC. *Am Rev Resp Dis* 1981; **123**: 434–9.

117. Zhang Y, Ramos BF, Jakschik BA. Augmentation of reverse Arthus reaction by mast cells in mice. *J Clin Invest* 1991; **88**: 841–6.

118. Sylvestre DL, Ravetch JV. A dominant role for mast cell Fc receptors in the Arthus reaction. *Immunity* 1996; **5**: 387–90.

119. Bozic CR, Lu B, Hopken UE et al. Neurogenic amplification of IC inflammation. *Science* 1996; **273**: 1722–5.

120. Rodwell JD, Tang LH, Schumaker VN. Antigen valence and Fc-localised secondary forces in antibody precipitation. *Molec Immunol* 1980; **17**: 1591–7.

121. Wilson CB, Dixon FJ. Renal response to immunological injury. In: Brenner BM, Rector FC, eds. *The Kidney*, 4th edn. Philadelphia: WB Saunders, 1986.

122. Ng YC. C3 nephritic factor and membranoproliferative glomerulonephritis. In: Pusey CD, ed. *Immunology of Renal Diseases*. Dordrecht: Kluwer Academic Publishers, 1991.

123. Verroust PJ, Wilson CB, Dixon FJ. Lack of nephritogenicity of systemic activation of the alternative complement pathway. *Kidney Int* 1974; **6**: 157–69.

124. Simpson IJ, Moran J, Evans DJ, Peters DK. Prolonged complement activation in mice. *Kidney Int* 1978; **13**: 467–71.

125. Baker PJ, Adler S, Yang Y, Couser WG. Complement activation by heat-killed human kidney cells: formation, activity and stabilization of cell-bound C3 convertases. *J Immunol* 1984; **133**: 877–81.

126. Chesney RW, Oregan S, Guyda HJ, Drummond KN. Candida endocrinopathy syndrome with membranoproliferative glomerulonephritis: demonstration of glomerular candida antigen. *Clin Nephrol* 1976; **5**: 232–8.

127. Wisnieski JJ, Baer AN, Christensen J et al. Hypocomplementemic urticarial vasculitis syndrome. Clinical and serologic findings in 18 patients. *Med Baltimore* 1995; **74**: 24–41.

128. Wisnieski JJ, Jones SM. Comparison of autoantibodies to the collagen-like region of C1q in hypocomplementaemic urticarial vasculitis syndrome and systemic lupus erythematosus. *J Immunol* 1992; **148**: 1396–403.

129. Uwatoko S, Gauthier VJ, Mannik M. Autoantibodies to the collagen-like region of C1q deposit in glomeruli via C1q immune deposits. *Clin Immunol Immunopathol* 1991; **61**: 268–73.

130. Halbwachs L, Leveille M, Lesavre P et al. Nephritic factor of the classical pathway of complement. Immunoglobulin autoantibody directed against the classical pathway C3 convertase enzyme. *J Clin Invest* 1980; **65**: 1249–56.

131. Daha MR, Hazavoet HM, van Es LA, Katz A. Stabilization of the classical pathway covertase C42 by a factor (F-42) isolated from sera of patients with SLE. *Immunology* 1980; **40**: 417–24.

132. Muta T, Kurosaki T, Misulovin Z et al. A 13-amino-acid motif in the cytoplasmic domain of Fcγ RIIB modulates B-cell receptor signalling. *Nature* 1994; **368**: 70–3.

133. Daeron M, Latour S, Malbec O et al. The same tyrosine-based inhibition motif in the intracytoplasmic domain of Fcγ RIIB, regulates negatively BCR-, TCR-, and FcR-dependent cell activation. *Immunity* 1995; **3**: 635–46.

134. Warmerdam PA, van de Winkel JG, Vlug A et al. A single amino acid in the second Ig-like domain of the human Fcγ receptor II is critical for human IgG2 binding. *J Immunol* 1991; **147**: 1338–43.

135. Wu J, Edberg JC, Redecha PB et al. A novel polymorphism of FcγRIIIa (CD16) alters receptor function and predisposes to autoimmune disease. *J Clin Invest* 1997; **100**: 1059–70.

136. Watanabe N, Akikusa B, Park SY et al. Mast cells induce autoantibody-mediated vasculitis syndrome through tumor necrosis factor production upon triggering Fcγ receptors. *Blood* 1999; **94**: 3855–63.

137. Salmon JE, Procop L. Human receptors for immunoglobulin G. *Arthritis Rheum* 2001; **44**: 739–50.

138. Lehrnbecher T, Foster CB, Zhu S et al. Variant genotypes of the low-affinity Fcγ receptors in two control populations and a review of low-affinity Fcγ receptor polymorphisms in control and disease populations. *Blood* 1999; **94**: 4220–32.

139. Ory PA, Clark MR, Kwoh EE et al. Sequences of complementary DNAs that encode the NA1 and NA2 forms of Fc receptor III on human neutrophils. *J Clin Invest* 1989; **84**: 1688–91.

140. Ory PA, Goldstein IM, Kwoh EE, Clarkson SB. Characterization of polymorphic forms of Fc receptor III on human neutrophils. *J Clin Invest* 1989; **83**: 1676–81.

141. Salmon JE, Edberg JC, Kimberly RP. Fc γ receptor III on human neutrophils. Allelic variants have functionally distinct capacities. *J Clin Invest* 1990; **85**: 1287–95.

142. Bredius RG, Fijen CA, De Haas M et al. Role of neutrophil Fc γ RIIa (CD32) and Fc γ RIIIb (CD16) polymorphic forms in phagocytosis of human IgG1- and IgG3-opsonized bacteria and erythrocytes. *Immunology* 1994; **83**: 624–30.

143. Salmon JE, Millard SS, Brogle NL, Kimberly RP. FcγRIIIb enhances FcγRIIa function in an oxidant-dependent and allele-sensitive manner. *J Clin Invest* 1995; **95**: 2877–85.

144. Salmon JE, Ng S, Yoo DH et al. Altered distribution of Fcγ receptor IIIA alleles in a cohort of Korean patients with lupus nephritis. *Arthritis Rheum* 1999; **42**: 818–19.

145. Koene HR, Kleijer M, Swaak AJ et al. The Fc γRIIIA-158F allele is a risk factor for systemic lupus erythematosus. *Arthritis Rheum* 1998; **41**: 1813–18.

146. Manger K, Repp R, Spriewald BM et al. Fcγ receptor IIa polymorphism in Caucasian patients with systemic lupus erythematosus: association with clinical symptoms. *Arthritis Rheum* 1998; **41**: 1181–19.

147. Song YW, Han CW, Kang SW et al. Abnormal distribution of Fc γ receptor type IIa polymorphisms in Korean patients with systemic lupus erythematosus. *Arthritis Rheum* 1998; **41**: 421–6.

148. Moser KL, Neas BR, Salmon JE et al. Genome scan of human systemic lupus erythematosus: evidence for linkage on chromosome 1q in African-American pedigrees. *Proc Natl Acad Sci USA* 1998; **95**: 14869–74.

149. Smyth LJ, Snowden N, Carthy D et al. Fc γ RIIa polymorphism in systemic lupus erythematosus. *Ann Rheum Dis* 1997; **56**: 744–6.

150. Oh M, Petri MA, Kim NA, Sullivan KE. Frequency of the Fc γ RIIIA-158F allele in African American patients with systemic lupus erythematosus. *J Rheumatol* 1999; **26**: 1486–9.

151. Norsworthy P, Theodoridis E, Botto M et al. Overrepresentation of the Fcγ receptor type IIA R131/R131 genotype in caucasoid systemic lupus erythematosus patients with autoantibodies to C1q and glomerulonephritis. *Arthritis Rheum* 1999; **42**: 1828–32.

152. Haseley LA, Wisnieski JJ, Denburg MR et al. Antibodies to C1q in systemic lupus erythematosus: characteristics and relation to Fc γ RIIA alleles. *Kidney Int* 1997; **52**: 1375–80.

153. Nieto A, Caliz R, Pascual M et al. Involvement of Fc γ receptor IIIA genotypes in susceptibility to rheumatoid arthritis. *Arthritis Rheum* 2000; **43**: 735–9.

154. Yee AM, Ng SC, Sobel RE, Salmon JE. Fc γRIIA polymorphism as a risk factor for invasive pneumococcal infections in systemic lupus erythematosus. *Arthritis Rheum* 1997; **40**: 1180–2.

155. Lehrnbecher TL, Foster CB, Zhu S et al. Variant genotypes of FcγRIIIA influence the development of Kaposi's sarcoma in HIV-infected men. *Blood* 2000; **95**: 2386–90.

156. Foster CB, Lehrnbecher T, Mol F et al. Host defense molecule polymorphisms influence the risk for immune-mediated complications in chronic granulomatous disease. *J Clin Invest* 1998; **102**: 2146–55.

157. Platonov AE, Kuijper EJ, Vershinina IV et al. Meningococcal disease and polymorphism of FcγRIIa (CD32) in late complement component-deficient individuals. *Clin Exp Immunol* 1998; **111**: 97–101.

158. Davies KA, Robson MG, Peters AM et al. Defective Fc-dependent processing of immune complexes in patients with systemic lupus erythematosus. *Arthritis Rheum* 2002; **46**: 1028–38.

5

Peripheral tolerance: the transplantation model

Bernd M Spriewald, Kathryn J Wood

Objectives • Overview • Introduction • Historical background • Tolerance • Principal mechanisms of peripheral tolerance • Rejection mechanisms • Application of antigen to induce transplantation tolerance • Chimerism: the balance between donor and recipient immune response? • Co-stimulation blockade • Concept of immune regulation • Outlook: from mouse to human • Glossary • References

OBJECTIVES

(1) To review the mechanisms of tolerance, peripheral and central, and how these break down in transplantation.
(2) To review how understanding the mechanisms which lead to transplant rejection and tolerance have shed light on basic immunological mechanisms and how, in turn, these might be used to design more effective immunosuppression.

OVERVIEW

Immunological tolerance is as a state of antigen-specific unresponsiveness induced by prior exposure to the antigen. Tolerance is most easily induced in developing lymphocytes in the central lymphoid organs, the thymus for T-cells and the bone marrow for B-cells, through the deletion of potentially harmful self-reactive lymphocytes. In addition, tolerance towards antigens not expressed in the thymus can be induced, under appropriate conditions, in mature lymphocytes at peripheral lymphoid and non-lymphoid sites. The main mechanisms of peripheral tolerance are deletion, anergy, ignorance and regulation/suppression. Tolerance induction can effectively be studied in transplantation models, since the introduction of allogeneic major histocompatibility (MHC) antigens expressed on the graft elicits a strong response of the recipient's immune system. Strategies for tolerance induction in transplantation that have so far proven successful in experimental models include the application of donor antigen under tolerogenic conditions, the application of T-cell-specific monoclonal antibodies and co-stimulation blockade. An exciting recent development has been the characterization of regulatory T-cells operating in peripheral tolerance that may be applicable in transplantation tolerance.

1. INTRODUCTION

The transplantation of cellular components, tissue or whole organs between genetically different individuals of the same species (allotransplantation) has uncovered many basic immunological principles, and over the past

40 years has become a routine clinical practice. Although not occurring naturally, a transplant causes a strong immune response that has to be suppressed by the continuous application of immunosuppressants. These drugs have many disadvantages such as toxicity, as well as an increased risk of infection and malignancy. However, even when these drugs are used, over time many grafts will succumb to the constant attacks made by the immune system. Only the induction of tolerance would allow the continued survival and function of the transplant without long-term non-specific immunosuppression. The study and development of strategies for the induction of tolerance is therefore a major goal, which not only fascinates the transplantation community but also broadens our knowledge about tolerance mechanisms. Many different strategies and efforts have been undertaken to achieve tolerance induction towards newly introduced antigens. In this chapter we will discuss the various forms of immunological tolerance, the immune response against allografts and the main approaches that have been investigated to overcome this immune response.

2. HISTORICAL BACKGROUND

The transplantation of organs between different individuals has long inspired peoples' imaginations. Yet it was not until the early twentieth century that the necessary surgical techniques were developed and the first proven transplants were carried out. It soon became clear that allotransplants do not usually survive and will be rejected by the recipient. The only exception to this is when the donor and recipient are genetically identical. The term histocompatibility was coined to describe the degree of compatibility, or indeed incompatibility, between the donor of the transplant and the recipient. On the basis of experimental work, Peter Gorer and George Snell identified the cell-surface molecules which were most important in determining whether a graft would 'take', in other words, be accepted or not.[1] These were called major histocompatibility complex (MHC) antigens. In the late 1950s, Jean Paul Dausset

discovered the first human MHC antigen on leucocytes, which is why they are still called human leucocyte antigens (HLA).[2] The second major barrier to successful clinical allotransplantation, apart from the MHC antigens, was identified as the ABO blood group system, which had been discovered in 1900 by Karl Landsteiner.[3]

Although it was obvious that the recipient usually rejected the transplanted organ, the mechanisms responsible remained largely unclear. It was not until the 1940s that Peter Medawar and colleagues proved that rejection was an immunological event.[4] Moreover, in the early 1950s, Medawar and his colleagues laid the foundation for tolerance research by demonstrating that tolerance towards foreign MHC antigens could be induced by injecting neonatal mice with allogeneic lymphocytes.[5] The mice subsequently accepted skin grafts from the same strain as the injected lymphocytes but would reject unrelated third-party grafts. These results were in accordance with the clonal selection theory formulated by Burnet[6] that stated that a lymphocyte specific for a certain antigen will, after activation, divide and give rise to daughter cells with the same specificity. In order to prevent autoimmunity, lymphocytes that recognize antigen before birth would be deleted whereas antigen recognition after birth would lead to activation.

In clinical transplantation, however, early attempts to prolong transplant (mainly kidney) survival by weakening the immune system through total body irradiation, occasionally followed by infusion of donor bone marrow, were less encouraging. This indicated that the prolongation of graft survival, let alone the induction of tolerance, in an adult human immune system would not be easy. It was not until reliable and predictable immunosuppression regimens were developed and introduced into the clinic that transplantation became an accepted standard therapy for end-stage organ failure. Such immunosuppression has led to very promising first-year graft survival rates, but long-term graft survival has not improved much over time, despite immunosuppression and the effort to match donor organ and recipient for their respective HLA antigens. Sporadic cases of long-term allograft survival without immunosuppression, demonstrating graft acceptance, remain the exception. Half a century after the key work of Burnet and Medawar, our understanding of the mechanisms behind tolerance has increased considerably, but we still seem quite far from translating this knowledge into clinically applicable strategies.

3. TOLERANCE

3.1 Definition

The prime task of the immune system is to prevent damage to the organism caused by harmful intruders from outside such as infectious agents. It also protects from cells derived from the organism itself that pose a risk, e.g. after malignant transformation. Usually the immune system does not react against the body itself, indicating that it must have means to distinguish self from non-self and dangerous from non-dangerous structures, and mechanisms to ensure unresponsiveness or tolerance towards self and non-dangerous antigens. Immunological tolerance can be defined as a state of antigen-specific non-responsiveness induced by prior exposure to the antigen.[7] This definition includes two key points of tolerance; firstly, that it is antigen specific, which means that the immune system can still mount an immune response towards other antigens; and secondly, that it has been actively acquired, requiring some form of T-cell activation as a result of the lymphocyte encountering its specific antigen.

This chapter focuses on mechanisms of T-cell tolerance, since T-cell responses play a central role in the adaptive immune response including rejection of allografts, either through direct cytotoxicity, cytokine secretion or by providing help for B-cells. However, it is noteworthy that similar mechanisms seem to operate in B-cell tolerance.[8] Anatomically, central tolerance, induced in the central lymphoid organs, the thymus for T-cells and bone marrow for B-cells, is distinguished from peripheral tolerance, induced in lymph nodes, spleen and non-lymphoid tissue.

3.2 Central tolerance

T-cell precursors originating from the bone marrow enter the thymus. The early precursors express neither the CD4 nor CD8 co-receptor (CD4-CD8-, double negative) and proliferate extensively. With maturation the thymocytes pass through a CD4+CD8+ double-positive stage before they become committed to either the CD4+ (MHC class II restricted) or CD8+ (MHC class I restricted) lineage. Through random rearrangement of their T-cell receptor (TCR) genes, thymocytes acquire a unique TCR with a certain avidity for the self-MHC plus peptide complexes expressed in the thymus. Only those thymocytes bearing a TCR that can interact with self-MHC plus peptide will be positively selected; the others die by neglect. The positively selected thymocytes undergo further scrutiny of the avidity of their TCR, and above a certain threshold, which would impose the risk of autoimmunity, they receive a death signal to undergo apoptosis and are negatively selected.[9] About 95% of all thymocytes die due to selection processes. It seems that the susceptibility for negative selection is not strictly defined to a specific stage in thymocyte development. Classically, bone-marrow-derived antigen-presenting cells (APC) mediate negative selection and thymic epithelium positive selection, but some other cell types can also mediate negative selection. There is increasing experimental evidence, however, that the thymus does not only delete self-reactive T-cells but is also important for the generation of regulatory T-cells, which seem to be part of the physiological repertoire of the exported T-cells.[10] Central tolerance towards newly introduced antigens can be induced by direct application of the antigen into the thymus (see section 5.2).

3.3 Peripheral tolerance

Central tolerance is of major importance for the induction of tolerance towards self-antigens. However, the question arises as to what happens to T-cells that are reactive to antigens that are not presented in the thymus and to those T-cells that are potentially self-reactive but evade thymic selection? Indeed, there is evidence that self-reactive T-cells are present in the periphery of normal individuals.[10] Thus, there must exist mechanisms to control these self-reactive lymphocytes in the periphery because somehow they are held in check and usually do not cause disease.

One experimental approach used to study peripheral tolerance was the use of transgenic mice engineered to express foreign antigens, including MHC alloantigens, under the control of tissue-specific promoters.[11] In theory, these mice express the transgene only at restricted extrathymic sites, such as the liver or pancreatic β-cells. If the mice expressed an allogeneic MHC antigen they did not show an inflammatory response towards the extrathymic antigen. Furthermore, they were able to accept skin grafts expressing the same alloantigen, whereas they rejected unrelated third-party grafts. Interestingly, this tolerance towards the extrathymic antigen was not broken when the mice expressing extrathymic MHC class I alloantigen were crossed with another strain expressing a transgenic TCR specific for this extrathymic antigen. This resulted in a T-cell repertoire in which all of the CD8+ T-cells were potentially able to recognize the extrathymic antigen, yet an immune response was not initiated.[12]

From these and other studies it became clear that the immune system does not rely on the deletion of self-reactive thymocytes alone but has additional mechanisms to induce and maintain peripheral tolerance. The understanding that tolerance is not only induced in the central lymphoid organs but also at peripheral sites is was an important achievement of recent years. The principal mechanisms of peripheral tolerance will be discussed in section 4.

3.4 Tolerance in transplantation

In the transplantation setting we have the graft and the presence or absence of an immune response against it that can be used to determine whether the recipient's immune system is unresponsive to the graft and its antigens or not. At a basic level, transplantation tolerance can be defined as the continuous survival and function of the transplant without long-term immunosuppression.[13] As we will see later, long-term graft survival without immunosuppression can be induced in various animal models. However, examination of long-term surviving allografts has shown that they are not inevitably free of immunological damage and changes typical of chronic rejection, demonstrating that long-term graft survival is not necessarily equivalent to tolerance.[14] An alternative definition of transplantation tolerance – the absence of a destructive immune response against the graft in an immunocompetent host – takes this into account.[15] In order to acknowledge a degree of uncertainty in determining whether true tolerance has been achieved in a transplantation model, the terms graft acceptance or operational tolerance are sometimes preferred.

The criteria of antigen specificity can be tested in transplantation tolerance by challenging the recipient's immune system with third-party grafts that carry alloantigens unrelated to the primary donor and recipient. If an antigen-specific mechanism is in operation towards the primary graft, the recipient will reject the third-party graft acutely.

For the evaluation of transplantation tolerance models it is important to consider whether they are strong enough to overcome the major or only the weaker minor histocompatibility antigen barriers. Furthermore, apart from its immunogenicity, the nature of the graft itself contributes to its susceptibility to rejection or tolerance induction.[16,17] A vascularized graft, such as heart and kidney, is more readily accepted than non-vascularized skin and pancreatic islet grafts.

4. PRINCIPAL MECHANISMS OF PERIPHERAL TOLERANCE

Upon encounter and cognate recognition of its antigen, a T-cell essentially has two options. It can become activated and initiate an immune response or it can be silenced. Whether the lymphocyte is activated or silenced depends on its stage of development, the affinity of its receptor for the antigen, the presence of co-stimulatory signals, characteristics of the respective antigen, such as its expression pattern, concentration and availability, and the presence of regulatory T-cells. The principal mechanisms that operate in immunological tolerance are deletion, anergy, ignorance and regulation/suppression.

4.1 Deletion

Deletion is the most profound and irreversible mechanism of tolerance induction and is the main mechanism of central tolerance (see section 3.2). However, deletion is also an important mechanism in peripheral tolerance.[18] The activation and repeated stimulation of mature T-cells leads to coexpression of Fas and Fas ligand (FasL) on their cell surface. Fas (CD95) belongs to the tumour necrosis factor

(TNF) receptor family and upon cross-linking through FasL can trigger apoptosis in any Fas-expressing cell it comes into contact with. Therefore, the coexpression of Fas and FasL in an expanding T-cell population leads to Fas/FasL interaction triggering apoptosis (Fig. 5.1). This mechanism of *activation-induced cell death* (AICD) can eliminate T-cells that are repeatedly stimulated through persistent (self-) antigen and is important for reducing the T-cell pool after an immune response. In its extreme form, AICD can lead to clonal exhaustion, the deletion of all cells of a particular antigen-reactive T-cell clone. Fas-mediated apoptosis of T-cells is also responsible for the protection of immune-privileged sites, including the testis and the eye. Cells in these organs express FasL, which enables them to kill T-cells reactive against them.

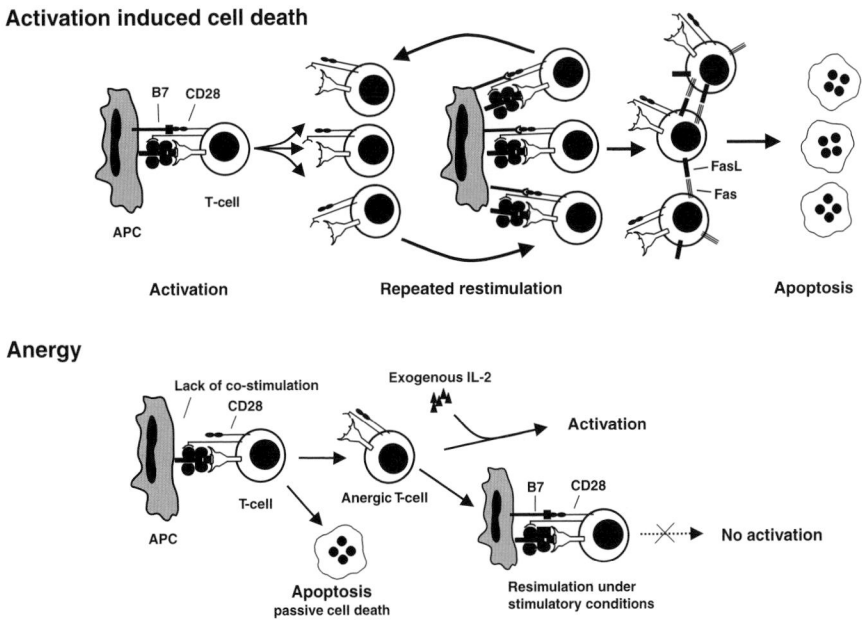

Fig. 5.1 Repeated restimulation of T-cells results in coexpression of Fas and Fas ligand (FasL) on the T-cell. Interaction of Fas/FasL leads to cell death via apoptosis. Since the process requires prior activation of the T-cell it is called activation-induced cell death (AICD). Engagement and signalling through the T-cell receptor in the absence of co-stimulatory signals, such as B7/CD28, can result in inactivation and anergy of the respective T-cell. The anergic state can be broken through exogenous addition of interleukin-2 (IL-2) but not through restimulation in the presence of appropriate co-stimulatory signals. Alternatively, the inappropriately stimulated T-cell may undergo apoptosis, which is called passive cell death to distinguish it from AICD.

Deletion, however, can also occur in form of so-called *passive cell death*, which is not mediated by Fas. Expression of T-cell survival factors, such as the cytokine interleukin (IL)-2 and anti-apoptotic proteins such as Bcl-2, are enhanced as a result of signalling through the co-stimulatory molecule CD28 (Fig. 5.1, section 8.1). Passive cell death, due to lack of survival factors, can occur if T-cells are inadequately stimulated or are in a non-permissive cytokine microenvironment.

4.2 Anergy

When a T-cell encounters its antigen but is insufficiently stimulated at the time of antigen recognition, the T-cell can be rendered unresponsive, or anergic. This inadequate stimulation can be due to the lack of co-stimulation or suboptimal signalling through the antigen receptor, as might be the case with altered peptide ligands. An anergized T-cell remains unresponsive even after subsequent exposure to the same antigen by fully stimulatory activated professional APC. However, a characteristic of the anergic state is that it can be broken by exogenous addition of IL-2 (Fig. 5.1). Anergy in T-cells was first discovered *in vitro*[19] and has mainly been investigated in *in vitro* systems. Although studies suggest that anergy can be induced *in vivo* and may play a role in tolerance towards peripheral antigens including transplants,[20,21] the dispute about its existence and role in tolerance *in vivo* is still not decided.

4.3 Ignorance

An antigen and the cell expressing it can be ignored by a lymphocyte specific for this antigen if lymphocyte and antigen are separated, e.g. through a physical barrier, as is the case for the lens of the eye. The antigen might also be ignored, even though the lymphocyte has encountered it when there is an insufficient concentration of antigen or MHC molecules to reach the threshold for signal transduction. However, in contrast to anergy, the state of the lymphocyte is not altered, and when the same antigen is presented later in an appropriate stimulatory context by professional APC the T-cell becomes activated and can also react against the previously ignored antigen-bearing cell. It should be noted though that ignorance is not strictly a mechanism of tolerance, because it is not actively acquired. Ignorance can potentially be exploited in transplantation by encapsulation of pancreatic islet allografts in order to prevent direct contact of recipient T-cells with the graft.

4.4 Regulation/suppression

The mechanisms described above deal primarily with the fate and decision made by a single lymphocyte encountering and recognizing its specific antigen. However, there is compelling evidence that tolerance towards peripheral self-antigens is also maintained by *regulation* of self-reactive lymphocytes through regulatory T-cells. One line of experiments suggesting the existence of regulatory T-cells showed that the removal of certain subsets of CD4+ T-cells, containing the putative regulatory cells, from the T-cell pool before transfer into T-cell-deficient mice resulted in autoimmune disease.[22] It has also been shown that at least some subsets of these regulatory T-cells are generated within the thymus but execute their regulatory function in the periphery. This finding also ascribes a new function to the thymus in that it not only deletes potentially self-destructive T-cells but can also generate regulatory T-cells that dominantly regulate self-reactive T-cells in the periphery, linking central and peripheral tolerance (Fig. 5.2). The role of regulatory T-cells in peripheral tolerance will be discussed in section 9.

4.5 Paradox of the fetal allograft

The fetus inherits a whole set of polymorphic genes from the father, most importantly the paternal MHC genes, which are expressed co-dominantly, making it a semi-allogeneic graft. However, somehow an immune response against the paternal alloantigens is suppressed and the fetus is tolerated by the mother's immune system throughout gestation. This immunological mystery of viviparity, a unique characteristic of mammals, is still not entirely solved and it seems that the mechanisms are not the same for all mammalian species.[23]

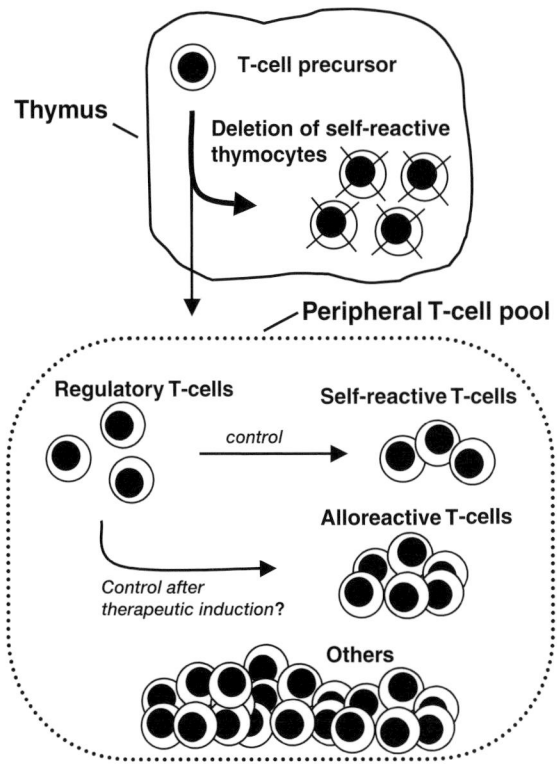

Fig. 5.2 The T-cells that are exported from the thymus and comprise the peripheral T-cell pool contain regulatory T-cells, which are able to control self-reactive T-cells that have escaped thymic selection, linking central and peripheral tolerance. It seems possible to induce regulatory T-cells against non-self antigens, such as allogeneic major histocompatibility complex (MHC) antigens, which are then able to control alloreactive T-cells present in the peripheral T-cell pool.

It has been suggested that a physical barrier between maternal T-cells and fetal antigens, as well as the antigenic immaturity of the fetus, contribute to maternal tolerance towards the fetal allograft. However, at least in murine pregnancy, it has been shown that the maternal T-cells are aware of the fetal alloantigens,[24] indicating the need for tolerogenic mechanisms in the maternal T-cell repertoire. Among these mechanisms are hormonal changes, such as T-cell inhibition through progesterone and a shift of the maternal immune system towards a type 2 helper T-cell (Th2) like cytokine milieu.

In humans, the trophoblast cells do not express MHC class I antigens, but this is not the case in mice. In both humans and rodents, however, there is no MHC class II expression, necessary for the activation of CD4+ T helper cells on trophoblast cells. Another contribution to this local immunosuppression has been reported recently in studies showing that the enzyme indoleamine-2,3-dioxygenase (IDO), expressed in trophoblasts and macrophages, can suppress T-cell activity by catabolizing tryptophan and starving them of an essential metabolite.[25] A unique feature in humans is the expression, preferentially on extravillous cytotrophoblasts, of the non-classical and relatively non-polymorphic MHC class I antigen HLA-G, which has been ascribed a T-cell and natural killer (NK) cell regulating function.[26] A recent report has shown that HLA-G expression in allografts may have a beneficial effect on the clinical outcome.[27] Also of interest with respect to transplantation is the finding that fetal cells can migrate into the maternal circulation and establish a fetal microchimerism that may affect the maternal immune system[28] (see section 5.2).

5. REJECTION MECHANISMS

If we want to understand why the induction of tolerance towards allogeneic grafts has proven such a challenging task, it is worth looking at the immune response that such antigens usually evoke. In principle, an allogeneic graft can activate all effector mechanisms of the immune system. Which one will be the leading cause of rejection depends on the experimental system or the clinical situation.

5.1 Allorecognition

The T-cells circulating in the periphery of the recipient have been selected on their ability to recognize recipient self-MHC. However, when the immune system encounters an allogeneic graft expressing foreign MHC antigens that were not involved in the selection of recipient T-cells, a vigorous T-cell response is initiated. It is estimated that 1–10% of the T-cell repertoire can recognize foreign MHC and contribute to cellular rejection.[29] There are two reasons for this high frequency. First, the recipient T-cells can cross-react with immunogenic epitopes formed either by the allogeneic MHC molecule itself or the complex of allogeneic MHC plus bound peptide. This is called the *direct pathway* of allorecognition (Fig. 5.3). It is mainly the donor-derived APC, so-called passenger leucocytes, that are being transferred with the transplant that can activate naive alloreactive T-cells via this pathway. The importance of the direct pathway of allorecognition is underlined by the strong response against MHC alloantigens in the mixed lymphocyte reaction, prolonged graft survival after depletion of donor APC from the transplant, and after matching donor and recipients for their MHC antigens.

Secondly, in the *indirect pathway* of allorecognition the MHC alloantigen is taken up by recipient APC and presented in the context of recipient MHC class I or class II molecules (Fig. 5.3).[30,31] This complex of recipient MHC class II plus

allogeneic peptide can then be recognized by recipient CD8+ or CD4+ T-cells, respectively. Indeed, CD4+ T-cells which can recognize only MHC class II molecules are sufficient to reject MHC class I disparate skin grafts.[32] Furthermore, non-MHC-derived peptides generated from other polymorphic donor proteins can be presented by the recipient APC. However, the resulting immune response involves a lower number of T-cells, and is therefore weaker, and can be overcome more easily than the one against allo-MHC-derived peptides. For this reason, these antigens are called minor histocompatibility antigens.

5.2 Acute cellular rejection

The pivotal role for T-cells in graft rejection is demonstrated experimentally by transplanting recipients carrying the *nude* gene defect, which do not have a thymus and therefore have no T-cells. These recipients accept allogeneic grafts but

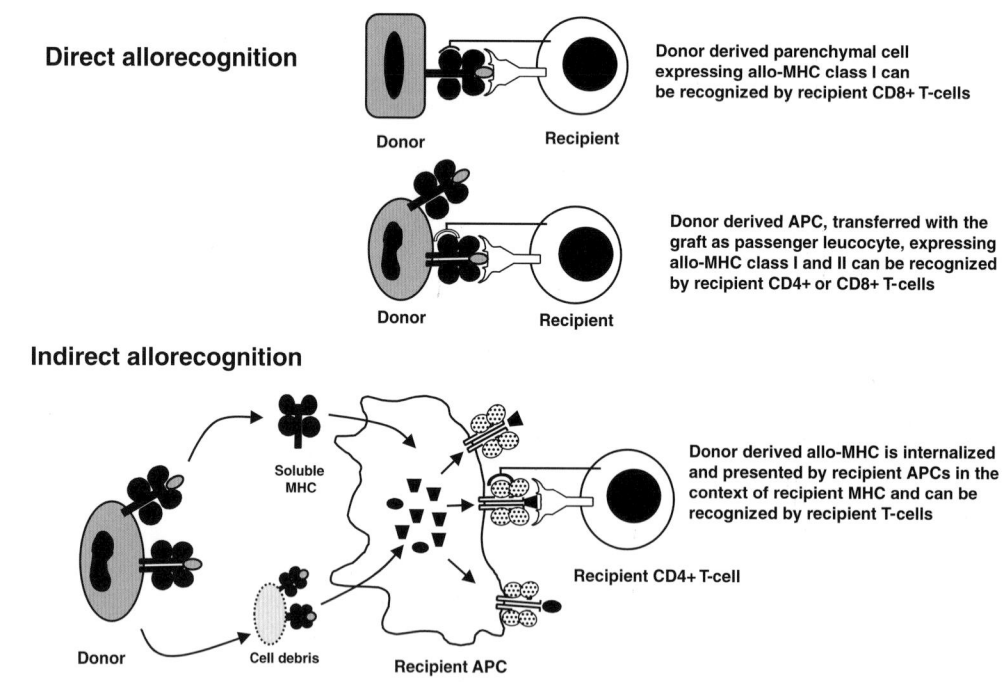

Fig. 5.3 Alloantigen carried on the transplant can be recognized by recipient T-cells via two possible pathways. In the direct pathway of allorecognition, recipient T-cells directly interact with the donor major histocompatibility complex (MHC) molecules expressed on donor-derived cells. In the indirect pathway of allorecognition, the donor alloantigen has to be processed and presented by recipient antigen-presenting cells.

reject the transplants rapidly when reconstituted with mature recipient-strain T-cells.[33] The activation of naïve recipient T-cells by donor-derived APC expressing MHC alloantigen shortly after transplantation can lead to acute cellular rejection, which represents the majority of all early rejection episodes in the clinic. This usually happens after the first week and most frequently in the first months after transplantation, and in general can be treated with increased immunosuppression or anti-lymphocyte globulin (ALG). The pathology of the graft undergoing acute cellular rejection is characterized by a massive cellular infiltrate that is comprised of T-cells, mononuclear cells such as macrophages, and also neutrophils that have been attracted to the graft site by chemokines and cytokines. The resulting effector mechanisms can comprise direct cytotoxicity by CD8+ T-cells but also a delayed-type hypersensitivity (DTH) reaction.

5.3 Antibody-mediated rejection

The first immunological barrier to allotransplantation was discovered when kidney transplants were lost within minutes after revascularization due to thrombosis and vascular occlusion. The reason for this *hyperacute rejection* was the presence of naturally occurring preformed antibodies of the immunoglobulin (Ig) M subtype against mismatched A or B antigens of the ABO blood group system (isoagglutinins). These antigens are not only expressed on red blood cells but also on the vasculature and parenchymal cells of the transplanted organ. Binding of isoagglutinins to their respective antigens expressed on donor endothelium results in the activation of the complement and coagulation systems, widespread thrombotic occlusion of the microvasculature and infarction of the whole organ. Although dramatic in its consequences, hyperacute rejection caused by isoagglutinins is easily avoided by transplanting organs between ABO-compatible individuals. IgG antibodies directed against other donor antigens, mainly HLA antigens, expressed on the graft endothelium can also cause hyperacute rejection.[34] Immunization of the recipient usually occurs through blood transfusion, pregnancy or a previous transplant. These antibodies can be detected, and hyperacute rejection avoided, by performing a cross-match in which donor lymphocytes are incubated with recipient serum. If present, donor-directed antibodies can be detected through flow cytometry or by the addition of complement which leads to lysis of the donor lymphocytes. In rare cases, preformed antibodies at a titre too low to be detected in a cross-match, lead to *accelerated rejection*, which is similar in its pathology to hyperacute rejection but develops more slowly over several days.

The transplant can also induce the *de novo* production of antibodies against the antigens it carries. This process requires 'help' from T-cells and it therefore does not occur before the first week after transplantation. The pathology of this *acute vascular rejection* is characterized by a vasculitis-like picture with antibodies binding to donor endothelial cells, cell necrosis of the vasculature and varying degrees of inflammation. However, as seen in clinical transplantation, the induction of donor-specific antibodies does not necessarily lead to graft loss.

5.4 Chronic rejection

Although the 1-year survival rates in clinical transplantation have improved, currently >80% for cadaver donor renal allografts, the rate of subsequent graft loss has hardly changed over the past two decades and the organ half-life for cadaver donor renal allografts remains 8–9 years.[35] A multifactorial process of progressive functional deterioration of the graft occurring months to years following transplantation is responsible. These events are usually subsumed under the descriptive term *chronic rejection*, although it has been suggested that the use of this terminology be restricted to immune-mediated late graft loss.[36] Antigen-independent factors contributing to chronic rejection include metabolic causes such as hyperlipidaemia, drug toxicity, infections and ischaemia–reperfusion injury of the graft. Antigen-dependent factors include the degree of MHC discrepancy between recipient and donor, previous acute rejection episodes and, possibly, ongoing immunological injury that can be cell or antibody mediated. Chronic rejection is characterized by transplant arteriosclerosis, and the gradual fibrosis and sclerosis of the graft. Overcoming at least the immune-mediated injury of chronic rejection is one of the main targets for tolerance-induction strategies.

6. APPLICATION OF ANTIGEN TO INDUCE TRANSPLANTATION TOLERANCE

The administration of donor antigen either before or at the time of transplantation has proven in various experimental models to be a powerful way of inducing non-responsiveness to alloantigens and donor-specific tolerance.[37] Although the application of antigen itself can be effective, it is usually combined with other immunomodulatory agents, such as anti-T-cell antibodies.

6.1 Intravenous infusion

Tolerance towards fully mismatched vascularized allografts can be achieved through the preoperative application of donor antigen in the form of a donor-specific blood transfusion (DST) under tolerogenic conditions such as co-administration with a T-cell-modulating agent. This strategy results in the induction of a regulatory T-cell population that can prevent rejection upon transfer into a naïve untreated recipient (Fig. 5.4).[38] Interestingly, in clinical transplantation it was observed that recipients who had received blood transfusions prior to transplantation had a better graft survival compared to untransfused patients.[39,40] This blood transfusion effect led to the deliberate transfusion of patients on the waiting list for an organ graft. However, the blood transfusion effect has become less prominent since the 1980s, mainly due to the introduction of the much more potent immunosuppressant cyclosporin into the clinic. Additionally, the introduction of erythropoietin, the growth hormone for erythrocyte precursors, has meant that transfusions are no longer required clinically, minimizing the risk of blood-borne infections.

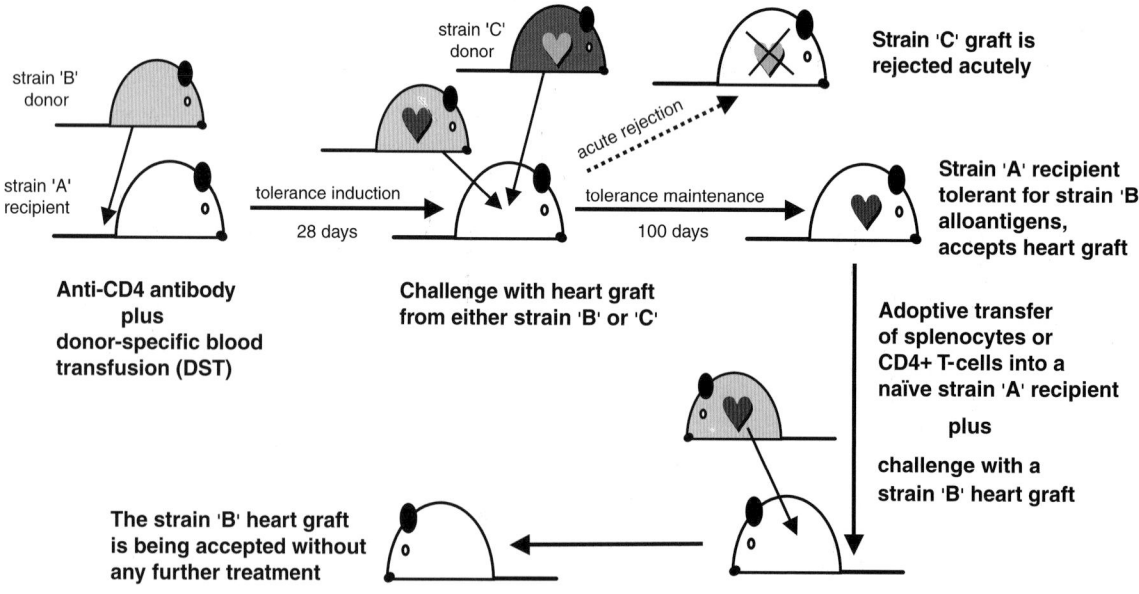

Fig. 5.4 Transplantation tolerance can be induced through the preoperative administration of a donor-specific blood transfusion (DST) in conjunction with a T-cell modifying agent such as anti-CD4 antibody. The tolerance induction is antigen specific in that only grafts from the same strain (B) as the pretreatment DST will be accepted, whereas unrelated third-party grafts (C) will be rejected acutely. This tolerance protocol induces regulatory T-cells as demonstrated by adoptive transfer of splenocytes or CD4+ T-cells from tolerant animals into naive recipients that will then accept a graft without further treatment.

The application of donor antigen on haematopoietic cells has some advantages over whole blood transfusions. It has been shown experimentally that tolerance induction towards a single MHC alloantigen is sufficient for the recipient to later accept a fully mismatched allograft,[41] exploiting the mechanism of linked epitope suppression (see section 9.3). Furthermore, the donor antigen that is used as tolerogen can be incorporated into donor-derived cells via gene transfer,[42] reducing the risk of graft versus host disease (GvHD) for the recipient, and providing an approach for gene therapy to tolerance induction.[43]

6.2 Intrathymic antigen application

Although the observation that intrathymic injection of antigen can result in tolerance was made in the 1960s, it was not until many years later that it was applied to a clinically relevant model, i.e. islet transplantation.[44] In this system, intrathymic injection of allogeneic islet cells, in combination with a single dose of ALG to deplete pre-existing alloreactive T-cells, led to graft acceptance. This direct approach to central tolerance induction has been extended to other sources of antigen such as donor-derived spleen cells,[45] complementary DNA encoding donor MHC[46] and synthetic peptides derived from allogeneic MHC molecules.[47]

Strategies that utilize synthetic peptides as tolerogens emphasize the importance of the indirect pathway of allorecognition for tolerance induction and are of interest for several reasons.[48] Peptides can be produced relatively easily and can be administered not only into the thymus but also intravenously or orally. Furthermore, it seems that not only peptides derived from polymorphic but also those from non-polymorphic regions of the MHC alloantigen can have immunomodulatory effects, possibly allowing a broader therapeutic effect. However, as far as the intrathymic route is concerned, the impaired accessibility of the thymus and the involution of the organ in adults are major obstacles to its use in any clinical setting.

6.3 Oral tolerance

The non-responsiveness of most individuals towards food antigens and their gut flora indicates the capacity to induce tolerance by administration of antigen via the oral route, and is a physiological mechanism of tolerance towards beneficial foreign antigens. Among the factors that seem to influence the induction of oral tolerance are the nature of the antigen, the bacterial gut flora and the antigen dose, whereby the administration of multiple low doses favours the generation of regulatory cells, in contrast to a single high dose which leads to deletion. On the other hand, very low doses of antigen and particulate antigens preferentially induce immunity.[49] The tolerizing effect of antigen application via the mucosa is not restricted to the gut, and is also seen after nasal application. The exact mechanisms of oral tolerance remain unclear, but it has been suggested that T-cell inactivation is caused by antigen presentation by either epithelial cells or APC in the gut-associated lymphoid tissue (GALT) without sufficient co-stimulatory signals.

Oral tolerance also involves the induction of regulatory CD4+ T-cells, which are characterized by the predominant expression of the cytokine transforming growth factor-beta (TGF-β).[50] Because of their unique cytokine expression pattern these cells have been termed Th3, indicating their phenotypic and functional difference from Th1 or Th2. Whether Th3 is related to, or even identical with, the recently described regulatory type 1 T-cell (Tr1; see section 9.4) is currently under debate.

The tolerizing effect of oral antigen administration has been demonstrated in several rodent models of autoimmune diseases and transplantation,[51] and assessed in humans with inflammatory autoimmune diseases such as multiple sclerosis and rheumatoid arthritis.[50]

7. CHIMERISM: THE BALANCE BETWEEN DONOR AND RECIPIENT IMMUNE RESPONSE?

7.1 Combined bone marrow and organ transplantation

The initial observation by Owen,[52] that dizygotic cattle twins sharing intrauterine blood circulation became permanent haematopoietic chimeras and subsequently accepted each other's skin grafts,[5] was followed by the experiments by Billingham et al showing that tolerance could be induced by injecting neonatal mice with donor-specific splenocytes. Following intrauterine or neonatal introduction of recipient splenocytes, haematopoietic chimerism, the coexistence of donor- and recipient-type blood cells, led to central tolerance by deleting recipient-derived thymocytes encountering MHC alloantigen expressed on donor-derived APC colonizing the recipient thymus. The question was whether central tolerance could also be induced in adult recipients.

Experiments using lethal total body irradiation (TBI) to destroy the recipient's haematopoiesis (myeloablation), followed by donor-type bone marrow transplantation (BMT) showed that subsequent donor-type grafts were accepted indefinitely, demonstrating that allogeneic BMT could lead to donor-specific tolerance. However, there are major problems with this approach that are even more severe in humans than in rodents and other animal models. First, allogeneic BMT can only be performed in a very narrow corridor of MHC disparity, in order to avoid the risk of severe graft-versus-host disease (GvHD). GvHD is mediated mainly by mature donor-derived T-cells, but depleting these T-cells from the bone marrow graft increases the risk of graft failure. Second, the discrepancy between the restriction of developing donor T-cells towards recipient MHC and the donor MHC expressed on the donor APC results in deficiencies in the T-cell repertoire and immunodeficiency. Third, the involution of the adult thymus and its further destruction through the myeloablation, reduces the capacity for reconstitution after T-cell depletion. Fourth, the procedure of myeloablation through irradiation and cytotoxic drugs itself poses risks that are unjustified for patients without haematopoietic diseases. For these and other reasons, early attempts in the 1950s of allogeneic BMT for the purpose of transplantation tolerance induction were not continued. However, a small number of patients who had undergone BMT from an HLA-identical sibling for malignant disease developed renal failure and received a kidney transplant from the same donor. Those patients not developing GvHD, and who therefore did not require immunosuppression, accepted their kidney graft,[53,54] thus demonstrating donor-specific non-responsiveness.

Further experiments have shown that the recipient could be treated with non-myeloablative conditioning consisting of lower dose irradiation so that a sufficient residual haematopoietic system can recover on its own. In this situation, the subsequent application of donor bone marrow resulted in stable haematopoietic chimerism and donor-specific tolerance.[55] This strategy also exploits central tolerance by providing space in the recipient bone marrow and thymus for repopulating donor cells.

7.2 Microchimerism

The concept that haematopoietic chimerism might facilitate transplantation tolerance was refuelled when it was discovered that, in transplant patients with long-term stable graft function, donor-derived cells could be detected in the blood, bone marrow, spleen, thymus and even skin.[56] This condition was termed microchimerism, because the frequency of donor-derived cells in the peripheral blood was <1%, the detection limit of flow cytometry. The source of the donor cells has been identified as passenger leucocytes that migrate out the graft soon after transplantation. Since the passenger leucocytes have a limited lifespan, it is assumed that haematopoietic precursor cells with the potential of self-renewal are being transferred with the graft. A potential working mechanism of microchimerism is the stimulation of alloreactive recipient T-cells through the donor-derived passenger leucocytes followed by activation-induced cell death and clonal exhaustion of the donor T-cells.

As a consequence, donor bone marrow infusion into otherwise unconditioned transplant recipients has been investigated as a means to augment microchimerism. Only minor GvHD was observed, and donor bone marrow augmentation may be of clinical benefit with respect to reduced rejection episodes compared to patients receiving no donor bone marrow.[57,58] The question, however, of whether microchimerism really facilitates donor-specific tolerance, remains to be answered. Microchimerism is not always associated with graft acceptance and may be the result rather than the cause of tolerance, or effective immunosuppression allowing the passenger leucocytes to survive in the periphery. Furthermore, the presence of the graft itself as a source for donor antigen is also important for tolerance induction.[59,60]

7.3 Liver as an immune-privileged organ graft

Soon after the first transplants it became apparent that liver grafts had a much better survival rate and that somehow the liver could protect not only itself against rejection but also a kidney transplanted simultaneously.[61] Liver-graft recipients are the majority among patients who accept their grafts, demonstrated by functioning grafts after withdrawal of immunosuppression. Several reasons may account for this effect. The high load of passenger leucocytes transferred with the graft facilitates microchimerism.[62] The mass of the liver can withstand rejection episodes more easily, has a certain ability for regeneration, and the parenchyma provides ample opportunity for recipient T-cells to encounter allo-MHC without co-stimulation and become silenced. Liver grafts can also shed soluble HLA molecules, which have an immunomodulatory effect and can bind alloantibodies if present.

8. CO-STIMULATION BLOCKADE

8.1 Co-stimulation in lymphocyte activation

In order to become activated, the lymphocyte requires engagement of its antigen receptor, so-called signal one, and additionally, a second, co-stimulatory signal. If the second signal is missing during the time a T-cell encounters its antigen, it undergoes an abortive activation, which can result in anergy or apoptosis (Fig. 5.1). The need for a second signal in addition to the one received through the antigen receptor was initially proposed by Bretscher and Cohn for B-cells[63] and by Lafferty and Cunningham[64] for T-cells. The second signal is not antigen

specific and is provided through co-stimulatory molecules expressed on the cell surface of professional APC, i.e. dendritic cells, macrophages and activated B-cells (Fig. 5.5). The expression of co-stimulatory molecules is regulated by, and usually restricted to, activated APC, ensuring the timely activation of T-cells at the site of inflammation and to prevent the aberrant activation of potentially harmful T-cells. The interaction of the co-stimulator with its ligand on the T-cell surface promotes T-cell activation through several mechanisms, including the enhanced expression of cytokines such as IL-2 and interferon gamma (IFN-γ), and the protection from apoptosis through expression of cell-survival genes such as *Bcl-2*.

The best characterized co-stimulatory pathway is that of the CD28/B7 pathway. Binding of T-cell-expressed CD28 to its two ligands CD80 (B7-1) and CD86 (B7-2) on the APC leads to activation of the T-cell. However, the pathway also contains a negative regulatory element in the form of the cytotoxic T-lymphocyte antigen-4, CTLA4 (CD152), which is only expressed on activated T-cells. It binds B7 family members with a higher affinity than CD28 and can therefore compete effectively with CD28 for B7 molecules. The downregulatory effect of CTLA4 on T-cell activation seems to be important in limiting T-cell responses and

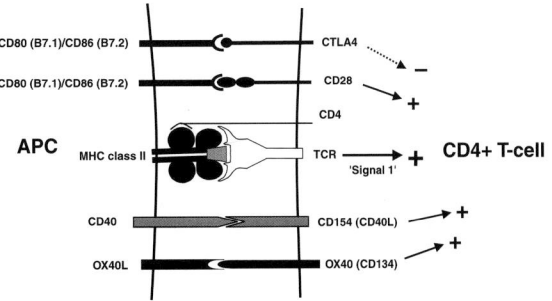

Fig. 5.5 Schematic representation of selected co-stimulatory ligand–receptor pairs that are of importance in the interaction between a T-cell and its antigen-presenting cell (APC), and that provide the necessary second signal for T-cell activation. Cytotoxic T-lymphocyte antigen (CTLA4) delivers inhibitory signals to the T-cell.

in regulating the initiation of responses under suboptimal co-stimulatory conditions. The latter may be important for autoreactive T-cells encountering self-antigen in the periphery and therefore contribute to the maintenance of peripheral tolerance.

Another important co-stimulatory pathway is the CD40/CD154 interaction.[65] CD154 (CD40 ligand) is expressed mainly on activated CD4+ T-cells and interacts with CD40, which is expressed on various cell types including APC. Although the CD40/CD154 interaction does seem to have a direct effect on T-cells, it primarily acts indirectly. Engagement of CD40 promotes the ability of the APC to induce and support T-cell responses through enhanced expression of co-stimulatory molecules, mainly B7, and adhesion molecules. Dendritic cells and macrophages are induced to produce proinflammatory cytokines. Ligation of CD40 has a very profound effect on B-cells, in that it provides cell-survival signals, augments immunoglobulin production and the Ig isotype switch from IgM to IgG. The latter role accounts for the phenotype of those individuals with a genetic defect in CD154, i.e. very high levels of IgM and an impaired humoral immune response. This condition is known as X-linked hyper-IgM syndrome.

8.2 Co-stimulation blockade and tolerance induction

If the lymphocyte receives only the first signal through its antigen receptor without co-stimulation it becomes anergic or undergoes apoptosis. Therefore, the interruption of co-stimulatory pathways can prevent T-cell activation, allograft rejection and may promote tolerance induction.[66] The CD28/B7 pathway can be blocked effectively using CTLA4–Ig, a fusion protein between CTLA4 and the constant part of the immunoglobulin IgG. CTLA4–Ig has a higher affinity for B7 and competes with CD28 for the B7 binding sites, preventing T-cell activation through CD28 signalling. The application of CTLA4–Ig has been shown to prolong allograft survival and even to induce donor-specific tolerance in various transplantation models.[67] Interestingly, CTLA4 is more effective if it is

administered after transplantation, but it fails to reverse acute rejection.[68] It has also been shown that it is necessary to block both B7-1 and B7-2, as either of the B7 molecules is effective in initiating graft rejection.[69] Another aspect to consider for CD28/B7 blockade is that reagents such as CTLA4–Ig also block the negative regulatory effect of CTLA4, which has been shown to prevent the induction of anergy.[70] It has been suggested that this effect might be responsible for the observed reduced efficacy of CTLAA4–Ig monotherapy in large animal models compared to rodents.[71] It might therefore be beneficial to develop strategies for blocking CD28 while enabling signalling through CTLA4.

Blocking the other major co-stimulatory pathway CD40/CD154 through anti-CD154 antibody has also been shown to induce long-term allograft survival, with or without the additional administration of donor antigen.[66] The mainly indirect action of the CD40/CD154 pathway suggested that anti-CD154 blockade would be more effective in a combination therapy. Indeed, the combined blockade of CD28/B7 and CD40/CD154 pathways did prove very effective in inducing donor-specific tolerance.[72] Anti-CD154 monotherapy has been shown to prolong allograft survival effectively in a primate model.[73] Potential limitations of anti-CD154 therapy have recently been reported: anti-CD154 did not target CD8+ T-cells[74–76] and the absence of the CD40/CD154 interaction promoted the development of transplant atherosclerosis.[77] Another interesting finding of co-stimulation blockade is that induction of peripheral tolerance across major MHC barriers using CTLA4–Ig and anti-CD154 treatment may require apoptosis of alloreactive T-cells. Where apoptosis was prevented either through administration of cyclosporin A,[78] or using transgenic recipients with impaired T-cell apoptosis,[79] tolerance induction was abrogated. Whether this requirement for T-cell apoptosis in peripheral tolerance induction is a unique characteristic of co-stimulation blockade or reflects a more general principle is currently unknown.

9. CONCEPT OF IMMUNE REGULATION

9.1 Suppressor cells

In the 1970s, studies were reported suggesting suppressor activity delivered through CD8+ T-cells.[80] Suppression means that potentially reactive T-cells are held in check as a result of other syngeneic T-cells, inhibiting their function. However, the tools to undertake a thorough characterization of the cell type and the mechanism of suppression were not available at that time. The existence of suppressor cells was therefore disregarded for some time. According to the network hypothesis proposed by Jerne, the antigen-specific antibodies or T-cells produced during an immune response constitute an idiotype against which anti-idiotype antibodies or T-cells are generated to control the initial immune response.[81] The T-cell, however, only recognizes peptide antigens presented via MHC and is unaware of the TCR, or TCR specificity, of other T-cells. Therefore, in order to function as an anti-idiotype, a T-cell must recognize peptides from the complementarity-determining region of the idiotypic TCR. This idiotype-specific suppression has been shown to exist and was used to prolong rat cardiac allograft survival through T-cell vaccination.[82]

It has also been proposed that suppression can be mediated in an antigen-specific way. In the latter case, the suppressor T-cell must recognize the same antigen, albeit not necessarily the same epitope, as the antigen-reactive T-cells it does suppress. Several possible mechanisms for suppressor activity have been suggested; however, most of these theories have never been proven experimentally.

9.2 Veto cells

Veto cells have been detected by their ability to suppress activation of naïve cytotoxic CD8+ T-cells.[83] Although first identified as CD8+ T-cells, veto cells probably consist of various cell populations, including NK and CD4+ T-cells. The veto cell causes inactivation or deletion of T-cells that recognize the MHC complex expressed on the veto cell, which for CD8+ T-cells has been shown to include negative signalling through the CD8 co-receptor (Fig. 5.6). The antigen-specific TCR of the veto cell is not involved in this interaction and the specificity of the veto cell is therefore unimportant. Veto cell activity has been implicated in graft prolongation following donor bone marrow infusion and the reduction of GvHD in BMT.[84] Whereas the original concept of a veto cell applied mainly to T-cells, the term is now being used more broadly to describe any cell type that can silence or delete T-cells. In this broader sense, veto cells can also be engineered genetically by transfecting recipient-derived cells with a target antigen, e.g. allogeneic MHC class I and a receptor molecule delivering a death signal to T-cells recognizing the antigen (Fig. 5.6).[85]

9.3 Infectious tolerance and linked epitope suppression

The depletion of recipient T-cells using polyclonal antiserum has been an important part of non-specific immunosuppressive treatment regimens. More sophisticated reagents to target individual T-cell subsets have become available with the development of monoclonal antibodies carrying a single defined specificity.[86] Monoclonal antibodies against the co-receptors CD4 and CD8 were amongst the first to be used successfully in tolerance induction. Grafts transplanted under the tolerogenic cover of non-depleting anti-CD4 and anti-CD8 antibodies were accepted without further treatment.[87]

The tolerant state exemplified important features, implying that tolerance was the result of active regulation and not due to deletion.[88] First, tolerance was dependent on the presence of recipient T-cells. Second, the tolerance could be adoptively transferred into several subsequent generations of naïve secondary recipients using T-cells of the tolerant individual. Thus, the primary tolerant T-cell population was able to render the secondary naïve T-cell population tolerant, even after the first generation of tolerant T-cells had specifically been eliminated. This transmission of tolerance from one generation of regulatory cells to the other was reminiscent of an infectious agent, hence the term infectious tolerance was applied to this system. Third, tolerance that has been induced towards a

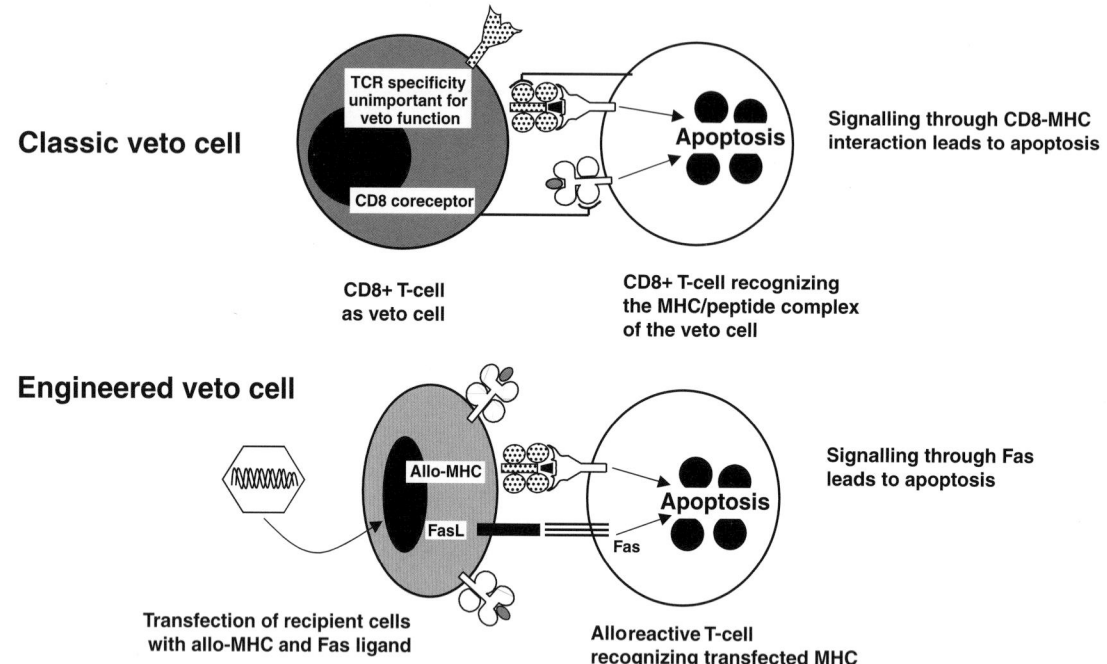

Fig. 5.6 A classic veto cell has been described as a CD8+ T-cell which inactivates another T-cell that recognizes the MHC antigen expressed on the veto T-cell. It is thought that the inhibitory function of the veto cell is mediated through its CD8 co-receptor binding to the MHC class I expressed on the silenced T-cell. The veto mechanism can be imitated by engineering recipient cells to express a target antigen such as allo-MHC and Fas ligand (FasL). Upon interaction of a responder T-cell with the transgenic allo-MHC antigen it will receive a death signal through the Fas/FasL interaction.

single antigen can spread towards newly introduced antigens, provided the new antigens are expressed on the same cell as the initial antigen. This phenomenon is called linked unresponsiveness or linked epitope suppression (Fig. 5.7). This mechanism allows for fully allogeneic grafts to be accepted, even though the recipient has been tolerized only against a single alloantigen expressed on the cell surface on the graft. From these and other studies, it became evident that T-cell regulation is a mechanism of peripheral tolerance *in vivo*.

9.4 Regulatory T-cells

Recent progress has been made to characterize immunomodulatory T-cell populations and their mode of action. In a model of autoimmune inflammatory bowel disease, it has been shown that the CD4+ T-cell population with low expression of the T-cell marker CD45RB (CD45RB[low] CD4+) is able to regulate the disease mediated by the T-cells with a high expression of this marker (CD45RB[high] CD4+) in an IL-10-dependent manner. In a model of long-term surviving cardiac allografts, alloantigen-specific regulatory T-cells were shown to be responsible for the maintenance of tolerance to donor alloantigens *in vivo*.[89] These murine regulatory T-cells were contained within the CD45RB[low] CD4+ or CD25+ CD4+ T-cell populations that had been made tolerant to donor alloantigens and required IL-10 for functional activity. *In vitro* studies have shown that repeated restimulation of T-cells in the presence of IL-10 induces a population of type 1 regulatory T-cells, i.e. Tr1.[90] Induction and activation of Tr1 cells is antigen dependent and therefore

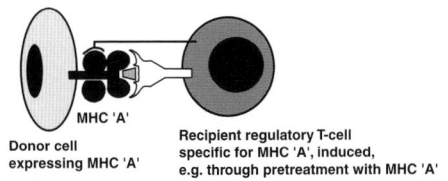

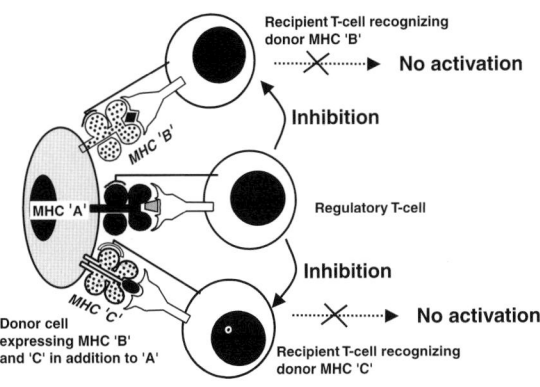

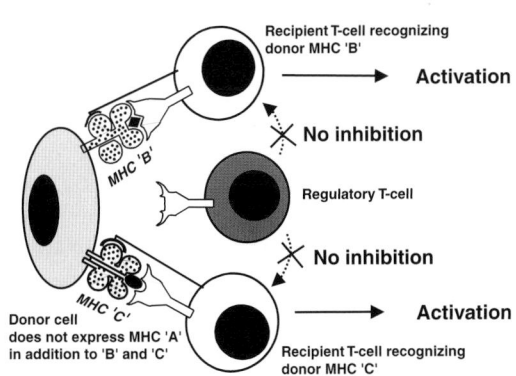

Fig. 5.7 This figure illustrates certain characteristics of linked unresponsiveness at the cellular level. When tolerance involving regulatory mechanisms has been induced towards a single major histocompatibility complex (MHC) antigen, this tolerance can extend towards newly introduced antigens, provided they are expressed on the same cell as the initial tolerogen. Linked unresponsiveness is thought to be mediated through regulatory T-cells that inhibit the T-cells recognizing the newly introduced alloantigens.

antigen specific. However, the regulatory effector function does not seem to be antigen-specific, a phenomenon which has been termed antigen-induced bystander suppression.[91]

Other T-cell markers that allow the separation of regulatory T-cells include CD25 and CD38. However, these T-cell markers are not directly associated with the regulatory T-cell function of the cell expressing it. The search for a T-cell marker that would allow the specific identification of regulatory T-cell subpopulation(s) is a focus of current research.

How exactly regulatory T-cells function is not yet elucidated. Several scenarios that do not have to be mutually exclusive are hypothesized (Fig. 5.8). First, the regulatory T-cell acts directly via cell–cell contact on naïve T-cells. Second, the regulatory function is provided through secretion of cytokines such as IL-10 and TGF-β. Third, the regulatory cells might act on APC to modify them so that naïve T-cells recognizing antigen presented on such APC are turned off.

The accumulating evidence shows that regulatory T-cells play an important role in the control of immune responses and are even functional in tolerance induced towards alloantigens. It should be noted that, to date, most studies have shown regulatory T-cells only in the CD4+ population and not in the CD8+ subset, as might have been suggested from the initial description of suppressor activity. Since regulatory T-cells in transplantation seem to be alloantigen specific, partial deletion of antigen-specific T-cells may perturb immune regulation. Indeed, this reciprocal relationship between deletion and regulation has been demonstrated in an experimental system, where a high dose of antigen has been shown to lead to deletion but not to regulation and vice versa, although in both scenarios the graft was accepted.[92]

9.5 Cytokines as mediators of transplant rejection and acceptance

After the discovery that T helper cells can be separated into distinct groups depending on their cytokine expression pattern,[93] it was shown that allograft rejection is usually associated with expression of the proinflammatory Th1 cytokines IL-2 and IFN-γ. On the other hand, the intragraft expression of the Th2 cytokines IL-4 and IL-10 may, in some circumstances, be beneficial and promote graft acceptance. This concept became

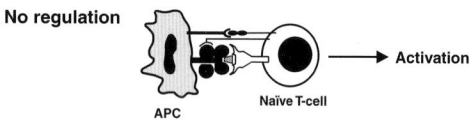

No regulation

Activation

APC   Naïve T-cell

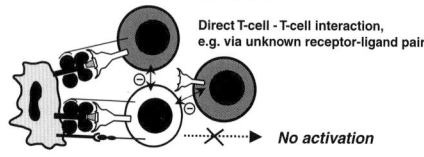

Regulation via direct T-cell - T-cell interaction

Direct T-cell - T-cell interaction, e.g. via unknown receptor-ligand pair

No activation

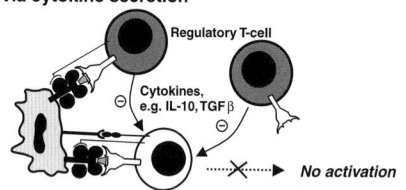

Regulation via cytokine secretion

Regulatory T-cell

Cytokines, e.g. IL-10, TGFβ

No activation

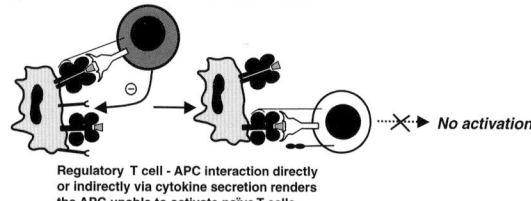

Regulation via T-cell - APC interaction

No activation

Regulatory T cell - APC interaction directly or indirectly via cytokine secretion renders the APC unable to activate naïve T cells

Fig. 5.8 Three potentially non-mutually exclusive mechanisms have been proposed for the function of regulatory T-cells. They may act through direct cell-cell contact, or the secretion of cytokines such as interleukin-10 or transforming growth factor (TGFβ). Alternatively, regulatory T-cells may alter the stimulatory potential of antigen presenting cells in such a way that the APC is rendered unable to activate naive T-cells.

known as the Th1/Th2 paradigm.[94] However, several studies have proven that this is too simplistic a model. Proinflammatory cytokines such as IFN-γ and IL-12 can play an essential role in tolerance induction or the prevention of GvHD,[95] whereas T-cell clones of the Th2 phenotype are able to reject cardiac allografts acutely.[96]

In transplantation, the picture gets more complicated if chronic rejection processes are also considered. The expression of cytokines such as IL-4 and TGF-β, which may be beneficial in the short term and even promote tolerance induction, can have negative effects in the long term and contribute to the development of transplant atherosclerosis. Therefore, manipulation of the cytokine milieu of the recipient's immune response in order to facilitate tolerance towards the allograft can increase the risk of long-term adverse effects.

However, the recent progress in identifying regulatory T-cells has demonstrated a clear role for cytokines, especially IL-10 and TGF-β, as differentiation factors for these regulatory T-cells and also as their effector molecules.[91] Strategies derived from these studies employ cytokines in order to induce antigen-specific regulatory T-cells, either *in vitro* or directly *in vivo*, that will then suppress unwanted responses.

10. OUTLOOK: FROM MOUSE TO HUMAN

Transplantation has provided useful tools to study the mechanisms underlying immunological tolerance over many years. Considerable progress has been made recently in our understanding of the mechanisms underlying tolerance, including the requirements for T-cell recognition and activation, and the substantiation of Tr activity. This basic science knowledge is continuously translated into experimental strategies for tolerance induction, the most promising of which will be further developed for testing in clinical trials.[97] This undertaking is labour and cost intensive. In most cases, these new strategies will need to be tested against already established therapies that have already proven very effective, at least in the short term. However, as experimental data suggest, conventional immunosuppression might not always be compatible with tolerance-induction protocols.[73,78] Thus, although the safest clinical trial approach might be to combine these strategies with conventional immunosuppression, it has yet to be determined whether this will be the most effective approach.[98] The potential reward from these complex studies in the future is prolonged graft survival or graft acceptance without the negative side effects of non-specific immunosuppression – a goal definitely worth aiming for.

GLOSSARY

Accelerated rejection
Rejection within days mediated by low levels of preformed, usually immunoglobulin (Ig) G, antibodies against donor endothelial antigens; similar pathology as hyperacute rejection.

Activation-induced cell death (AICD)
Repeated stimulation of T-cells by antigen present in high doses can lead to the programmed cell death, or apoptosis, of T-cells specific for this antigen.

Acute cellular rejection
T-cell mediated and can occur several days after transplantation; represents the majority of clinical rejection episodes and is characterized by cellular graft infiltration and parenchymal necrosis.

Acute vascular rejection
Caused by newly induced antibodies requiring T-cell help; occurs after the first week post-transplant and is characterized by a vasculitis-type of pathology.

Allotransplantation
Transplantation of an organ (allograft) between genetically non-identical members of the same species.

Anergy
If T-cells encounter antigen on antigen-presenting cells that do not express co-stimulatory signals, the T-cells can become unresponsive, or anergic, and remain so, even after proper restimulation with antigen.

Central tolerance
Induction of tolerance in generative lymphoid organs (thymus for T-cells, bone marrow for B-cells) through deletion of immature lymphocytes recognizing self-antigens.

Chimerism
The existence of more than one genetically distinct stable cell line in one individual; in transplantation used to describe the presence, outside the graft itself, of donor-derived cells in the recipient organism.

Chronic rejection (delayed graft loss)
Describes the multifactorial process of gradual decrease in function, and finally loss, of a graft that occurs over years following transplantation; characterized by fibrosis and arteriosclerosis of the graft.

Clonal exhaustion
An extreme form of activation-induced cell death (AICD), when all T-cells of a clone specific for a particular antigen have been eliminated.

Hyperacute rejection
Rejection of vascularized organs within minutes to hours by preformed antibodies, mainly against ABO blood group antigens or human leucocyte antigens (HLA) binding to donor endothelium and causing thrombosis.

Ignorance
Lymphocytes encounter antigen that they can recognize but are neither activated nor rendered tolerant, or lymphocytes are unable to encounter their antigen; not strictly a mechanism of tolerance.

Infectious tolerance
Tolerance that is transferable through more than

one generation of recipients in the absence of the original antigen; is associated with linked epitope suppression.

Linked epitope suppression
Tolerance that has been induced towards a particular antigen is extended towards newly encountered antigens if they are expressed on the same (antigen-presenting) cell as the initial tolerated antigen.

Microchimerism
Presence of genetically non-identical cells in the peripheral blood, below the detection level by flow cytometry (~ 0.1 %).

Peripheral tolerance
Induction of unresponsiveness in peripheral sites as a result of mature lymphocytes encountering self- or foreign antigen under tolerogenic conditions resulting in deletion, anergy or the induction of immunoregulation.

Polymorphism
Discretely different forms of a gene that exist in the population in at least two phenotypes, neither of which occurs at a frequency of <1%.

Tolerance
A state of antigen-specific unresponsiveness induced by prior exposure to the antigen.

Veto cell
A cell that causes death or inactivation of a T-cell that recognizes the major histocompatibility complex (MHC)/peptide complex expressed on the veto cell.

REFERENCES

Scientific papers

1. Brent L. *A History of Transplantation Immunology.* London: Academic Press, 1997.
2. van Rood JJ. The history of the discovery of HLA. In: Lechler R, Warrens A, eds. *HLA in Health and Disease.* Second edn. London: Academic Press, 2000.
3. Tagarelli A, Piro A, Lagonia P, Tagarelli G. Karl Landsteiner: a hundred years later. *Transplantation* 2001; **72**: 3–7.
4. Medawar PB. The behaviour and fate of skin autografts and skin homografts in rabbits. *J Anat* 1944; **78**: 176.
5. Billingham RE, Brent L, Medawar PB. Actively acquired tolerance of foreign cells. *Nature* 1953; **172**: 603–6.
6. Burnet FM. *The Clonal Selection Theory of Acquired Immunity.* Cambridge: Cambridge University Press, 1959.
7. Miller JF, Morahan G. Peripheral T cell tolerance. *Annu Rev Immunol* 1992; **10**: 51–69.
8. Goodnow CC. Transgenic mice and analysis of B-cell tolerance. *Annu Rev Immunol* 1992; **10**: 489–518.
9. Goldrath AW, Bevan MJ. Selecting and maintaining a diverse T-cell repertoire. *Nature* 1999; **402**: 255–62.
10. Shevach EM. Regulatory T cells in autoimmunity. *Annu Rev Immunol* 2000; **18**: 423–49.
11. Morahan G, Allison J, Miller JF. Tolerance of class I histocompatibility antigens expressed extrathymically. *Nature* 1989; **339**: 622–4.
12. Schonrich G, Kalinke U, Momburg F et al. Down-regulation of T cell receptors on self-reactive T cells as a novel mechanism for extrathymic tolerance induction. *Cell* 1991; **65**: 293–304.
13. Bushell A, Wood KJ. Permanent survival of organ transplants without immunosuppression: experimental approaches and possibilities for tolerance induction in clinical transplantation. *Exp Rev Molec Med* 1999; **29 October**. (http://www-ermm.cbcu.cam.ac.uk/99001179h.htm.)
14. Russell PS, Chase CM, Winn HJ, Colvin RB. Coronary atherosclerosis in transplanted mouse hearts. I. Time course and immunogenetic and immunopathological considerations. *Am J Pathol* 1994; **144**: 260–74.
15. Suthanthiran M. Transplantation tolerance: fooling mother Nature. *Proc Natl Acad Sci USA* 1996; **93**: 12072–5.
16. Steinmuller D. Passenger leukocytes and the immunogenicity of skin allografts. *J Invest Dermatol* 1980; **75**: 107–15.

17. Jones ND, Turvey SE, Van Maurik A et al. Differential susceptibility of heart, skin, and islet allografts to T cell-mediated rejection. *J Immunol* 2001; **166**: 2824–30.

18. van Parijs L, Perez VL, Abbas AK. Mechanisms of peripheral T cell tolerance. *Novartis Found Symp* 1998; **215**: 5–14; discussion 14–20, 33–40.

19. Lamb JR, Skidmore BJ, Green N et al. Induction of tolerance in influenza virus–immune T lymphocyte clones with synthetic peptides of influenza hemagglutinin. *J Exp Med* 1983; **157**: 1434–47.

20. Lechler R, Chai JG, Marelli-Berg F, Lombardi G. T-cell anergy and peripheral T-cell tolerance. *Phil Trans R Soc Lond B Biol Sci* 2001; **356**: 625–37.

21. Charlton B, Auchincloss H, Fathman CG. Mechanisms of transplantation tolerance. *Annu Rev Immunol* 1994; **12**: 707–34.

22. Sakaguchi S. Regulatory T cells: key controllers of immunologic self-tolerance. *Cell* 2000; **101**: 455–8.

23. Mellor AL, Munn DH. Immunology at the maternal–fetal interface: lessons for T cell tolerance and suppression. *Annu Rev Immunol* 2000; **18**: 367–91.

24. Tafuri A, Alferink J, Moller P et al. T cell awareness of paternal alloantigens during pregnancy. *Science* 1995; **270**: 630–3.

25. Munn DH, Zhou M, Attwood JT et al. Prevention of allogeneic fetal rejection by tryptophan catabolism. *Science* 1998; **281**: 1191–3.

26. Carosella ED, Paul P, Moreau P, Rouas-Freiss N. HLA-G and HLA-E: fundamental and pathophysiological aspects. *Immunol Today* 2000; **21**: 532–4.

27. Lila N, Carpentier A, Amrein C et al. Implication of HLA-G molecule in heart-graft acceptance. *Lancet* 2000; **355**: 2138.

28. Lo YM, Corbetta N, Chamberlain PF et al. Presence of fetal DNA in maternal plasma and serum. *Lancet* 1997; **350**: 485–7.

29. Sherman LA, Chattopadhyay S. The molecular basis of allorecognition. *Annu Rev Immunol* 1993; **11**: 385–402.

30. Shoskes DA, Wood KJ. Indirect presentation of MHC antigens in transplantation. *Immunol Today* 1994; **15**: 32–8.

31. Gould DS, Auchincloss Jr, H. Direct and indirect recognition: the role of MHC antigens in graft rejection. *Immunol Today* 1999; **20**: 77–82.

32. Auchincloss H, Lee R, Shea S et al. The role of 'indirect' recognition in initiating rejection of skin grafts from major histocompatibility complex class II-deficient mice. *Proc Natl Acad Sci USA* 1993; **90**: 3373–7.

33. Bolton EM, Gracie JA, Briggs JD et al. Cellular requirements for renal allograft rejection in the athymic nude rat. *J Exp Med* 1989; **169**: 1931–46.

34. Kissmeyer-Nielsen F, Olsen S, Petersen VP, Fjeldborg O. Hyperacute rejection of kidney allografts, associated with pre-existing humoral antibodies against donor cells. *Lancet* 1966; **2**: 662–5.

35. Tilney NL. Chronic rejection. In: Ginns LC, Cosimi AB, Morris PJ, eds. *Transplantation*. Oxford: Blackwell Science, 1999.

36. Libby P, Pober JS. Chronic rejection. *Immunity* 2001; **14**: 387–97.

37. Wood KJ, Jones ND, Bushell AR, Morris PJ. Alloantigen-induced specific immunological unresponsiveness. *Phil Trans R Soc Lond B Biol Sci* 2001; **356**: 665–80.

38. Bushell A, Niimi M, Morris PJ, Wood KJ. Evidence for immune regulation in the induction of transplantation tolerance: a conditional but limited role for IL-4. *J Immunol* 1999; **162**: 1359–66.

39. Morris PJ, Ting A, Stocker J. Leukocyte antigens in renal transplantation. 1. The paradox of blood transfusions in renal transplantation. *Med J Aust* 1968; **2**: 1088–90.

40. Opelz G, Terasaki PI. Prolongation effect of blood transfusions on kidney graft survival. *Transplantation* 1976; **22**: 380–3.

41. Wong W, Morris PJ, Wood KJ. Pretransplant administration of a single donor class I major histocompatibility complex molecule is sufficient for the indefinite survival of fully allogeneic cardiac allografts: evidence for linked epitope suppression. *Transplantation* 1997; **63**: 1490-4.

42. Madsen JC, Superina RA, Wood KJ, Morris PJ. Immunological unresponsiveness induced by recipient cells transfected with donor MHC genes. *Nature* 1988; **332**: 161–4.

43. Wood KJ. Gene therapy and allotransplantation. *Curr Opin Immunol* 1997; **9**: 662–8.

44. Posselt AM, Barker CF, Tomaszewski JE et al. Induction of donor-specific unresponsiveness by intrathymic islet transplantation. *Science* 1990; **249**: 1293–5.

45. Jones ND, Fluck NC, Roelen DL et al. Deletion of alloantigen-reactive thymocytes as a mechanism of adult tolerance induction following intrathymic antigen administration. *Eur J Immunol* 1997; **27**: 1591–600.

46. Knechtle SJ, Wang J, Graeb C et al. Direct MHC class I complementary DNA transfer to thymus induces donor-specific unresponsiveness, which involves multiple immunologic mechanisms. *J Immunol* 1997; **159**: 152–8.

47. Saborio DV, Chowdhury NC, Jin MX et al. Regulatory T cells maintain peripheral tolerance to islet allografts induced by intrathymic injection of MHC class I allopeptides. *Cell Transplant* 1999; **8**: 375–81.

48. Magee CC, Sayegh MH. Peptide-mediated immunosuppression. *Curr Opin Immunol* 1997; **9**: 669–75.

49. Strobel S, Mowat AM. Immune responses to dietary antigens: oral tolerance. *Immunol Today* 1998; **19**: 173–81.

50. Weiner HL. Oral tolerance: immune mechanisms and treatment of autoimmune diseases. *Immunol Today* 1997; **18**: 335–43.

51. Niimi M, Witzke O, Bushell A et al. Nondepleting anti-CD4 monoclonal antibody enhances the ability of oral alloantigen delivery to induce indefinite survival of cardiac allografts: oral tolerance to alloantigen. *Transplantation* 2000; **70**: 1524–8.

52. Owen RD. Immunogenetic consequences of vascular anastomoses between bovine twins. *Science* 1945; **102**: 400-1.

53. Sayegh MH, Fine NA, Smith JL et al. Immunologic tolerance to renal allografts after bone marrow transplants from the same donors. *Ann Intern Med* 1991; **114**: 954–5.

54. Dey B, Sykes M, Spitzer TR. Outcomes of recipients of both bone marrow and solid organ transplants. A review. *Medicine (Baltimore)* 1998; **77**: 355–69.

55. Sykes M. Chimerism and central tolerance. *Curr Opin Immunol* 1996; **8**: 694–703.

56. Starzl TE, Demetris AJ, Murase N et al. Cell migration, chimerism, and graft acceptance. *Lancet* 1992; **339**: 1579–82.

57. Salgar SK, Shapiro R, Dodson F et al. Infusion of donor leukocytes to induce tolerance in organ allograft recipients. *J Leukoc Biol* 1999; **66**: 310–14.

58. Ciancio G, Miller J, Garcia-Morales RO et al. Six-year clinical effect of donor bone marrow infusions in renal transplant patients. *Transplantation* 2001; **71**: 827–35.

59. Hamano K, Rawsthorne MA, Bushell AR et al. Evidence that the continued presence of the organ graft and not peripheral donor microchimerism is essential for maintenance of tolerance to alloantigen *in vivo* in anti-CD4 treated recipients. *Transplantation* 1996; **62**: 856–60.

60. Wood K, Sachs DH. Chimerism and transplantation tolerance: cause and effect. *Immunol Today* 1996; **17**: 584–7.

61. Calne RY, Sells RA, Pena JR et al. Induction of immunological tolerance by porcine liver allografts. *Nature* 1969; **223**: 472–6.

62. Schlitt HJ, Raddatz G, Steinhoff G et al. Passenger lymphocytes in human liver allografts and their potential role after transplantation. *Transplantation* 1993; **56**: 951–5.

63. Bretscher PA, Cohn M. Minimal model for the mechanism of antibody induction and paralysis by antigen. *Nature* 1968; **220**: 444–8.

64. Lafferty KJ, Cunningham AJ. A new analysis of allogeneic interactions. *Aust J Exp Biol Med Sci* 1975; **53**: 27–42.

65. Grewal IS, Flavell RA. CD40 and CD154 in cell-mediated immunity. *Annu Rev Immunol* 1998; **16**: 111–35.

66. Billing JS, Gilot BJ, Wood KJ. Tolerance induction in cardiac transplantation. *Curr Opin Organ Transplant* 1999; **4**: 219–226.

67. Sayegh MH, Turka LA. The role of T-cell costimulatory activation pathways in transplant rejection. *N Engl J Med* 1998; **338**: 1813–21.

68. Perico N, Imberti O, Bontempelli M, Remuzzi G. Toward novel antirejection strategies: *in vivo* immunosuppressive properties of CTLA4Ig. *Kidney Int* 1995; **47**: 241–6.

69. Zheng XX, Sayegh MH, Zheng XG et al. The role of donor and recipient B7-1 (CD80) in allograft rejection. *J Immunol* 1997; **159**: 1169–73.

70. Perez VL, Van Parijs L, Biuckians A et al. Induction of peripheral T cell tolerance *in vivo* requires CTLA-4 engagement. *Immunity* 1997; **6**: 411–7.

71. Harlan DM, Kirk AD. Promise of costimulatory pathway modifying reagents for transplantation. *Curr Opin Organ Transplant* 2000; **5**: 90–5.

72. Larsen CP, Alexander DZ, Hollenbaugh D et al. CD40–gp39 interactions play a critical role during allograft rejection. Suppression of allograft rejection by blockade of the CD40–gp39 pathway. *Transplantation* 1996; **61**: 4–9.

73. Kirk AD, Burkly LC, Batty DS et al. Treatment with humanized monoclonal antibody against CD154 prevents acute renal allograft rejection in nonhuman primates. *Nature Med* 1999; **5**: 686–93.

74. Trambley J, Bingaman AW, Lin A et al. Asialo GM1(+) CD8(+) T cells play a critical role in costimulation blockade-resistant allograft rejection. *J Clin Invest* 1999; **104**: 1715–22.

75. Honey K, Cobbold SP, Waldmann H. CD40 ligand blockade induces CD4+ T cell tolerance and linked suppression. *J Immunol* 1999; **163**: 4805–10.

76. Jones ND, Van Maurik A, Hara M et al. CD40–CD40 ligand-independent activation of CD8+ T cells can trigger allograft rejection. *J Immunol* 2000; **165**: 1111–18.

77. Ensminger SM, Spriewald BM, Sorensen HV et al. Critical role for IL-4 in the development of

transplant arteriosclerosis in the absence of CD40–CD154 costimulation. *J Immunol* 2001; **167**: 532–41.

78. Li Y, Li XC, Zheng XX et al. Blocking both signal 1 and signal 2 of T-cell activation prevents apoptosis of alloreactive T cells and induction of peripheral allograft tolerance. *Nature Med* 1999; **5**: 1298–302.

79. Wells AD, Li XC, Li Y et al. Requirement for T-cell apoptosis in the induction of peripheral transplantation tolerance. *Nature Med* 1999; **5**: 1303–7.

80. Gershon RK, Mokyr MB, Mitchell MS. Activation of suppressor T cells by tumour cells and specific antibody. *Nature* 1974; **250**: 594–6.

81. Jerne NK. Towards a network theory of the immune system. *Ann Immunol* 1974; **125C**: 373–89.

82. Shapira OM, Mor E, Reshef T et al. Prolongation of survival of rat cardiac allografts by T cell vaccination. *J Clin Invest* 1993; **91**: 388–90.

83. Miller RG, Muraoka S, Claesson MH et al. The veto phenomenon in T–cell regulation. *Ann NY Acad Sci* 1988; **532**: 170–6.

84. Fink PJ, Shimonkevitz RP, Bevan MJ. Veto cells. *Annu Rev Immunol* 1988; **6**: 115–37.

85. Lau HT, Yu M, Fontana A, Stoeckert CJ. Prevention of islet allograft rejection with engineered myoblasts expressing FasL in mice. *Science* 1996; **273**: 109–12.

86. Kohler G, Milstein C. Continuous cultures of fused cells secreting antibody of predefined specificity. *Nature* 1975; **256**: 495–7.

87. Qin S, Cobbold SP, Pope H et al. Infectious transplantation tolerance. *Science* 1993; **259**: 974–7.

88. Waldmann H, Cobbold S. How do monoclonal antibodies induce tolerance? A role for infectious tolerance? *Annu Rev Immunol* 1998; **16**: 619–44.

89. Hara M, Kingsley CI, Niimi M et al. Il-10 is required for regulatory T cells to mediate tolerance to alloantigens *in vivo*. *J Immunol* 2001; **166**: 3789–96.

90. Groux H, O'Garra A, Bigler M et al. A CD4+ T-cell subset inhibits antigen-specific T-cell responses and prevents colitis. *Nature* 1997; **389**: 737–42.

91. Groux H, Powrie F. Regulatory T cells and inflammatory bowel disease. *Immunol Today* 1999; **20**: 442-5.

92. Bemelman F, Honey K, Adams E et al. Bone marrow transplantation induces either clonal deletion or infectious tolerance depending on the dose. *J Immunol* 1998; **160**: 2645–8.

93. Mosmann TR, Coffmann RL. TH1 and TH2 cells: different patterns of lymphokine secretion lead to different functional properties. *Annu Rev Immunol* 1989; **7**: 145–73.

94. Strom TB, Roy-Chaudhury P, Manfro R et al. The Th1/Th2 paradigm and the allograft response. *Curr Opin Immunol* 1996; **8**: 688–93.

95. Spriewald BM, Billing JS, Wood KJ. Cytokines as mediators in immunological tolerance. *Curr Opin Organ Transplant* 2001; **6**: 7–13.

96. VanBuskirk AM, Wakely ME, Orosz CG. Transfusion of polarized TH2-like cell populations into SCID mouse cardiac allograft recipients results in acute allograft rejection. *Transplantation* 1996; **62**: 229–38.

97. Kirk AD. Transplantation tolerance: a look at the nonhuman primate literature in the light of modern tolerance theories. *Crit Rev Immunol* 1999; **19**: 349–88.

98. Calne R, Moffatt SD, Friend PJ et al. Campath IH allows low-dose cyclosporine monotherapy in 31 cadaveric renal allograft recipients. *Transplantation* 1999; **68**: 1613–16.

6

Tumour immunology

Hans J Stauss, Ilaria Bellantuono, Shiou Chih Hsu, Francisco Ramirez

Objectives • Overview • Introduction • Role of cytotoxic T-lymphocytes • Role of helper T-cells • Role of B-cells in tumour immunity • Role of natural killer cells • Conclusions • References

OBJECTIVES

(1) To review the contribution of the different arms (cytotoxic T-lymphocytes, CD4+ T-cells, B-cells and natural killer cells) of the adaptive immune system in stimulating and suppressing tumour development.
(2) To review how knowledge of immune responses to tumours can lead to therapeutic interventions to enhance tumour elimination.

Overview

The concept of immunosurveillance of cancer, formulated approximately three decades ago, provided a framework for experimentation to test whether the immune system does indeed play a critical role in the protection against cancer. In the past 10 years, numerous antigens recognized by human tumour-reactive T-lymphocytes have been identified, and tetramer technology provided a means to demonstrate that these T-lymphocytes are present in cancer patients. Whether they fight an active battle against resident cancer cells or whether they have been rendered inactive by the tumour and by regulatory cells remains to be determined. Indeed, regulatory CD4 T-cells and natural killer T-cells have been shown to interfere with effective tumour immunity in animal models. The

knowledge of T-cell-recognized tumour antigens, together with a better understanding of the interplay between regulatory and effector cells of the immune system, provides hope for the design of effective antigen-specific immunotherapy protocols for the treatment of cancer.

1. Introduction

Historic immunization experiments with irradiated tumour cells have clearly demonstrated the existence of rejection antigens expressed by carcinogen-induced murine tumours.[1] The demonstration of T-cell-recognized tumour antigens led Burnett[2] to postulate that a major function of the immune system was early recognition and elimination of transformed cells, thus preventing the development of overt malignancies. This concept of immunological surveillance is clearly relevant for virus-associated malignancies, such as Epstein-Barr virus (EBV) lymphomas, which frequently develop in immune-suppressed individuals.

However, the existence of T-cell-recognized antigens in human tumours that do not contain viral sequences has remained controversial for a long time. Indeed, there was a worry that such antigens might be present in experimental tumours induced with high doses of mutation-inducing carcinogens but not in human cancers that arise spontaneously. The cloning of tumour antigens recognized by autologous cytotoxic T-lymphocytes in melanoma patients was done successfully for the first time in 1989, showing that tumour antigens are not an artefact of experimental tumours.[3] This seminal work was followed by the identification of a large number of cytotoxic-T-lymphocyte-(CTL)-recognized human tumour antigens, some of which are now in clinical vaccination trials. In contrast, the identification of antigens recognized by CD4 helper T-cells (Th) is still in its infancy, and only few CD4 T-cell antigens have been molecularly cloned to date. New technologies have been developed to identify tumour antigens that are recognized by antibodies present in the serum of cancer patients. Thus, the tools are now available to study the target antigens recognized by both components of the adaptive immune system, i.e. B- and T-cells.

Finally, it has been known for a long time that natural killer (NK) cells can reject major histocompatibility complex (MHC) class-I-deficient tumour cells in murine model experiments.[4] It took a long time to understand the mechanisms by which these NK cells recognize the absence of MHC molecules. In the last few years a number of inhibitory and activation receptors have been identified which tune the activity of NK cells. We are now getting a glimpse of how NK cells can recognize and kill tumour cells.

2. ROLE OF CYTOTOXIC T-LYMPHOCYTES (CTL)

2.1 Antigens recognized by human CTL

In the past 10 years a large number of CTL-recognized antigens have been identified in human tumours.[5] These antigens can be divided into two major categories. The first category are tumour-specific antigens that are present in tumours only, i.e. not in normal cells. The major advantage of these antigens is that they provide targets for CTL with exquisite tumour specificity, since there is no danger of CTL attack of normal cells. Examples of tumour-specific antigens are virus-encoded proteins present in

malignancies that are associated with infection by viruses with transforming activity such as EBV, human papilloma virus and hepatitis B virus. Indeed, the first successful prophylactic cancer vaccine was the vaccine against hepatitis B, which resulted in a reduction of liver cell carcinomas in Southeast Asia, where the incidence of cancer promoting chronic hepatitis B infection was high prior to the vaccination programme.[6,7]

Mutated cellular proteins can also function as tumour-specific antigens. CTL recognition of mutated oncogenes was first demonstrated in a murine model showing that CTL recognized a point mutation in the Ras protein, leading to specific CTL killing of tumour cells harbouring the mutated *Ras* gene.[8] However, mutations are infrequently recognized by CTL isolated from cancer patients. This was surprising, considering that mutational alterations are commonly found in tumours, resulting in the expression of proteins with altered amino acid composition, or in fusion proteins with novel joining sequences. Why is it that CTL do not commonly recognize such mutated sequences? One reason lies in the mechanism by which antigens need to be processed to produce peptide fragments that are presented on the cell surface for recognition by CTL. Peptide sequences are CTL targets only if the intracellular protein breakdown results in the production of the relevant peptide sequence, and if this peptide is transported into the lumen of the endoplasmic reticulum (ER) and if it binds to MHC class I molecules. MHC class I molecules travel from the ER to the cell surface where they present peptides for recognition by CTL. There are several reasons why mutated proteins may escape CTL recognition: (1) peptides containing the mutation are not generated in the process of protein breakdown; (2) the mutation-containing peptides are not transported into the ER; (3) the peptides fail to bind with high affinity to MHC class I molecules. Hence, although mutated proteins are commonly present in tumours, they are frequently invisible for CTL.

The majority of CTL isolated from cancer patients recognize tumour-associated antigens. These antigens are present in tumour cells but also in normal cells. In some cases, these antigens are expressed at high levels in tumours and at low levels in normal cells of the same tissues, which can lead to selective CTL killing of tumour cells. In other cases, the genes encoding these antigens are abnormally switched on in cancer cells, whilst they are silent in non-malignant cells of the same tissue. For example, the testis cancer antigens are usually silent in most tissues except testis, but are switched on in various malignancies including melanoma, lung and colon cancer.[5,9] The advantage of these tumour-associated antigens is that the whole protein sequence is available for CTL recognition, allowing selection of those peptides that are efficiently produced inside the cell, transported and bind with high affinity to MHC class I molecules. The disadvantage is that the proteins are present in normal tissues that may induce immunological tolerance or, in cases where tolerance is incomplete, may lead to the activation of CTL that cause autoimmunity. Indeed, CTL against tumour-associated melanoma antigens can sometimes also kill normal melanocytes, leading to depigmentation and the clinical symptoms of vitiligo.[10]

2.2 Evidence that CTL can mediate tumour protection

The first clear demonstration that CTL can eliminate tumours came from experiments in tumour-bearing, T-cell-deficient nude mice. The infusion of CTL clones specific for a virus-encoded tumour antigen resulted in complete regression of large tumours.[11] Depletion experiments and adoptive transfer of purified T-cell populations have demonstrated that CD8 T-cells are important for tumour protection in many murine models. The evidence in humans, however, is more difficult to obtain. The most convincing demonstration of T-cell-mediated tumour protection comes from immunotherapy experiments in immune-suppressed transplant patients suffering from B-cell lymphomas. These lymphomas are caused by the transforming activity of EBV, and EBV-specific T-cell lines infused prophylactically were shown to eliminate existing tumours and prevent

lymphomas.[12,13] Since the infused T-cell lines are typically a mixture of CD4-expressing Th and CD8-expressing CTL, it is difficult to determine the relative tumour protective effect of the two T-cell populations. The adoptively transferred EBV-specific T-cells can mediate long-term protection and can be found in patients years after the infusion. This is in contrast to the relatively short lifespan of infused cells when pure CD8 T-cell lines were used for adoptive T-cell therapy. There is now evidence that CD4 T-cells are required for long-term CD8 T-cell survival,[14] providing an explanation of how they enhance the tumour protective effect of CTL. In addition, CD4 T-cells can contribute to tumour immunity by mechanisms that are independent of CD8 T-cells (see below).

2.3 Danger of autoimmunity

In melanoma patients, tumour regression is sometimes associated with vitiligo, suggesting that tumour immunity resulted in autoimmune destruction of normal melanocytes. Similarly, a recent study suggested that CTL responses against a neuronal antigen that is abnormally expressed in gynaecological cancers may cause paraneoplastic cerebellar degeneration, a condition that is sometimes seen in patients with gynaecological malignancies.[15] It has been demonstrated that these patients harbour antibodies and CTL against the neuronal antigen, cdr-2, which is abnormally expressed in ovarian and breast cancer cells. It is difficult, however, to establish a link between the observed CTL and the paraneoplastic neurological symptoms in these patients.

Therefore, transgenic animal models have been developed to explore the risk of autoimmunity when T-cell-recognized tumour antigens are also expressed on normal host tissues. From these studies it is emerging that the risk of autoimmunity is determined by the frequency and avidity of the CTL, and by the tissue microenvironment that may promote or inhibit CTL infiltration.

Transgenic mice that express virus antigens in the pancreatic islet cells were challenged with tumours expressing the same viral antigens. In one series of experiments, immunization of such mice resulted in tumour protection without autoimmune damage to the pancreatic islet cells.[16] This protection was mediated by low-avidity CTL. High-avidity CTL had been rendered tolerant as a consequence of antigen expression in the pancreas. In a similar transgenic model, repeated dendritic cell vaccination stimulated CTL that prevented tumour growth but also caused autoimmune diabetes.[17] In this case, there was no detectable tolerance prior to vaccination, because the CTL ignored antigen expression in the pancreas. Hence, it is likely that the repeated vaccination triggered a large number of high-avidity CTL recognizing not only tumour cells but also pancreatic islet cells.

There is good evidence showing that the tissue microenvironment can determine whether the presence of autoreactive CTL results in the attack of tissues expressing the auto-antigen. Murine experiments showed that circulating autoreactive CTL did not enter healthy tissues, but did enter infected or irradiated tissues leading to tissue damage.[18] It has been suggested that a healthy tissue microenvironment does not promote T-cell extravasation, and that inflammatory and other stress signals can lead to the activation of endothelial cells, promoting T-cell access to the target tissue.

2.4 Problems of CTL tolerance

CTL in melanoma patients most frequently recognize melanocyte-specific differentiation antigens. Tetramer analysis has demonstrated that such CTL can be present in melanoma patients and vaccination studies showed that immunization can further increase the CTL number. The presence of such CTL suggest that tolerance to these melanocyte-specific differentiation antigens is incomplete. However, so far, there is no correlation between the presence of CTL and the regression of melanoma. One possible explanation is that partial tolerance causes inactivation of high-avidity CTL, leaving only low-avidity CTL to mount antimelanoma responses in patients. Partial tolerance has been confirmed in murine studies comparing CTL responses against a melanocyte-specific

differentiation antigen, tyrosinase, in normal and tyrosinase-deficient mice.[19] This comparison has demonstrated that the physiological expression of tyrosinase resulted in a substantial diminution of the CTL response.

Tolerance is even more profound to overexpressed tumour antigens that are more widely expressed in normal tissues than the melanocyte antigens. This interferes with the immunological targeting of proteins that are frequently overexpressed in human malignancies. For example, the p53 and mdm-2 transcription factors are present at elevated levels in a substantial proportion of solid cancers and leukaemias, and the overexpression is probably required for the malignant phenotype. Immunological targeting of proteins that are linked to transformation is particularly attractive, because tumours cannot escape CTL attack by switching off antigen expression. Recently, new approaches have been developed allowing CTL targeting of antigens independent of immunological tolerance.

2.5 Avoiding CTL tolerance

Two major strategies have been developed to generate CTL responses against antigens to which the autologous immune system is tolerant. One approach uses transgenic mice expressing human leucocyte antigen (HLA)-A0201 class I molecules, which are also expressed in approximately 45% of Caucasian individuals. In these mice, it is possible to generate CTL against peptide epitopes of p53, provided the peptide sequence is different between human and murine p53. In this case, the mice are only tolerant to the murine but not the human sequence. CTL specific for p53 have been isolated from these mice and shown to selectively recognize human tumour cells expressing elevated p53 levels, but not normal cells with physiological p53 expression.[20]

Another strategy is based on the observation that tolerance is MHC restricted.[21,22] Thus, HLA-A0201-expressing individuals are tolerant to self-peptides presented by this HLA allele. However, individuals expressing a different set of HLA alleles will not be tolerant to peptide epitopes presented by the A0201 molecule. Hence, A0201-negative individuals can be used to generate CTL against peptide epitopes that are presented by A0201, irrespective of immunological tolerance. This opens the opportunity to direct CTL responses against any cellular protein that is expressed at elevated levels in tumour cells. The feasibility of this strategy was first demonstrated in mice[23] and then in humans by generating CTL against the cell cycle protein, cyclin D1, that is overexpressed in various tumours.[24] These CTL showed selective killing of cyclin-D1-expressing tumours.

More recently, this approach was used to direct CTL against a transcription factor, WT-1, that is overexpressed in various leukaemias and solid cancers.[25] The overexpression is likely to be required for the abnormal growth and differentiation of malignant cells.[26,27] *In vitro* studies have shown that WT-1-specific CTL can recognize and kill malignant bone marrow stem cells from leukaemia patients but not normal bone marrow cells from healthy controls. It is likely that the selective killing of leukaemic cells is due to the observation that CD34-positive stem cells from leukaemia patients express higher levels of WT-1 than CD34-positive stem cells from normal donors.[25] Considering the exquisite specificity of WT-1-specific CTL, they provide exciting reagents for immunotherapy of leukaemia. In HLA-A0201-expressing leukaemia patients who received a bone marrow transplant (BMT) from an HLA-mismatched donor, it would be possible to isolate WT-1-specific donor CTL for adoptive therapy. Alternatively, it will be possible to exploit allogeneic WT-1-specific CTL as a source of T-cell receptors (TCR) with tumour specificity. It has been shown that viral vectors can be used to transfer TCR into human CD8 T-cells.[28] This gene therapy approach can be used to introduce cloned WT-1-specific TCR into patients' CD8 T-cells, and equip them with a tumour specificity that they do not naturally possess.

3. ROLE OF HELPER T-CELLS (Th)

The immunosurveillance hypothesis proposes that the immune system can recognize and eliminate tumour cells. CD4 Th play a central role in the regulation of most antigen-specific immune responses. However, in the study of tumour immunity, much more attention has been given to the role of cytotoxic CD8 T-cells. CD8 T-cells recognize epitopes presented by MHC class I molecules while CD4 T-cells recognize peptides presented by MHC class II molecules. The fact that most tumours express MHC class I molecules but do not express MHC class II molecules may explain this disproportionate interest. In addition, cytotoxic CD8 T-cells are considered the main effector mechanism in tumour killing. Many human and rodent antigens recognized by cytotoxic CD8 T-cells have been characterized. The ability of CTL to recognize and kill tumour cells, and eradicate tumour cells *in vivo*, has been extensively reported. In contrast, few antigens recognized by CD4 T-cells have been described. In recent years, the study of mouse models has emphasized the importance of both CD4 and CD8 T-cells in establishing an optimal immune response to tumours. These experiments have revealed two important facts: CD4 T-cells are required to provide help for optimal CD8 T-cell responses and CD4 T-cells can act as effector cells in tumour eradication. Ultimately, the ideal effective tumour-specific immunotherapies will induce immune responses against a panel of epitopes recognized by both CD4 and CD8 T-cells.

3.1 Antigens recognized by human Th

The methodology for identifying MHC class-II-restricted antigens is more limited than for class I and no standard methodology exists. CD4 T-cell responses specific for unidentified tumour antigens have been described in several tumours, including melanomas, lymphomas, colon cancers, breast cancer and others.[29] Responses of Th to defined tumour-specific peptide sequences have also been described. These epitopes include sequences from mutated Ras proteins from different cancers; the joining sequence of bcr–abl fusion proteins resulting from chromosomal translocation characteristic of chronic myeloid leukaemia; human papillomavirus E7 oncoprotein, characteristic of cervical cancer; idiotypic immunoglobulin (Ig)M sequences expressed by B-cell lymphomas; and several epitopes from different proteins from melanoma cells.[29,30] In the previous examples, CD4 T-cell responses were tested against potential tumour antigen candidates that are lineage specific, overexpressed or mutated. Classical fractionation techniques, together with new technical developments such as peptide elution, serological identification of antigens (SEREX) and antigen expression targeted to the MHC class II presentation pathway, have permitted the identification of new epitopes in human tumours. In particular, several epitopes from melanoma and oesophageal cancer have been described.[29–31] In some of these examples there was a direct correlation between the response of CD4 T-cells to the peptides and pathology.

3.2 CD4 T-cells provide help for CD8 effector cells

MHC class-I-restricted responses are initiated after antigen-presenting cells (APC) take up exogenous antigens, process them and present short fragments of the antigens via MHC class I to CD8 T-cells. This phenomenon is called cross-priming, as the APC presents antigens synthesized by other cells, and is the main pathway to prime CTL *in vivo* against tumour and other antigens.[32] The main APC in the body is the dendritic cell. Dendritic cells exist in a range of functional states with different capabilities to initiate immune responses. It has been shown in several experimental systems that, for optimal CTL priming, Th must recognize antigen on the same APC that stimulates CTL. Th requirement is based on two functions: synthesis of lymphokines that promote CTL responses, interleukin (IL)-2 being one of the most relevant,[33] and conditioning of dendritic cells to stimulate CTL.[34] In the latter case, dendritic cells are intermediaries between Th and CTL. CD4 T-cells provide signals that induce the differentiation of dendritic cells; two molecules are central in this role: CD40, expressed by dendritic cells, and its ligand CD40L, expressed on activated T-cells.[34] Direct stimulation of CD40 molecules on dendritic cells by anti-CD40 antibody bypasses the need for T-cell help. Additionally, CD4

T-cells are able to condition dendritic cells from mice lacking CD40, suggesting that CD4 T-cells also employ a CD40-independent pathway to condition dendritic cells.[35] Dendritic cells also differentiate to optimal APC in response to signals characteristic of inflammation. This may explain why Th are not always required to prime CTL. Certain conditions may induce an inflammatory environment in which dendritic cells can differentiate in the absence of CD4 T-cells. This is not the case in most cancers, where there is no inflammation, suggesting a strong dependence of antitumour CTL responses on CD4 T-cell help.[30]

Th do not only play an important role in the induction of CTL responses, they may also help to maintain the CTL memory response, as shown in the response against certain viruses.[14] The mechanism by which CD4 T-cells sustain memory CTL is unclear.

3.3 CD4 T-cells can protect in the absence of CD8 cells

In addition to their involvement in optimal CTL priming, CD4 T-cells also display effector functions against tumours. This has been shown in several murine models. Adoptively transferred tumour-specific CD4 T-cells can eradicate tumours in animals.[36] Vaccination with tumour cells transfected with MHC class II molecules activates CD4 T-cells. These effector cells do not only eradicate the genetically modified tumour cell but also the wild-type MHC class-II-negative tumour cell.[37] Vaccination with tumour cells genetically modified to secrete granulocyte–macrophage colony-stimulating factor (GM-CSF) induces a protective CD4 T-cell response.[38] Two effector mechanisms based on cytokine secretion have been implicated, activation and recruitment of macrophages and eosinophils, mediated by Th1 and Th2, respectively. Other possible effector mechanisms described include CD4 T-cell cytotoxicity[29] and, recently, eradication of tumours by CD4 T-cells has been shown to be provoked by interferon-gamma (IFN-γ) release-mediated inhibition of angiogenesis.[39]

Importantly, in some of the experimental systems where effector CD4 T-cells are generated, tumour cells do not express MHC class II molecules. This shows that CD4 T-cells do not need to recognize antigen directly on the tumour cells. The most probable model is that tumour antigens are released in a particular site and are ingested by APC which, after processing and presentation by MHC class II molecules, activate CD4 T-cells. These activated CD4 T-cells will orchestrate the other effector mechanisms involved: macrophages, eosinophils and CTL.

3.4 Regulatory CD4 T-cells can inhibit tumour responses

Many tumour antigens recognized by T-cells are normal self-constituents. In fact, it has been reported that immunotherapy against tumours elicits autoimmunity as a harmful side effect.[10] It is believed that in this case, the response against tumour antigens cross-reacts with normal self-antigens. These observations suggest that tumour immunity is a form of autoimmunity. This has important implications, in particular that the same mechanisms that maintain self-tolerance may inhibit the development of effective antitumour responses.

The two main mechanisms invoked to maintain self-tolerance are clonal deletion and anergy of self-reactive cells. There is accumulating evidence for another mechanism of self-tolerance in which Tr control self-reactive T-cells;[40] this is an active regulatory mechanism in contrast to deletion and anergy which are passive. It is more feasible to disrupt active mechanisms than passive ones. It has long been recognized that treatment with the cytotoxic drug cyclophosphamide increases the generation of effective antitumour responses in certain murine tumour models; it was proposed that this phenomenon was due to the existence of cyclophosphamide-sensitive suppressor (regulatory) T-cells.[41]

CD4 T-cells with regulatory function have been characterized by the expression of several membrane molecules, including specific CD45 isoforms, CD25, CTLA-4, CD38 and others. Interestingly, elimination of CD4 T-cells with a putative regulatory phenotype induces a range

of autoimmune diseases in rodents.[40] Additionally, the elimination of regulatory CD4+CD25+ T-cells elicits potent tumour-specific immune responses to syngeneic tumours *in vivo* and eradicates them. The absence of regulatory CD4 T-cells allows the priming of tumour-specific CD8 T-cells and the activation of tumour-non-specific NK cells.[42] These results suggest that autoimmunity and tumour immunity share a common regulatory basis, and this is of major importance for the design of immunotherapies against tumours.

4. ROLE OF B-CELLS IN TUMOUR IMMUNITY

4.1 Immune responses by B-cells

The role of B-cells in tumour immunity is poorly understood. The presence of increased levels of tumour-specific antibodies in 10–30% of cancer patients provides evidence of B-cell involvement in tumour immunity.[43] The response is often directed against testis cancer antigens (HOM-MEL-40 in melanoma and NY-ESO1 in oesophageal carcinoma),[44,45] or against proteins that are overexpressed in the tumour, such as HOM-RCC3.1.3 in renal cell carcinoma,[44] or against proteins derived from mutated genes such as p53.[46] However, in some cases, an antibody response is observed although the antigen is present in equal amounts in the tumour and in normal tissue, as in the case of HOM-MEL-2-4. The ability to evoke a response only in tumour patients may be due to different post-translational modifications of the antigen in tumour cells or differences in antigen processing and presentation.[47]

The most obvious mechanism by which B-cells could mediate tumour elimination is the production of tumour-specific antibodies. The antibody binds to the tumour cell and mediates the elimination of the tumour cells by antibody-dependent cell-mediated cytotoxicity (ADCC). Immunoglobulin present on tumour cells can also fix complement, activating the complement cascade that leads to lysis of the target cell. Alternatively, the antibody may bind receptors that are vital for the function and growth of the tumour cells, leading to cell death by blocking of the receptor or inducing apoptosis.

Anti-idiotypic antibodies in B-cell lymphoma recognize unique idiotypic determinants in the variable region of the membrane immunoglobulin and, in doing so, have been shown to cause tumour cell apoptosis.[48]

For some antigens, such as Her2/neu or mutated Ras, the humoral response does not correlate with the clinical outcome, suggesting that antibody production is unlikely to play a major role in tumour rejection.[49,50] Only one study, in lung cancer, demonstrated a correlation between the humoral response against autologous tumour cell protein extracts and a better prognosis.[51] In this study, two of 36 patients with good prognosis had antibodies against p53. However, in most studies, a response to p53 was associated with a poor prognosis. This may be due to the requirement of an extended tumour mass to release enough p53 to stimulate an immune response. This is often associated with more aggressive tumour types such as oestrogen and/or progesterone receptor negative breast cancers.

An alternative mechanism by which B-cells could intervene in tumour immunity is via interaction with CD4 Th. Several lines of evidence point to an integrated response of CD4 T-cells, CD8 and B-cells to tumour antigens. Indeed, tyrosinase, Her2/neu, mutated Ras and NYESO-1 elicit both a humoral and cytotoxic T-cell response.[49,52–54] However, there is evidence that B-cells both enhance and diminish tumour immunity.

B-cells play a role in tumour immunity by interacting with Th. Tumour antigen-specific B-cells can act as APC for Th responses when the tumour antigens are present at very low levels.[55] Indeed, B-cells are very effective in capturing the antigen recognized by surface immunoglobulin and present the antigen fragment by MHC class II molecules to Th.[56] Antigen-activated B-cells upregulate expression of co-stimulatory molecules and adhesion molecules such as LFA-1, allowing B-cells to cluster around Th. The most important interaction is between CD40 on B-cells and CD40L on Th. The effect of CD40 on resting B-cells is particularly important when the antigen–antibody interaction is moderate and not very effective.

Depending upon the circumstances, B-cell responses can enhance or inhibit tumour elimination. For instance, immunization with activated B-cells can stimulate cytotoxic T-cells that are usually dependent upon Th1 responses and are important for tumour elimination. However, Th2 CD4+ cells produce IL-4 that promotes B-cell maturation into antibody-secreting plasma cells. Where the T-cell response is skewed towards a predominantly Th2 response, cytotoxic T-cell responses tend to be inhibited, which may favour tumour growth. Uptake of tumour antigens via pinocytosis by resting B-cells can also lead to inhibition of tumour rejection, as the resting B-cells present antigen in the absence of upregulation of co-stimulatory molecules. This leads to delivery of an anergic signal to Th.[57] Indeed, a recent study in BALB/c mice, where B-cells were not present, showed that B-cells inhibited the generation of tumour immunity via inhibition of CD4 Th activity.[58]

4.2 Tumour-specific antibodies in cancer patients

The antibody repertoire of cancer patients can be used for the identification of new tumour antigens using a new technology called SEREX that is based on recombinant expression cloning.[43] A cDNA library is constructed from fresh tumour cells, packaged in lambda phage vectors and expressed in *Escherichia coli*. Bacteria producing tumour antigens are screened for their reactivity with antibody present in the sera of the patient bearing the tumour. The positive bacterial colonies are then expanded and the cDNA sequenced. With this technology it is possible to detect antigens that are unique to the tumour or overexpressed in the tumour cells. One limitation is that antigens that undergo post-translational modifications, not possible in bacteria, may be lost. Antigens that are sequenced with the SEREX system can then be used to elicit B- and T-cell responses.

4.3 Antibody therapy

In principle, monoclonal antibody therapy can be an effective cancer treatment and the level of tumour specificity is determined by the expression pattern of the target antigen. Antibody therapy can exploit the natural mechanism of action of antibodies such as in the case of anti-CD20 (Rituximab) for non-Hodgkin's B-cell lymphoma or anti-Her2/neu (Trastuzamab) for breast cancer.[59,60] CD20 is a B-cell-specific marker involved in cellular growth and differentiation. The molecule is expressed only on B-cell malignancies and normal B-cells. It is an attractive target as it is not shed from cells, and hence will not be mopped up by circulating antigen. Moreover, it does not internalize when bound by anti-CD20 antibody, which can fix complement and mediate ADCC. CD20 promotes survival and proliferation of the tumour cells, and binding of the anti-CD20 antibody can induce cell death by apoptosis.

Several phase I/II clinical trials have demonstrated CD20-specific antibodies to be safe and of low toxicity. A phase III trial showed a initial response rate of 73% but the mean time to relapse was <1 year.[60] Earlier intervention, repetitive treatments, possibly in conjunction with adjuvant surgical therapy or chemotherapy, may improve long-term outcomes.

To enhance the cytotoxicity of anti-CD20 antibodies, antibodies have been designed that carry chemotherapy molecules or radioactive isotopes to the tumour and increase antibody cytotoxicity, decreasing damage to the adjacent organs. Clinical trials of anti-CD20 combined with ^{131}I or ^{90}Y, to take advantage of non-Hodgkin's lymphoma radiosensitivity, resulted in 60–80% response rates, with a median duration of response ranging from 6 to 18 months, although some complete remissions lasted over >5 years.[62]

Novel strategies being explored include the development of antibodies to block angiogenesis in order to 'starve' tumour cells and thus prevent tumour growth. An alternative approach is to use antibodies to potentiate weak ineffective antitumour responses by stimulating receptors on cells of the immune system. For example, the use of anti-CD40 antibodies to activate CD40 molecules on APC, thus promoting more efficient antigen presentation and stimulation of CD8 T-cells, which in turn may eliminate the tumour.[63]

5. ROLE OF NATURAL KILLER (NK) CELLS

5.1 Activating and inhibitory receptors

NK cell activity is controlled by the balance of activating and inhibitory signals.[64,65] The NK inhibitory receptors have immunoreceptor tyrosine-based inhibitory motifs (ITIM) in their cytoplasmic domains that recruit tyrosine phosphatases.[66] The recruitment of phosphatases can lead to the blockade of activating signalling pathways that depend upon intracellular phosphorylation events. The activating receptors of NK cells do not contain ITIM motifs in their cytoplasmic domain. They can associate with adapter proteins that bear immunoreceptor tyrosine-based activation domains (ITAM), and are therefore capable of initiating stimulatory signalling events. Interestingly, inhibitory receptors also exist as activating isoforms with a shortened cytosolic tail, resulting in the loss of inhibitory ITIM motifs (see Table 6.1).

In combination, the balance of inhibitory signals from ITIM receptors and stimulatory signals from ITAM-associated receptors determines the response of NK cells. Most of the inhibitory receptors expressed by NK cells recognize MHC class I molecules and so

Table 6.1 Activating and inhibitory receptors of natural killer (NK) cells

Activating receptors	Inhibitory receptors	Binding ligands
KIR2DS (Short cytosolic tail)	KIR2DL (Long cytosolic tail)	HLA-C
KIR3DS (Short cytosolic tail)	KIR3DL (Long cytosolic tail)	HLA-A3 and -A11 HLA-Bw4
CD94/NKG2C	CD94/NKG2A	HLA-E
NKG2D		MICA, MICB

prevent the lysis of healthy cells that express normal amounts of class I molecules on the cell surface. Downregulation of class I molecules on the target cell surface, by viral infection or transformation, can lead to NK cell activation.[67]

Several activating and inhibitory NK receptors interact with the same MHC molecules on target cells. In these cases, the balance between activating and inhibitory signals is determined by variations in the level of MHC expression, or differences in the affinity of the receptors for MHC, or in the receptor expression levels on NK cells. In addition, activating NK receptors such as NKG2D bind to the non-classical MHC-like molecules, MICA and MICB, which are not recognized by inhibitory NK receptors.[68] Interestingly, these non-classical MHC class I molecules are upregulated on stressed cells and are frequently overexpressed by tumours.[69] This may account for the observation that NK cells sometimes kill tumour cells even if they express normal levels of HLA-A, -B and -C class I molecules.

5.2 Protective immunity mediated by NK cells

The importance of NK-cell-mediated protection against growth of tumour cells with low levels of MHC expression has been clearly demonstrated in elegant murine experiments.[4] It has also been recognized for a long time, again from murine experiments, that NK cells are critical contributors to the rejection of MHC class I mismatched bone marrow grafts.[70] These observations raise the question of whether the role of human NK cells in protection against malignancies and in the outcome of BMT has been underestimated so far. This issue is particularly relevant for the treatment of leukaemia, which frequently involves allogeneic BMT and the infusion of donor leucocytes, including T-cells and NK cells.

The expression pattern of KIR genes can vary considerably among individuals,[71] and KIR epitope mismatches lead to NK alloreactivity.[72] It is possible that alloreactive NK cells may kill normal and leukaemia cells after infusion into KIR-epitope-incompatible patients. Indeed, transplants from KIR-epitope-incompatible donors had higher engraftment rates compared with KIR-epitope-matched donor recipient

combinations.[73] It will be interesting to see if NK cells can display graft versus leukaemia (GvL) effects as well as engraftment-facilitating functions in KIR-epitope-mismatched patients. The use of NK cell populations expressing NK receptors of defined specificity might lead to the development of antigen-specific NK treatment in the context of allogeneic BMT.

5.3 Regulatory NK T-cells (NKT)

Murine studies have identified a population of NKT, characterized by the expression of CD3 molecules and NK markers.[74,75] Unlike classical T-cells, NKT express intermediate amounts of TCR (TCRαβ) molecules and exhibit a very restricted TCR usage ($V_\alpha 14$-$J_\alpha 281$, $V_\beta 2$, $V_\beta 7$ or $V_\beta 8$). NKT account for only 2–3% of the total T-cell population in peripheral lymphoid organs. The function and development of NKT is restricted by the MHC class-I-like molecule CD1. For example, CD1-deficient mice showed a severe diminution in number of NKT.[37–40] CD4+ NKT produce large quantities of IL-4 following *in vivo* stimulation,[76] suggesting that they may downregulate immune responses by Th1. Indeed, NKT were shown to function as suppressor cells through the secretion of IL-4.[77] This raises the possibility that NKT may inhibit Th1-dependent immune responses against tumours. Recent experiments have confirmed this possibility.

Animals exposed to subcarcinogenic doses of UV radiation are immune suppressed, which facilitates the outgrowth of highly antigenic UV-induced skin cancer.[78] It was shown some time ago, that the immunosuppression of UV-irradiated animals is transferable to normal recipients by CD4+ T-cells.[79] The identity of the cells and the detailed mechanisms that mediate the immunosuppression remained unclear, though IL-4 was involved. The critical role of NKT in enhancing the growth of UV-induced skin cancers has now been demonstrated.[80] In a murine UV-induced tumour model, CD1-restricted NKT were shown to inhibit the tumour-protective immune response by CD8+ cytotoxic T-cells. These studies point to a possible involvement of regulatory NKT in human skin cancer.

6. CONCLUSIONS

Many of the basic mechanisms by which the immune system can recognize malignant cells have been revealed and tumour antigens have been identified at the molecular level. There is hope that this new knowledge will help to realize the dream of tumour immunologists – the development of cancer vaccines. At present, most immunotherapy and vaccination protocols exploit primarily one effector arm of the immune system. Protocols that can harness the protective effects of Th, CTL and antibody-producing B-cells need to be developed to reduce the risk of tumour escape from immuno-logical attack.

The uncovering of the mechanisms by which certain NK subpopulations can recognize and kill tumour cells may allow us to exploit these populations for adoptive immunotherapy. Finally, NK cells as well as CD4 T-cells display regulatory activities that can prevent effective tumour immunity. The concept of removing such negative regulators to enhance tumour immunity has already been validated in animal experiments.

ACKNOWLEDGEMENTS

The authors were funded by the Leukaemia Research Fund and by Cancer Research UK.

REFERENCES

Scientific papers

1. Foley EJ. Antigenic properties of methylcholan-threne-induced tumours in mice of the strain of origin. *Cancer Res* 1953; **13**: 835–7.
2. Burnet FM. The concept of immunological surveillance. *Prog Exp Tumour Res* 1970; **13**: 1–27.
3. van der Bruggen P, Traversari C, Chomez P et al. A gene encoding an antigen recognized by cytolytic T lymphocytes on a human melanoma. *Science* 1991; **254**: 1643–7.
4. Ljunggren HG, Karre K. Host resistance directed selectively against H-2-deficient lymphoma variants. Analysis of the mechanism. *J Exp Med* 1985; **162**: 1745–59.
5. Boon T, van der Bruggen P. Human tumour antigens recognized by T lymphocytes. *J Exp Med* 1996; **183**: 725–9.

6. Huang K, Lin S. Nationwide vaccination: a success story in Taiwan. *Vaccine* 2000; **18**: S35–S38.
7. Safary A, Beck J. Vaccination against hepatitis B: current challenges for Asian countries and future directions. *J Gastroenterol Hepatol* 2000; **15**: 396–401.
8. Skipper J, Stauss HJ. Identification of two cytotoxic T lymphocyte-recognized epitopes in the Ras protein. *J Exp Med* 1993; **177**: 1493–8.
9. Lucas S, De Plaen E, Boon T. MAGE-B5, MAGE-B6, MAGE-C2, and MAGE-C3: four new members of the MAGE family with tumour-specific expression. *Int J Cancer* 2000; **87**: 55–60.
10. Rosenberg SA, White De. Vitiligo in patients with melanoma: normal tissue antigens can be targets for cancer immunotherapy. *J Immunother* 1996; **19**: 81–4.
11. Kast WM, Offringa R, Peters PJ et al. Eradication of adenovirus E1-induced tumours by E1A-specific cytotoxic T lymphocytes. *Cell* 1989; **59**: 603–14.
12. Rooney CM, Smith CA, Ng CY et al. Infusion of cytotoxic T cells for the prevention and treatment of Epstein-Barr virus-induced lymphoma in allogeneic transplant recipients. *Blood* 1998; **92**: 1549–55.
13. Rooney CM, Smith CA, Ng CY et al. Use of gene-modified virus-specific T lymphocytes to control Epstein-Barr-virus-related lymphoproliferation. *Lancet* 1995; **345**: 9–13.
14. Matloubian M, Concepcion RJ, Ahmed R. CD4+ T cells are required to sustain CD8+ cytotoxic T-cell responses during chronic viral infection. *J Virol* 1994; **68**: 8056–63.
15. Albert ML, Darnell JC, Bender A et al. Tumour-specific killer cells in paraneoplastic cerebellar degeneration. *Nature Med* 1998: **4**: 1321–4.
16. Morgan DJ, Krewel HT, Fleck S et al. Activation of low avidity CTL specific for a self epitope results in tumour rejection but not autoimmunity. *J Immunol* 1998; **160**: 643–51.
17. Ludewig B, Ochsenbein AF, Odermatt B et al. Immunotherapy with dendritic cells directed against tumour antigens shared with normal host cells results in severe autoimmune disease. *J Exp Med* 2000; **191**: 795–804.
18. Ganss R, Limmer A, Sacher T et al. Autoaggression and tumour rejection: it takes more than self-specific T-cell activation. *Immunol Rev* 1999; **169**: 263–72.
19. Colella TA, Bullock TN, Russell LB et al. Self-tolerance to the murine homologue of a tyrosi-nase-derived melanoma antigen: implications for tumour immunotherapy. *J Exp Med* 2000; **191**: 1221–32.

20. Theobald M, Biggs J, Hernandez J et al. Tolerance to p53 by A2.1-restricted cytotoxic T lymphocytes. *J Exp Med* 1997; **185**: 833–41.

21. Matzinger P, Zamoyska R, Waldmann H. Self tolerance is H-2-restricted. *Nature* 1984; **308**: 738–41.

22. Rammensee HG, Bevan MJ. Evidence from *in vitro* studies that tolerance to self antigens is MHC-restricted. *Nature* 1984; **308**: 741–4.

23. Sadovnikova E, Stauss HJ. Peptide-specific cytotoxic T lymphocytes restricted by nonself major histocompatibility complex class I molecules: reagents for tumour immunotherapy. *Proc Natl Acad Sci USA* 1996; **93**: 13,114–18.

24. Sadovnikova E, Jopling LA, Soo KS, Stauss HJ. Generation of human tumour-reactive cytotoxic T cells against peptides presented by non-self HLA class I molecules. *Eur J Immunol* 1998; **28**: 193–200.

25. Gao L, Bellantuono I, Elsasser A et al. Selective elimination of leukemic CD34(+) progenitor cells by cytotoxic T lymphocyes specific for WT1. *Blood* 2000; **95**: 2198–203.

26. Yamagami T, Sugiyama H, Inoue K et al. Growth inhibition of human leukemic cells by WT1 (Wilms tumour gene) antisense oligodeoxynucleotides: implications for the involvement of WT1 in leukemogenesis. *Blood* 1996; **87**: 2878–84.

27. Oji Y, Ogawa H, Tamaki H et al. Expression of the Wilms' tumour gene WT1 in solid tumours and its involvement in tumour cell growth. *Jpn J Cancer Res* 1999; **90**: 194–204.

28. Clay TM, Custer MC, Sachs J et al. Efficient transfer of a tumour antigen-reactive TCR to human peripheral blood lymphocytes confers antitumour reactivity. *J Immunol* 1999; **163**: 507–13.

29. Pardoll DM, Topalian SL. The role of CD4+ T cell responses in antitumour immunity. *Curr Opin Immunol* 1998; **10**: 588–94.

30. Toes REM, Ossendorp F, Offringa R, Melief CJM. CD4 T cells and their role in antitumour immune responses. *J Exp Med* 1999; **189**: 753–6.

31. Wang RF, Wang X, Atwood AC et al. Cloning genes encoding MHC class II-restricted antigens: mutated CDC27 as a tumour antigen. *Science* 1999; **284**: 1351–4.

32. Huang AY, Golumbek P, Ahmadzadeh M et al. Role of bone marrow-derived cells in presenting MHC class I-restricted tumour antigens. *Science* 1994; **264**: 961–5.

33. Keene JA, Forman J. Helper activity is required for the *in vivo* generation of cytotoxic T lymphocytes. *J Exp Med* 1982; **155**: 768–82.

34. Schoenberger SP, Toes REM, van der Voort EIH et al. T cell help for cytotoxic T lymphocytes is mediated by CD40–CD40L interactions. *Nature* 1998; **393**: 490–3.

35. Lu Z, Yuan L, Zhou X et al. CD40-independent pathways of T cell help for priming of CD8+ cytotoxic T lymphocytes. *J Exp Med* 2000; **191**: 541–50.

36. Greenberg PD, Cheever MA, Fefer A. Eradication of disseminated murine leukaemia by chemoimmuno-therapy with cyclophosphamide and adoptively transferred immune syngeneic Lyt1+2- lymphocytes. *J Exp Med* 1981; **154**: 952–63.

37. Ostrand-Rosenberg S, Thakur A, Clements V. Rejection of mouse sarcoma cells after transfectionof MHC class II genes. *J Immunol* 1990; **144**: 4068–71.

38. Hung K, Hayashi R, Lafond-Walker A et al. The central role of CD4+ T cells in the antitumour immune response. *J Exp Med* 1998; **188**: 2357–68.

39. Qin Z, Blankenstein T. CD4+ T cell-mediated tumour rejection involves inhibition of angiogenesis that is dependent on IFNg receptor expression by nonhematopoietic cells. *Immunity* 2000; **12**: 677–86.

40. Mason D, Powrie F. Control of immune pathology by regulatory T cells. *Curr Opin Immunol* 1998; **10**: 649–55.

41. North RJ. Cyclophosphamide-facilitated adoptive immunotherapy of an established tumour depends on elimination of tumour-induced suppressor T cells. *J Exp Med* 1982; **155**: 1063–74.

42. Shimizu J, Yamazaki S, Sakaguchi S. Induction of tumour immunity by removing CD25+ CD4+ T cells: a common basis between tumour immunity and autoimmunity. *J Immunol* 1999; **163**: 5211–18.

43. Sahin U, Tureci O, Pfreundschuh M. Serological identification of human tumour antigens. *Curr Opin Immunol* 1997; **9**: 709–16.

44. Sahin U, Tureci O, Schmitt H et al. Human neoplasms elicit multiple specific immune responses in the autologous host. *Proc Natl Acad Sci USA* 1995; **92**: 11,810–13.

45. Chen YT, Scanlan MJ, Sahin U et al. A testicular antigen aberrantly expressed in human cancers detected by autologous antibody screening. *Proc Natl Acad Sci USA* 1997; **94**: 1914–18.

46. Angelopoulou K, Diamandis EP, Sutherland DJ et al. Prevalence of serum antibodies against the p53 tumour suppressor gene protein in various cancers. *Int J Cancer* 1994; **58**: 480–7.

47. Skipper JC, Hendrickson RC, Gulden PH et al. An HLA-A2-restricted tyrosinase antigen on

melanoma cells results from posttranslational modification and suggests a novel pathway for processing of membrane proteins. *J Exp Med* 1996; **183**: 527–34.

48. Vuist WM, Levy R, Maloney DG. Lymphoma regression induced by monoclonal anti-idiotypic antibodies correlates with their ability to induce Ig signal transduction and is not prevented by tumour expression of high levels of bcl-2 protein. *Blood* 1994; **83**: 899–906.

49. Disis ML, Calenoff E, McLaughlin G et al. Existent T-cell and antibody immunity to HER-2/neu protein in patients with breast cancer. *Cancer Res* 1994; **54**: 16–20.

50. Disis ML, Cheever MA. Oncogenic proteins as tumour antigens. *Curr Opin Immunol* 1996; **8**: 637–42.

51. Winter SF, Sekido Y, Minna JD et al. Antibodies against autologous tumour cell proteins in patients with small-cell lung cancer: association with improved survival. *J Natl Cancer Inst* 1993; **85**: 2012–18.

52. Topalian SL, Gonzales MI, Parkhurst M et al. Melanoma-specific CD4+ T cells recognize nonmutated HLA-DR-restricted tyrosinase epitopes. *J Exp Med* 1996; **183**: 1965–71.

53. Jager E, Gnjatic S, Nagata Y et al. Induction of primary NY-ESO-1 immunity: CD8+ T lympho-cyte and antibody responses in peptide-vaccinated patients with NY-ESO-1+ cancers. *Proc Natl Acad Sci USA* 2000; **97**: 12,198–203.

54. Abrams SI, Stanziale SF, Lunin SD et al. Identification of overlapping epitopes in mutant ras oncogene peptides that activate CD4+ and CD8+ T cell responses. *Eur J Immunol* 1996; **26**: 435–43.

55. Metlay JP, Pure E, Steinman RM. Control of the immune response at the level of antigen-presenting cells: a comparison of the function of dendritic cells and B lymphocytes. *Adv Immunol* 1989; **47**: 45–116.

56. Lanzavecchia A. Receptor-mediated antigen uptake and its effect on antigen presentation to class II-restricted T lymphocytes. *Annu Rev Immunol* 1990; **8**: 773–93.

57. Zhong G, Sousa CR, Germain RN. Antigen-unspecific B cells and lymphoid dendritic cells both show extensive surface expression of processed antigen-major histocompatibility complex class II complexes after soluble protein exposure *in vivo* or *in vitro*. *J Exp Med* 1997; **186**: 673–82.

58. Qin Z, Richter G, Schuler T et al. B cells inhibit induction of T cell-dependent tumour immunity. *Nature Med* 1998; **4**: 627–30.

59. Stebbing J, Copson E, O'Reilly S. Herceptin (trastuzamab) in advanced breast cancer. *Cancer Treat Rev* 2000; **26**: 287–90.

60. Green MC, Murray JL, Hortobagyi GN. Monoclonal antibody therapy for solid tumours. *Cancer Treat Rev* 2000; **26**: 269–86.

61. Colombat P, Salles G, Brousse N et al. Rituximab (anti-CD20 monoclonal antibody) as single first-line therapy for patients with follicular lymphoma with a low tumour burden: clinical and molecular evaluation. *Blood* 2001; **97**: 101–6.

62. Kaminski MS, Estes J, Zasadny KR et al. Radioimmunotherapy with iodine (131)I tositumomab for relapsed or refractory B-cell non-Hodgkin lymphoma: updated results and long-term follow-up of the University of Michigan experience. *Blood* 2000; **96**: 1259–66.

63. French RR, Chan HT, Tutt AL, Glennie MJ. CD40 antibody evokes a cytotoxic T-cell response that eradicates lymphoma and bypasses T-cell help. *Nature Med* 1999; **5**: 548–53.

64. Lanier LL. NK cell receptors. *Annu Rev Immunol* 1998; **16**: 359–93.

65. Lanier LL. On guard – activating NK cell receptors. *Nat Immunol* 2001; **2**: 23–7.

66. Long EO. Regulation of immune responses through inhibitory receptors. *Annu Rev Immunol* 1999; **17**: 875–904.

67. Algarra I, Cabrera T, Garrido F. The HLA cross-road in tumour immunology. *Hum Immunol* 2000; **61**: 65–73.

68. Bahram S, Bresnahan M, Geraghty DE, Spies T. A second lineage of mammalian major histocompatibility complex class I genes. *Proc Natl Acad Sci USA* 1994; **91**: 6259–63.

69. Groh V, Rhinehart R, Secrist H et al. Broad tumour-associated expression and recognition by tumour-derived gamma delta T cells of MICA and MICB. *Proc Natl Acad Sci USA* 1999; **96**: 6879–84.

70. Cudhowicz G, Bennett M. Peculiar immunobiology of bone marrow allografts. II. Rejection of parental grafts by resistant F 1 hybrid mice. *J Exp Med* 1971; **134**: 1513–28.

71. Uhrberg M, Valiante NM, Shum BP et al. Human diversity in killer cell inhibitory receptor genes. *Immunity* 1997; **7**: 753–63.

72. Moretta A, Bottino C, Pende D et al. Identification of four subsets of human CD3-CD16+ natural killer (NK) cells by the expression of clonally distributed functional surface molecules: correlation between subset assignment of NK clones and ability to mediate specific alloantigen recognition. *J Exp Med* 1990; **172**: 1589–98.

73. Ruggeri L, Capanni M, Casucci M et al. Role of natural killer cell alloreactivity in HLA-mismatched hematopoietic stem cell transplantation. *Blood* 1999; **94**: 333–9.

74. Bendelac A, Rivera MN, Park SH, Roark JH. Mouse CD1-specific NK1 T cells: development, specificity, and function. *Annu Rev Immunol* 1997; **15**: 535–62.

75. Mendiratta SK, Martin WD, Hong S et al. CD1d1 mutant mice are deficient in natural T cells that promptly produce IL-4. *Immunity* 1997; **6**: 469–77.

76. Yoshimoto T, Bendelac A, Watson C et al. Role of NK1.1+ T cells in a TH2 response and in immunoglobulin E production. *Science* 1995; **270**: 1845–7.

77. Sonoda KH, Exley M, Snapper S et al. CD1-reactive natural killer T cells are required for development of systemic tolerance through an immune-privileged site. *J Exp Med* 1999; **190**: 1215–26.

78. Fisher MS, Kripke ML. Suppressor T lymphocytes control the development of primary skin cancers in ultraviolet-irradiated mice. *Science* 1982; **216**: 1133–4.

79. Ullrich SE, Kripke ML. Mechanisms in the suppression of tumour rejection produced in mice by repeated UV irradiation. *J Immunol* 1984; **133**: 2786–90.

80. Moodycliffe AM, Nghiem D, Clydesdale G, Ullrich SE. Immune suppression and skin cancer development: regulation by NKT cells. *Nat Immunol* 2000; **1**: 521–5.

Section B

Infection

7

Genetic susceptibility to infection

Jeremy Hull

Objectives • Overview • Introduction • Aim of studies of genetic susceptibility • Available methods for study • Interpretation of positive disease association studies • Interpetation of negative disease association studies • Examples where a genetic component of susceptibility to infection has been shown • General comments • The future • Glossary • References

OBJECTIVES

(1) To introduce the concept of genetic susceptibility to infection with the normal population.
(2) To indicate the power of this approach as a tool for understanding disease pathogenesis.
(3) To discuss the methods currently available for studying genetic susceptibility, their aims, interpretations and limitations, and some of the findings.

OVERVIEW

Infections are diseases that arise in any given individual as a result of complex interactions between the environment, the pathogen and the host. An understanding of the host response component of this interaction is important for the development and targeting of novel therapies and vaccines. Investigations of host responses have indicated that large numbers of mediators are likely to be involved. Molecular genetics provides a new tool to study these complicated interactions. It has the potential to identify true susceptibility and therefore the causal mechanisms in the disease pathogenesis.

1. INTRODUCTION

The use of genetic susceptibility studies as a way of understanding complex interactions in disease processes (not just infectious diseases) has expanded over the last five years, largely as a result of the rapidly rising number of useful DNA markers that have emerged as a spin-off of the Human Genome Project. There are now many examples where convincing association between genetic variants and infection has been demonstrated. Instances where this knowledge has led to novel insights into pathogenesis or to new therapeutic approaches are much less common. In this review, the methods currently available, their aims, interpretations and limitations, and some of the findings, will be discussed. Others have reviewed the evidence for genetic susceptibility to specific infections in more detail.[1,2]

There is no doubt that some individuals are more likely to suffer from infectious disease than others. This increased risk may be due to many reasons, including contributions from the environment, which may increase exposure to pathogens (e.g. poor sanitation or overcrowding), ard from the host, such as the presence of other illnesses [e.g. human immunodeficiency virus (HIV) infection or malnutrition], as well as genetic defects in innate and acquired immunity. In the majority of the cases where genetic defects have been identified, they arise as a result of mutations of a single gene. An example of a genetic defect is seen in boys with agammaglobulinaemia. These boys have a high incidence of bacterial sepsis and few or no B-cells. The condition occurs because of mutation of the B-cell cytoplasmic tyrosine kinase gene (*btk*).[3] In this disease, and others like it that affect T-cells, neutrophils and complement, the mechanism which leads to increased susceptibility to infection is well understood and individually the diseases are rare. In this chapter, the more general concept of differing susceptibility to infections as a consequence of genetically determined variations in immune responses of different individuals within a normal population is explored.

Two assumptions are made. Firstly, the known variation seen in most measurable biological parameters (e.g. height, hair colour, plasma sodium level) extends to the host response against pathogens. It would be more remarkable if there were no variation; nevertheless, evidence for this type of variation is not available for many immune responses. Secondly, at least some of this variability occurs as a consequence of differences in the DNA sequence. At the simplest level, these DNA differences may affect the structure of a protein and interfere with its function. More subtle differences might affect the expression of these genes, e.g. one individual may be a high responder to a particular stimulus whereas another individual may produce a lesser amount of the same gene product. That different individuals have different and unique genomic DNA sequences is not in doubt. Indeed, they form the basis of forensic DNA testing – it has been estimated that there are at least three million DNA differences between any two individuals. There is now good evidence that genetic variability can influence susceptibility to a number of infectious diseases. The suggestion that the phenomenon is at work in all common infections is open to question. Nor can we be sure that understanding the basis of susceptibility will lead to important advances in treatment of infections.

2. AIMS OF STUDIES OF GENETIC SUSCEPTIBILITY

2.1 Increased understanding of pathogenesis of infection

Most infectious diseases occur as a consequence of a complex series of events. As mentioned, some of these are environmental, such as the risk of exposure, others relate to virulence of the pathogen and to the host response. For example, the likelihood of becoming ill with malaria will be higher in those who sleep near a marsh in the Gambia or get bitten by a mosquito carrying a multidrug-resistant *Plasmodium falciparum* parasite or who have never had malaria before and therefore have no immunity to the parasite.

The traditional approach to studying host responses involves generating a model of the pathogenesis and then measuring immunomodulatory responses in secretions or blood. Concentrations of these modulators are then correlated with outcome and compared to those found in controls. There are a number of difficulties with this analysis. The most important is whether what is measured is responsible for the disease process or is a consequence of it. If it is the latter, attempts to target that component of the immune response with the hope of altering outcome would be fruitless. There are also technical problems; e.g. tests frequently need to be performed soon after the sample has been collected, the specimen volume limits the number of different indicators which can be measured and what can be measured is limited by the availability of appropriate assays.

Genetic studies avoid many of these problems. A genetic disease association indicates that the gene variant predisposes to *susceptibility* to the disease as defined in the index cases. Once the index case has been identified and DNA collected, several thousand assays can be performed, if necessary several years after the sample is taken, and any gene can be studied.

In practice, it is likely that these two approaches will complement each other, one providing corroborative evidence for the other. Once particular mechanisms have been shown to be important in the pathogenesis, they can provide targets for intervention. For example, if a variant of gene A leads to increased activity of protein A, and the gene variant was associated with a specific infection, then it is reasonable to conclude that protein A is important in the pathogenesis of that disease. Monoclonal antibodies to block the activity of protein A may then modulate the disease process. This approach has been used in the development of new drugs for HIV infection. It has been found that a variant of the chemokine receptor CCR5 leads to more rapid progression of the disease, presumably by enhancing viral entry into cells.[4] This highlighted the importance of these receptors in HIV disease pathogenesis and have recently led to the development of chemokine-receptor blocking drugs.[5] These drugs are now in the clinical trial phase of development.

Improved understanding of disease pathogenesis may also aid vaccine development. For example, vaccines which elicit a host response known to be associated with good outcome from infection would be favoured over those which elicited responses associated with poor outcomes.

2.2 Increased understanding of genes and gene regulation

DNA variants with well-defined functional effects are the variants of choice for genetic association studies. They have the advantage that should a positive association be found, the mechanism of the disease association will be readily apparent. Unfortunately, the number of such variants is small and most studies use markers with no known function. If a particular DNA variant is convincingly shown to be associated with susceptibility to a disease, then it follows that there must be some functional effect linked with that variant. Understanding the nature of the functional variation can lead to increased knowledge of the activity of the gene product or the regulation of expression of the gene. For example, Knight et al[6] have shown

that a polymorphic variant in the promoter of tumour necrosis factor (TNF) is associated with a four-fold increased risk of developing cerebral malaria. Further analysis of the DNA sequence containing the polymorphism has revealed a previously undiscovered region of DNA–protein interaction, which influences the expression of TNF, and has led to efforts to isolate and clone a novel transcription factor.

2.3 Identification of at-risk individuals

In future, it may be possible to determine an individual's genotype in order to determine their likelihood of suffering from a particular infection. Susceptible individuals could then be offered specific intervention. For example, palivizumab, a monoclonal antibody directed against respiratory syncytial virus (RSV), provides protection against developing the lower respiratory tract infection bronchiolitis caused by this virus. Palivizumab needs to be given by monthly injection for 5 months. Although bronchiolitis is common, and results in 20,000 admissions to hospital each winter in the UK,[7] within the population the incidence is only 1%. It is well known that infants with pre-existing heart and lung disease or prematurity are more at risk of suffering from bronchiolitis, but the majority of disease occurs in previously well infants. It is not practical to provide passive immunization on a population basis. If it were possible to genetically identify the 1% with a high risk of developing bronchiolitis, then these infants could be offered the treatment.

3. AVAILABLE METHODS FOR STUDY

Usually, when a causative pathogen is common there will be widespread exposure. The incidence of clinical disease will be much lower and it is reasoned that it is the susceptible individuals who become ill. The first step in undertaking genetic susceptibility studies is to define the disease to be investigated. It is essential to have a precise definition of the disease; it is the phenotype by which affected individuals are identified. The second step is to collect DNA samples from cases, controls and/or family members depending on the type of study being carried out. DNA can be extracted from blood (1 ml is sufficient) or from buccal smears – the latter approach is especially useful in children. The third step is to identify the genotypes present and carry out linkage or association analysis.

3.1 Linkage versus association

3.1.1 Linkage methods

Until recently, most methods for identifying the genetic elements responsible for disease have used linkage analysis.[8] The methods require DNA samples from families in which there are either three or more generations of affected individuals, or parents and at least two affected siblings. Linkage analysis then determines whether affected individuals within a family share specific fragments of DNA more often than expected by chance. The fragments of DNA are tracked through the families using DNA markers spread evenly across the genome (most studies use about 300–400 markers). If it is found that the same region of DNA is inherited by affected individuals more often than expected in many different families, a susceptibility gene is likely to reside somewhere in that DNA fragment. When the affects of the susceptibility gene are strong, as in monogenetic disorders like cystic fibrosis, linkage is likely to be successful. Even so, the size of DNA fragment identified will be very large, often several million bases long and containing hundreds of genes. A great deal more work is then necessary to find the specific gene responsible for the effect. Although linkage methods have been used for mapping genetic effects for susceptibility to tuberculosis and schistosomiasis,[9,10] in general, the contribution of each genetic element to complex diseases like infections will be too small for this method to be generally useful for identifying causal mechanisms. Furthermore, there are practical problems in collecting sufficient numbers of parents and affected siblings for many infectious diseases.

3.1.2 Association methods

Association studies are thought to be more appropriate for identifying genetic susceptibility in complex diseases like infections.[11] These studies are not concerned with inheritance of regions of DNA; rather, they compare allele frequencies at specific genetic loci between affected individuals and controls. An allele is said to be associated with the disease if it occurs more frequently in affected individuals. Put simply, if the entire population is sampled and it is found that an allele occurs twice as often in affected individuals as non-affected, it follows that individuals possessing this allele have a two-fold increased risk of getting the disease.

3.2 Genomewide searches

Association studies can be used either for genomewide or candidate gene studies. A genomewide search for genetic susceptibility is attractive because it requires no assumptions of pathogenesis. Previously unknown genes may be implicated in susceptibility. Once the function of the genes is established, new and unexpected insight into the pathogenesis of the disease may be gained. The difficulty is that it has been estimated that as many as 500,000 DNA markers would be needed to achieve genomewide coverage with a reasonable chance of finding true positive associations where they exist.[12] This number of markers was derived from theoretical calculation of linkage disequilibrium (LD; see Box 7.1), which suggested that LD is likely to extend over only 3 kilobases (kb). This means that each marker would only provide information about the 3 kb of surrounding DNA and thus 500,000 markers would be needed to cover the three billion bases in the human genome. The estimate of 3 kb may turn out to be an underestimate of the true extent of LD (there are increasing numbers of loci where LD has been shown to extend tens or even hundreds of kilobases; see Koch et al[13]), but even if 10 times fewer markers were required, with current technology, a genomewide approach using 50,000 markers would not be feasible for most laboratories. Nevertheless, DNA collections being undertaken at present should be sufficiently large to allow genomewide studies when the necessary advances in methodology have been made.

Box 7.1 Linkage disequilibrium (LD)

To understand LD a recap on cell biology, long forgotten by most of us is needed. Each nucleated human cell has two copies of each chromosome (apart from the X and Y chromosomes in males). Although each pair of homologous chromosomes are identical in basic structure (e.g. which genes are present), many loci will possess different alleles. During meiosis, homologous chromosomes line up together and swap bits of DNA, a process called *recombination*. Once this process is complete the chromosomes are despatched to the daughter cells. Which of the two homologous chromosomes ends up in which daughter cell is entirely random (so-called *random segregation*). Thus, if two markers are located on different chromosomes there is a 50:50 chance they will end up in the same offspring. The situation is obviously going to be different for two markers on the same chromosome. If there was no recombination between the two markers they would always end up together. These markers are then said be in *complete linkage*. The likelihood of a recombination event occurring that would separate the markers is dependent on how far apart the markers are on the chromosome. The probability of a recombination event occurring within one generation is about 1% for markers separated by about 1 million bases, so a degree of linkage will therefore exist over very large chromosomal distances. In a population where, say, there have been 100 generations, there will have been 100 opportunities for the two markers to be separated and the likelihood of two markers on the same chromosome occurring together will be much lower. For markers a long way apart the probability of this happening will be the same as if they were on different chromosomes and equal to the product of the frequencies of each marker in the population. These markers are then said to show *random association*. For markers that remain linked, the frequency at which they occur together will be greater than this, and the random association or equilibrium will be lost, hence the term *linkage disequilibrium* (*LD*). The distance over which linkage, and hence LD, extends seems to vary considerably, both in terms of chromosomal location and ethnic origin of the population studied. The extent of LD is critical in understanding the results of disease-association studies. If LD extends for only 2 or 3 kilobases, then if a marker shows a positive disease association, the disease-causing gene is very nearby. On the other hand if LD extends tens or even hundreds of kilobases, then the functional variant may lie anywhere in the intervening sequence. Extensive LD would, however, be advantageous for genome-wide approaches, since it would mean that fewer markers were needed to cover the genome. It is also important to realize that just because a marker is close to the disease-causing DNA variant (and in complete LD with it), that it will not necessarily be efficient in detecting the disease susceptibility effect (see Fig. 7.3) later.

3.3 Candidate gene analysis

Analysis of candidate genes is more practical but requires a model of pathogenesis. This may be derived from animal work or by measuring immune modulators, such as cytokines, in affected individuals and correlating the results with outcome. Once a model has been generated, specific genes can be identified as key players and their involvement tested by genetic association methods. It is possible to use single nucleotide polymorphisms (SNP) or microsatellites (Box 7.2) in candidate gene studies.

Box 7.2 Types of DNA variant

Single nucleotide polymorphisms (SNP)

These are single base differences that are identified by comparing the same sequence between different individuals. For example, at a given base position, one chromosome may carry an adenine (A base) and another chromosome may carry a cytosine (C base). SNPs probably arise as the result of an error made during replication in a single individual. With time, the SNP may become more common within a population. For neutral SNPs to have risen to frequencies above a few per cent, it is likely that they arose several thousand years ago. SNPs have the advantage of being stable DNA changes. It is extremely rare for a second error to be made at the same position that corrects the original mistake. This stability is one of the major advantages of the use of SNPs as DNA markers. They also occur frequently throughout the genome (one occurs every 500–1000 bases or so), and so it is always likely one will be present near the gene of interest. Over 800,000 SNPs have been registered by the SNP consortium, http://snp.csh1.org although population frequencies are available for only a very small proportion. Finally, SNPs are relatively easy to type (i.e. to work out which variant is present in a given individual) and amenable to high-throughput automated technology. The vast majority of SNPs will be neutral (non-functional).

Their major disadvantage is that they only have two alleles (e.g. a chromosome can carry either an A or a C). This limits their usefulness in dividing a population to look for association, since only two groups can be identified with a single SNP. Combining several SNP together and constructing *haplotypes* (a set of markers on a chromosome) gets around this problem.

Microsatellites

This is the second major type of DNA variant used in genetic association studies. These markers are repeats of usually of two, three or four bases that occur in clusters. For example, a trinucleotide repeat would look like this: ACG ACG ACG ACG ACG. It is the *number* of repeats that differs on different chromosomes (in this example there are five). Microsatellites probably also arise due to errors made in copying DNA during cell division. Microsatellites often have four or more different repeat lengths, making them a more informative marker than bi-allelic SNPs. Like SNPs they are relatively easy to type and occur frequently throughout the genome. The major disadvantage of microsatellites is that they are thought to be relatively unstable and the number of repeat lengths could change in a few generations.

Conceptually, the simplest study design is a case-control study (Fig. 7.1). DNA is collected from precisely defined cases and from carefully matched, unaffected controls. The frequency of a DNA variant in the cases is then compared with that in controls. From this data an odds ratio (OR) is calculated. This is a powerful approach and the simple design means it is relatively easy to collect large numbers of cases and controls. The major disadvantage is that it is difficult to be certain that positive results do not reflect undetected differences between cases and controls other than

disease state. The commonest pitfall reflects ethnic differences. For example, if cases are acquired using a definition of smear-positive tuberculosis (TB) and controls are routine blood donors, it is possible that the ethnic mix in each group will differ. Since most allele frequencies differ according to ethnicity, any apparent association may simply reflect differences in the population structure rather than susceptibility to TB. Differences in ethnicity can be subtle and difficult to detect, yet they can produce both false-positive and false-negative results.

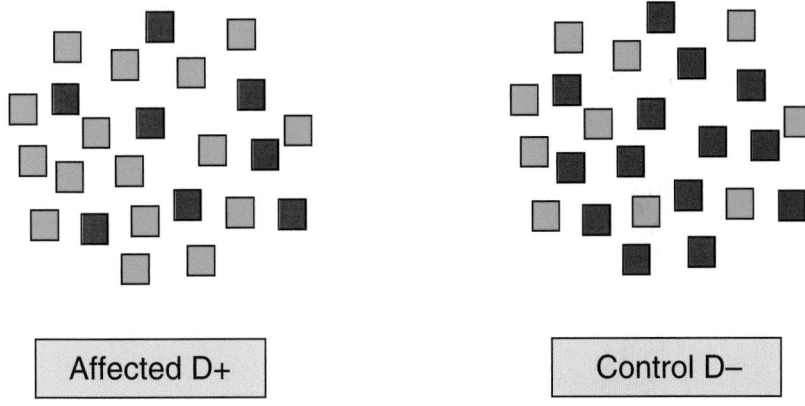

Affected D+   Control D−

Fig. 7.1 Case-control study. Cases are selected by a given phenotypic characteristic, e.g. blood-culture-proven pneumococcal septicaemia. At least an equal number of carefully matched controls are identified. Allele frequencies are then compared between the two groups. For relatively rare diseases (affecting < 10% of the population), odds ratio (OR) gives the best estimate of true relative risk (RR) within the population. In this example:

	Affected (D+)	Control (D−)
Blue allele	16	10
Red allele	8	14

OR = (16/8) / (10/14) = 2.8.

Note the OR is the same whether it is calculated as the odds of being affected if carrying the blue variant or the odds of carrying the blue variant if affected. It estimates the true population risk of being affected if carrying the allele of interest. The probability (*P* value) is calculated by the chi-square test or Fisher's exact test. In this example, *P* = 0.08

A family-based design gets around this problem. In this study design, DNA samples are collected from the index case and both parents (case–parent triads). The frequency of alleles in the offspring is compared to what would be expected given the parental genotype (Fig. 7.2). The results are often reported as percentage transmission, i.e. is the allele of interest transmitted from the parents to the offspring significantly more or less often than the expected 50%? A positive result implicates the allele as a susceptibility (or protective) factor. Although this result does not give a direct indication of relative risk (RR) compared to the general population, an estimate can be obtained using the same data. It turns out that the frequency of the non-transmitted alleles in each case–parent

triad is a true measure of the population frequency of that allele.[14] Therefore by using this frequency as a comparator to that found in index cases, an estimate of disease RR for possession of the allele of interest can be given.

3.4 Sample size

The size of the study population is one of the most important factors determining the likelihood of obtaining meaningful results from genetic association studies. A number of parameters influence sample size calculations, including:

(1) *Frequency of the DNA variant in the population.* If the variant of interest is present at a frequency of 1%, only a very small

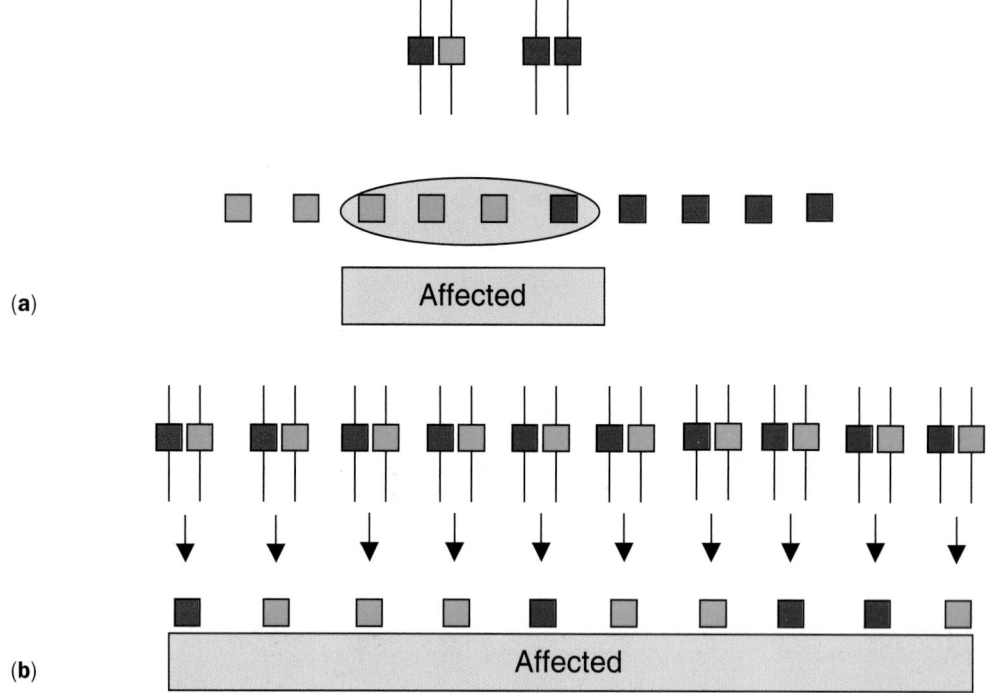

(a)

(b)

Fig. 7.2 Family-based study. This design can be easily understood by considering the hypothetical family in (**a**). One of the parents is heterozygous for the marker of interest and carries a blue and a red allele. The other parent is homozygous for the red allele and therefore not informative. When we look at whether the red or blue allele is transmitted from the heterozygote parent to the 10 offspring, as expected, five offspring have the red allele and five have the blue allele. If it turns out that the blue allele predisposes to the infection being studied, then more offspring carrying the blue allele will be affected (in this example three blue versus one red). If we now select families on the basis of having an affected offspring, we notice that, because we are now selecting for those offspring who are more likely to carry the blue allele, there is an apparent excess of transmission of this allele from heterozygote parents to their offspring. In the example shown in (**b**), instead of the 50% transmission expected if there were no effect, we observe the blue allele being transmitted on six out of 10 occasions (transmission of 60%). This distortion of expected transmission forms the bases of the transmission disequilibrium test (TDT) used in most family-based designs. The probability of this being a non-random variation (*p* value) is calculated using the Chi-square test, with 50% transmission giving the 'expected' values.

proportion of the cases are likely to carry the variant, so significant differences between cases and controls are only going to be found if the original sample is large (several hundreds of cases).

(2) *Size of effect to be detected*. If the DNA variant increases the likelihood of having the disease by a factor of four, the sample size needed to detect the effect would be smaller than if it only doubled the risk of the disease.

(3) *Disease model*. Whether it is assumed that the risk of disease is different in individuals who have two copies (homozygotes) for the DNA variant compared to those that carry only one copy (heterozygotes). The risk may be dominant, additive, multiplicative or recessive.

(4) *Number of markers to be studied*. Any estimate of probability will need to be corrected for the effects of multiple comparisons.

(5) *Study design*. (E.g. sib-pair, case-control or family).

The following example gives an indication of the sort of sample size needed when these factors are taken into account. To identify an effect of a two-fold increased susceptibility using a marker present at a frequency of 0.1, assuming an additive model (i.e. homozygotes have double the risk of heterozygotes) and correcting for 10^6 multiple comparisons, a family-based study would need 800 case–parent triads,[15] and a case-control study would require 425 cases and the same number of unaffected controls. The numbers required for dominant and multiplicative models are similar, but detection of recessive effects requires several thousand cases (45,000 families in this example!).

4. INTERPRETATION OF POSITIVE DISEASE ASSOCIATION STUDIES

When a positive association (susceptibility or protection) is found between a DNA variant and a disease, the first question to ask is whether the study design was robust enough for the association to be considered valid. Ideally, the association should be highly significant and confirmed by an independent study and be observed using both population-based and family-based methods. Once it seems likely that the association is genuine the next question is: what does it mean?

4.1 Relative risk

At one level the answer is easy. Individuals who carry the DNA variant are at increased risk of the disease, often expressed as an OR (see Fig. 7.1). OR are statistical parameters which can be used as estimates of the true RR, i.e. the frequency of the disease in those who carry the DNA variant divided by the frequency of the disease in those who do not carry the DNA variant. OR are only a good estimate of true RR if the disease is rare (affecting <10% of the population sampled). Once an estimate of RR has been calculated, it is tempting to assign an attributable fraction to the risk, meaning the proportion of cases that appear to be caused by the DNA variant. The method used is simply based on RR and the population frequency of

the DNA marker. Thus, DNA variants that confer modest increased RR but which occur frequently in a population can produce population-attributable fractions >30%. For example, 32% of meningococcal disease has been attributed to polymorphisms of mannose-binding lectin (MBL).[16] Using the same calculations, we have identified an interleukin (IL)-8 polymorphism with an apparent attributable fraction of 43% for RSV bronchiolitis.[17] Given the complex nature of these diseases and the contribution of both environmental and genetic effects, such high values of attributable fraction are surprising. In truth, these calculations are misleading. For example, in our study of the IL-8 gene region, an additional polymorphism was found near the gene. This polymorphism is also associated with RSV bronchiolitis and gives an attributable fraction of 40%. Taken together, these two polymorphisms would apparently account for nearly all bronchiolitis. This is obviously not true. The reason why these simple calculations cannot be applied to these types of data is that they assume that each factor is independent of all the others, and that all the contributory factors, genetic and non-genetic, have been identified. In the example used it seems very likely that both IL-8 polymorphisms are acting as markers for the same functional effect, and, in fact, it turns out that they are in strong linkage disequilibrium and therefore not independent of each other. Even for DNA variants which are not linked there may well be unknown interactions with other genetic factors and with environmental influences. Thus, assumptions that each identified factor is acting independently of all other influences on susceptibility simply cannot be made for genetic associations, therefore, quoted attributable fractions should be interpreted with caution.

4.2 Disease mechanisms

Perhaps of more interest than simply the RR associated with the variant is the mechanism by which it confers susceptibility. The interpretation will depend to some extent on what types of variants have been studied. In some instances there is no doubt that the DNA variants themselves are functional. For example, base changes with the MBL gene directly affect circulating plasma concentrations of MBL.[18] Thus, the straightforward explanation of an association between MBL gene variants and disease (e.g. meningococcal disease)[16] is that low levels of circulating MBL are responsible for the susceptibility. The situation becomes more difficult when a DNA marker with no known function is used. If a genuine association exists between the marker and the disease, this must indicate that the fragment of DNA identified by the marker possesses a functional element which influences disease susceptibility. In other words, the DNA marker is in linkage disequilibrium with a functionally important gene variant. In many ways this result is more exciting than when using functional markers, since it may lead to the discovery of novel gene variants.

The difficulty then is knowing how far to look upstream and downstream from the DNA variant to find the functional element, i.e. to determine the extent of LD. Although on average, with randomly mating populations, it has been estimated that LD only extends for 3 kb,[12] it is quite clear that this distance is highly variable and in some regions, such as the major histocompatibility complex (MHC) locus, LD extends over hundreds of kilobases. Thus, the disease-associated DNA variant could in fact, be acting as a marker for a gene tens of thousands of bases away. In order to be certain of the genes to which the association applies, it is important to determine the extent of LD for the region under study. All candidate genes within that region could then be considered. It could be argued that this degree of stringency should be applied even to apparently functional variants since the effect observed may be unrelated to the presumed function and instead to some other linked element.

5. INTERPRETATION OF NEGATIVE DISEASE ASSOCIATION STUDIES

The opposite result, where a disease association is not found, is even more difficult to interpret. Once again, it is important to ensure that the study is adequately designed, but even with very large studies a negative result for a single DNA variant has little meaning unless the DNA variant is itself functional. This problem is illustrated in Fig. 7.3. It can been seen that even markers very close to functional DNA variants can fail to show positive associations with the disease. This is because even though they are in complete LD with the functional variant, they are poor markers for it. This problem can be overcome by the use of haplotypes rather than single DNA variants. Haplotypes more precisely identify particular chromosomal variants and are less prone to false-negative results. Since by definition they are made up of a number of markers, their use requires more resources and time. Even with extensive haplotypes, unless one or more of the haplotypes is known to be linked to functional elements, a negative result cannot be interpreted as indicating that a particular gene is not involved in the disease pathogenesis, since it may simply be that there are no functional variants of the gene, or that the effects of the variants are too small to be detected. The gene in question may still be critical in the development of the disease.

6. EXAMPLES WHERE A GENETIC COMPONENT OF SUSCEPTIBILITY TO INFECTION HAS BEEN SHOWN

6.1 Increased risk in family members

Since there can be many reasons why a particular individual develops an infectious disease, it has been difficult to separate out the genetic influences on susceptibility. A study from Denmark has tried to distinguish the genetic from the environmental factors by looking at the causes of premature death amongst adults who were placed early in life with adoptive parents who were unrelated to them.[19] This study showed that if either of the biological parents died from infection before the age of 70, there was a five-fold increased risk that the adoptee had also died from infection. There was no increased risk to the adoptee related to death of an adoptive parent. These results suggest that there is a strong genetic influence on the risk of premature death from infection.

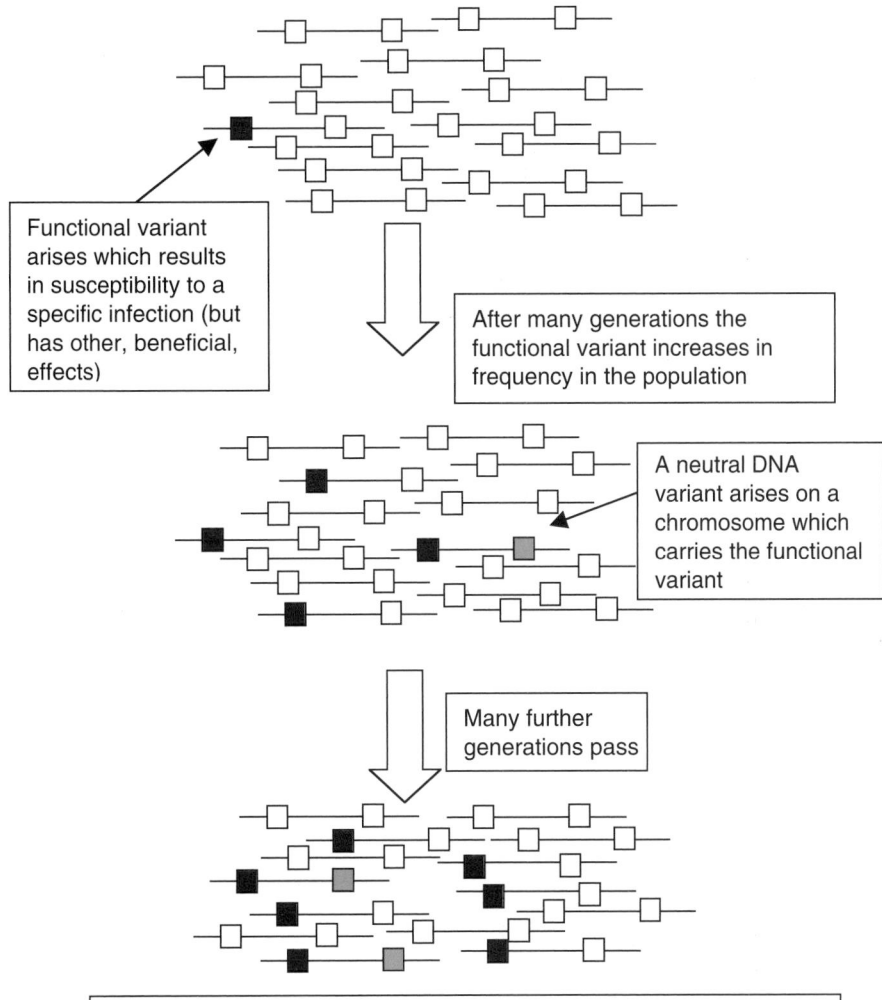

Functional variant arises which results in susceptibility to a specific infection (but has other, beneficial, effects)

After many generations the functional variant increases in frequency in the population

A neutral DNA variant arises on a chromosome which carries the functional variant

Many further generations pass

The neutral variant is close to and in complete linkage disequilibrium with the functional variant. Nevertheless, since it only occurs on one third of the chromosomes carrying the functional variant, much of the effect of the functional variant on disease susceptibility would not be detected in studies using just the neutral marker. The same effect is observed if the rare variant is functional and the commoner variant is neutral. In this scenario many of the controls would carry the marker without the functional variant, again diluting the effect.

Fig. 7.3 Efficiency of markers to detect disease effects. Imagine a population in which disease-causing variant (D; red box) is present. When this variant is used in an association study it is found to confer a three-fold increased risk of the disease. A second neutral variant (M; blue box) also occurs in the population. M is found on 28% of chromosomes which carry D, and is only found when D is also present. Thus, there is no evidence of recombination (which would have separated M from D), and M is therefore in complete linkage disequilibrium (LD) with D. However, since M only detects 28% of D chromosomes, when M is used in a disease association study, most of the effect of D is lost [in the case shown the relative risk (RR) of disease associated with M would be 1.6]. Thus, simply using markers that are close to the gene of interest does not guarantee that effects due that gene will be detected.

The concept of increased risk of disease amongst relatives (another use of the term relative risk) has been used as a crude measure of the influence of inheritance on susceptibility, sometimes referred to as λ_R. An increased risk of some infectious diseases has been shown to be higher for monozygotic twins than for dizygotic twins. This is particularly powerful if it can be demonstrated that monozygotic twins reared apart have a higher concordance for the infection than dizygotic twins reared apart. Since monozygotic twins are genetically identical, the inference is that the higher concordance has a genetic basis. There is evidence of a genetic effect from this type of twin study for TB,[20] malaria,[21] leprosy[22] and *Helicobacter pylori* infection.[23] Where there are no data on twins reared apart (e.g. in the malaria study), some caution is needed with this interpretation since identical twins tend to be treated more similarly than non-identical twins and thus have a more similar environment.

6.2 Positive linkage and/or association with specific infections

Single gene variants have been implicated as susceptibility or protective factors in at least 11 different infectious diseases (TB, malaria, HIV, disseminated BCG, RSV bronchiolitis, hepatitis B, leprosy, leishmaniasis, shistosomiasis, meningococcal septicaemia, Creuztfeldt–Jakob disease). One of the best-known examples is the relationship between sickle cell anaemia and severe malaria. Individuals who are heterozygous for the sickle cell mutation (a single base change in the β-globin gene) have a 10-fold protection against developing severe malaria (H Akerman, personal communication). Although this association was described well before the broad concept of genetic susceptibility was developed, it does give proof of principle. In fact malaria is a disease that is well suited to genetic susceptibility studies. The *Plasmodium* parasite infects nearly 100% of individuals in endemic regions, but only a small proportion develops severe disease. Nevertheless, severe malaria is sufficiently common in these regions to allow large sample collections (1000–2000 cases) to be amassed. It is hoped that by understanding what is it different in the immune response made by individuals that are susceptible, more can be learned of the pathogenesis and new therapies developed. Using this approach a number of other gene variants have now been associated with severe disease in malaria (Table 7.1).

RSV bronchiolitis is a disease in the UK where there is widespread exposure to the infecting organism. RSV is a highly infectious virus and nearly all infants become infected during their first winter. Most develop a minor cough and cold only. One to two per cent, however, go on to develop severe disease requiring hospital treatment. As with malaria, research has gone on for many years trying to determine which aspects of the host response is protective and which leads to severe disease. Traditional approaches have led to the development of a number of different models. Genetic association studies can now be used to assess the involvement of candidate genes to determine which model is most likely to be correct. Using a family-based approach this method has already implicated gene variants in the region of the IL-8 gene (IL-8 is a proinflammatory cytokine), in susceptibility to RSV disease.[17] Table 7.1 gives other examples of single gene associations with infectious diseases.

7. GENERAL COMMENTS

Although there are now several infectious diseases in which genetic susceptibility appears to play an important role (see Table 7.1), there are still those who express doubts over the value of this approach. Most investigators agree that genetic variance leading to disease susceptibility will be encoded by alleles at several genes. How many 'several' turns out to be is hard to know. The most common criticism is that so many genes will be involved that it will impossible to unravel the effect of any one in isolation. This, in turn, would make it impossible to modify the cause of the disease by direct intervention with, for example, immunomodulators. Of course, it will never be known whether this is the case unless the possibility is examined. It is hoped that some factors will have large enough effects on susceptibility to some infections to be worth attempting specific

Table 7.1 Examples where DNA variants have been associated or linked with susceptibility to infectious disease (adapted from Kwiatkowski[1])

Disease	Implicated gene regions	Selected references
Tuberculosis (TB)	HLA-DR, NRAMP1, vitamin D receptor	29, 30
Malaria	Alpha and beta globin, DARC, TNF, G6PD, HLA class I and II	6, 31–35
HIV and AIDS	Chemokine receptors CCR2 and CCR5, HLA class I	4, 36
Disseminated BCG	INF-γ receptor	37
Respiratory syncytial virus (RSV) bronchiolitis	IL-8	17
Hepatitis B	HLA class II	38
Leprosy	HLA class II, TNF	39, 40
Shistosomiasis	5q31–q33	10
Meningococcal septicaemia	MBL plasminogen activating factor	16, 41
Creutzfeldt–Jakob disease	Host prion protein	42

DARC. Duffy antigen receptor; HLA, human leucocyte antigen; IL, interleukin; INF-γ, interferon-gamma; TNF, tumour necrosis factor.

therapies. Even if most genetic susceptibility to infection arises as a consequence of the combined action of many gene variants, each with relatively minor effects, the increased understanding of disease pathogenesis is still likely to yield valuable information for therapeutic intervention or vaccine design.

It has been proposed that genetic association studies should only use DNA variants which are known to be functional.[24] The advantage would be that it would be more straightforward to interpret the results. However, there are several disadvantages. At present, the number of available known functional variants is tiny compared to the total genetic variability and would severely limit the genes which could be investigated. The evidence required to demonstrate physiologically relevant variation in a gene's function is very hard to produce. Any polymorphisms that are shown to be associated with a disease will, by definition, occur in the normal population and only confer an increased risk, probably of the order of 1.5–2-fold, of being affected. It would not be surprising if this increased risk were the result of a relatively subtle effect on gene function. For example let's say a promoter variant of interferon-gamma (INF-γ) results in a 15% increased production of INFγ by CD8+ T-cells following exposure to hepatitis B virus *in vivo*. With current technologies it is impossible to reliably detect this size of difference using *in vitro* systems and there is too much biological noise to hope to be able to detect it from blood taken from individuals with and without the polymorphism. Nevertheless, a well-planned and appropriately powered genetic association study would be able to identify an increased risk of hepatitis B in individuals carrying the promoter variant. This would implicate INF-γ in the pathogenesis and stimulate functional studies to unravel the mechanism.

There have also been criticisms of the study designs used and their interpretation. Over-enthusiastic reports of questionable associations derived from small sample sizes, which subsequently fail to be replicated by other studies, have undermined the used of genetic association techniques.[25] The underlying difficulty for the investigator faced with a modest but encouraging probability (P) value is knowing how to differentiate between a real, but small, effect from that caused by random statistical fluctuation. The best way is to repeat the study using an independent set of samples, and the ability to perform this check should be built into study design.

8. THE FUTURE

What will underpin all successful studies is a large and phenotypically robust DNA collection. For this, at least 1000 index cases, including family samples where appropriate, with carefully matched controls will be needed. This type of sample collection needs multicentre cooperation, a great deal of planning and close attention to detail. There are two broad approaches. One is to collect DNA from everybody (say one million people) and then to follow them as a cohort and record who suffers from what disease. After 20 years or so there should be sufficient numbers of cases for many different diseases to allow detailed analysis. The alternative is to collect DNA from index cases and controls. This will certainly be achieved more rapidly (provided the disease is relatively common) but the study will be limited to the disease by which the index cases were identified. The DNA in either archive could be subject to SNP and microsatellite typing using several thousand markers spread across the genome. Alternatively, for specific diseases, candidate gene approaches could be used.

Both of the investigations mentioned above are technically possible now. Some large sample collections are being assembled for specific infections (e.g. for malaria, TB and bronchiolitis), and a few population-based collections already exist, with larger ones being planned. At present, very few collections are large enough or robust enough to give unequivocal results. The difficulties with screening these DNA collections with large numbers of markers are financial, ethical and legal, as well as technical. At present, most genotyping methods cost at least £0.3 per genotype, so to screen 1000 cases and 1000 controls would cost £600. A genomewide screen, even with a modest number of markers, say 300, on this number of samples would be expensive (£180,000). Markers as widely spaced as these (one every 10 million bases) are also quite likely to miss important associations. The high cost of using large numbers of markers is a strong incentive to using a candidate gene approach. The candidate gene approach is restricted to testing genes that are already suspected to be involved, therefore results of these studies are less likely to come up with novel insights into disease pathogenesis.

There are a number of potential new developments which will allow high throughput genotyping at reasonable cost. Most of the new high throughput technologies are designed for typing SNP rather than microsatellites. Nearly all require the genomic fragment of DNA containing the SNP to be amplified using the polymerase chain reaction (PCR). The SNP is then detected either directly by minisequencing,[26] through its effect on changing the overall mass of the fragment detected using a mass spectrometer,[27] or through changes in binding affinity for complementary oligonucleotides often detected using fluorochromes. The latter approach may eventually become the most efficient. It is now possible to spot several thousand different oligonucleotides on a small DNA chip (usually an etched silicon surface).[28] Fluorescent-labelled DNA from one individual is then incubated with the chip and the pattern of binding, analysed by computer, indicates the SNP carried by that individual. Current chip technology means that the chips can only be used a few times before they become unreliable; they are also very expensive to produce. If these problems can be overcome, this technology has the potential of allowing analysis of vast numbers of genotypes everyday. As with all high throughput methods, robots are used to handle the samples and, once set up, will run 24 hours per day.

Once a positive association has been found, it will be necessary to localize the effect. This process is sometimes called fine mapping. It requires a high density of markers, and knowledge of haplotypes in the population being studied. At present, these high-density markers and haplotype information are not available for most loci. With high-throughput genotyping, these types of data will be available at the beginning of a study, rather than being acquired during the study, as is currently the case. This will allow more rapid and efficient interpretation of positive associations. These, in turn, will lead to functional assays to determine the underlying biological mechanism for the observed effect on disease susceptibility.

GLOSSARY

Allele	One of a series of different forms of the same gene or DNA marker. For example, if a car was a gene or marker, then a Mini would be one allele and a Rolls Royce another. Single nucleotide polymorphisms have two alleles, whereas microsatellites can have several, depending on the number of repeats.
Diploid	A state in which each chromosome is represented twice. This is the situation for all the cells in the body apart from gametes.
Gene	Generally meant to mean units of DNA that encodes proteins. Genes occupy a fixed position (or locus) within the genome.
Genome	All the DNA sequence from all the chromosomes in the nucleus. The total length of the human genome is thought to be around three billion bases and contains an estimated 40,000 genes. The genes occupy only 0.1% of the genome.
Haploid	A state in which each chromosome is represented once. This state is only found in gametes. When male and female gametes fuse, a diploid state is re-established.
Haplotype	A symbolic representation of linked alleles. In other words, the collection of alleles that occur together on one chromosome and which have not been separated by recombination.
Homologous chromosomes	Chromosomes that contain the same linear sequence of genes. In a diploid cell, all chromosomes (apart from the X and Y chromosomes) occur in homologous pairs, one chromosome is inherited from the mother and one from the father.
Linkage and linkage disequilibrium (LD)	See Box 7.1.
Meiosis	A process of cell division that results in the formation of haploid gametes. During meiosis, recombination between homologous chromosomes occurs.
Microsatellite	See Box 7.2
Single nucleotide polymorphism (SNP)	See Box 7.2.

REFERENCES

Scientific papers

1. Kwiatkowski D. Susceptibility to infection. *Br Med J* 2000; **321**: 1061–5.
2. Hill AV. Genetics and genomics of infectious disease susceptibility. *Br Med Bull* 1999; **55**: 401–13.
3. Conley ME. Molecular approaches to analysis of X-linked immunodeficiencies. *Annu Rev Immunol* 1992; **10**: 215–38.

4. Martin MP, Dean M, Smith MW et al. Genetic acceleration of AIDS progression by a promoter variant of CCR5. *Science* 1998; **282**: 1907–11.

5 Dorn CP, Finke PE, Oates B et al. Antagonists of the human CCR5 receptor as anti-HIV-1 agents. Part 1: discovery and initial structure–activity relationships for 1-amino-2-phenyl-4-(piperidin-1-yl) butanes. *Bioorg Med Chem Lett* 2001; **11**: 259–64.

6 Knight JC, Udalova I, Hill AV et al. A polymorphism that affects OCT-1 binding to the TNF promoter region is associated with severe malaria. *Nature Genet* 1999; **22**: 145–50.

7 Allport TD, Davies EG, Wells C et al. Ribavirin and bronchiolitis: variation in use in the UK [letter]. *Arch Dis Child* 1997; **76**: 385.

8 Mein CA, Esposito L, Dunn MG et al. A search for type 1 diabetes susceptibility genes in families from the United Kingdom. *Nature Genet* 1998; **19**: 297–300.

9 Bellamy R, Beyers N, McAdam KP et al. Genetic susceptibility to tuberculosis in Africans: a genome-wide scan. *Proc Natl Acad Sci USA* 2000; **97**: 8005–9.

10 Marquet S, Abel L, Hillaire D et al. Genetic localization of a locus controlling the intensity of infection by *Schistosoma mansoni* on chromosome 5q31-q33. *Nature Genet* 1996; **14**: 181–4.

11. Risch N, Merikangas K. The future of genetic studies of complex human diseases. *Science* 1996; **273**: 1516–17.

12. Kruglyak L. Prospects for whole-genome linkage disequilibrium mapping of common disease genes. *Nature Genet* 1999; **22**: 139–44.

13. Koch HG, McClay J, Loh EW et al. Allele association studies with SSR and SNP markers at known physical distances within a 1 Mb region embracing the ALDH2 locus in the Japanese, demonstrates linkage disequilibrium extending up to 400 kb. *Hum Molec Genet* 2000; **9**: 2993–9.

14. Thomson G. Mapping disease genes: family-based association studies. *Am J Hum Genet* 1995; **57**: 487–98.

15. Schaid DJ. Likelihoods and TDT for the case-parents design. *Genet Epidemiol* 1999; **16**: 250–60.

16. Hibberd ML, Sumiya M, Summerfield JA et al. Association of variants of the gene for mannose-binding lectin with susceptibility to meningococcal disease. Meningococcal Research Group. *Lancet* 1999; **353**: 1049–53.

17. Hull J, Thomson A. Kwiatkowski D. Association of respiratory syncytial virus bronchiolitis with the interleukin 8 gene region in UK families. *Thorax* 2000; **55**: 1023–7.

18. Sumiya M, Super M, Tabona P et al. Molecular basis of opsonic defect in immunodeficient children. *Lancet* 1991; **337**: 1569–70.

19. Sorensen TI, Nielsen GG, Andersen PK et al. Genetic and environmental influences on premature death in adult adoptees. *N Engl J Med* 1988; **318**: 727–32.

20. Comstock GW. Tuberculosis in twins: a re-analysis of the Prophit survey. *Am Rev Respir Dis* 1978; **117**: 621–4.

21. Jepson AP, Banya WA, Sisay-Joof F et al. Genetic regulation of fever in *Plasmodium falciparum* malaria in Gambian twin children. *J Infect Dis* 1995; **172**: 316–19.

22. Fine PE. Immunogenetics of susceptibility to leprosy, tuberculosis, and leishmaniasis. An epidemiological perspective. *Int J Lepr Other Mycobact Dis* 1981; **49**: 437–54.

23. Malaty HM, Engstrand L, Pedersen ML et al. *Helicobacter pylori* infection: genetic and environmental influences. A study of twins. *Ann Intern Med* 1994; **120**: 982–6.

24. Editor. Freely associating. *Nature Genet* 1991; **22**: 1–2.

25. Roberts SB, MacLean CJ, Neale MC et al. Replication of linkage studies of complex traits: an examination of variation in location estimates. *Am J Hum Genet* 1999; **65**: 876–84.

26. Pastinen T, Kurg A, Metspalu A et al. Minisequencing: a specific tool for DNA analysis and diagnostics on oligonucleotide arrays. *Genome Res* 1997; **7**: 606–14.

27. Haff LA, Smirnov IP. Single-nucleotide polymorphism identification assays using a thermostable DNA polymerase and delayed extraction MALDI-TOF mass spectrometry. *Genome Res* 1997; **7**: 378–88.

28. Wang DG, Fan JB, Siao CJ et al. Large-scale identification, mapping, and genotyping of single-nucleotide polymorphisms in the human genome. *Science* 1998; **280**: 1077–82.

29. Bellamy R, Ruwende C, Corrah T et al. Variations in the NRAMPI gene and susceptibility to tuberculosis in West Africans. *N Engl J Med* 1998; **338**: 640–4.

30. Singh SP, Mehra NK, Dingley HB et al. Human leukocyte antigen (HLA)-linked control of susceptibility to pulmonary tuberculosis and association with HLA-DR types. *J Infect Dis* 1983; **148**: 676–81.

31. Hill AV, Allsopp CE, Kwiatkowski D et al. Common west African HLA antigens are associated with protection from severe malaria. *Nature* 1991; **352**: 595–600.

32. Miller LH, Mason SJ, Clyde DF et al. The resistance factor to *Plasmodium vivax* in blacks. The Duffy-blood-group genotype, FyFy. *N Engl J Med* 1976; **295**: 302–4.

33. Tournamille C, Colin Y, Cartron JP et al. Disruption of a GATA motif in the Duffy gene promoter abolishes erythroid gene expression in Duffy-negative individuals. *Nature Genet* 1995; **10**: 224–8.

34. Ruwende C, Khoo SC, Snow RW et al. Natural selection of hemi- and heterozygotes for G6PD deficiency in Africa by resistance to severe malaria. *Nature* 1995; **376**: 246–9.

35. Flint J, Hill AV, Bowden DK et al. High frequencies of alpha-thalassaemia are the result of natural selection by malaria. *Nature* 1986; **321**: 744–50.

36. Carrington M, Nelson GW, Martin MP et al. HLA and HIV-1: heterozygote advantage and B*35-Cw*04 disadvantage [see comments]. *Science* 1999; **283**: 1748–52.

37. Newport MJ, Huxley CM, Huston S et al. A mutation in the interferon-gamma-receptor gene and susceptibility to mycobacterial infection. *N Engl J Med* 1996; **335**: 1941–9.

38. Thursz MR, Kwiatkowski D, Allsopp CE et al. Association between an MHC class II allele and clearance of hepatitis B virus in the Gambia [see comments]. *N Engl J Med* 1995; **332**: 1065–9.

39. Todd JR, West BC, McDonald JC. Human leukocyte antigen and leprosy: study in northern Louisiana and review. *Rev Infect Dis* 1990; **12**: 63–74.

40. Roy S, McGuire W, Mascie-Taylor CG et al. Tumor necrosis factor promoter polymorphism and susceptibility to lepromatous leprosy. *J Infect Dis* 1997; **176**: 530–2.

41. Hermans PW, Hibberd ML, Booy R et al. 4G/5G promoter polymorphism in the plasminogen-activator-inhibitor-1 gene and outcome of meningococcal disease. Meningococcal Research Group. *Lancet* 199; **354**: 556–60.

42. Deslys JP, Jaegly A, d'Aignaux JH et al. Genotype at codon 129 and susceptibility to Crutzfeldt-Jakob disease [letter]. *Lancet* 1998; **351**: 1251.

8

Toll-like receptors and the host response to infection

David H Wyllie, Robert C Read

OBJECTIVES

(1) To review the structure, specificity and mechanism by which Toll-like receptors (TLR) influence innate immune responses.
(2) To consider the implications of TLR in human infectious disease pathogenesis.

OVERVIEW

Animals can respond rapidly to infection even if they have not previously encountered the invading microbe. This innate response occurs in plants and insects, as well as mammals, and includes the secretion of antimicrobial molecules and proinflammatory cytokines. The mechanism of pathogen detection has been clarified by the recent identification of Toll-like receptors (TLR) as essential components of the innate pathogen recognition system. Several TLR-dependent systems mediate the immediate response of vertebrates to invading bacteria. Current concepts of TLR structure, specificity and mechanism of action are reviewed. It is suggested that integration of TLR-dependent signals provide the host with its first perception of the presence and nature of an invading microbe. Implications for future research into human infectious disease pathogenesis are discussed.

1. INTRODUCTION

The immune system of vertebrates can initiate very rapid responses to infecting pathogens. The responses include fever, changes in the peripheral blood leucocyte count and release of acute phase proteins. This article concerns Toll-like receptors (TLR), transmembrane receptors shown to be essential for the initiation of the host response to infection, which are conserved throughout the animal kingdom. Recent work on TLR has revealed much about the strategy used by mammals to detect pathogens; implications for the understanding of human disease susceptibility are discussed.

2. RECOGNITION OF PATHOGEN BY SPECIFIC RECEPTORS

Systemic microbial invasion is detected by the immune system, which then initiates a response. That the detection event occurs

Box 8.1 Innate and adaptive immunity

Plants, insects and vertebrates generate an immune response when infected

Innate immunity relies on germline receptors for conserved microbial components

Adaptive immunity selects receptors, such as antibodies, on the basis of antigen exposure

Innate immunity is found in plants and animals, being phylogenetically ancient

Adaptive responses are found in higher vertebrates only

implies the existence of some sort of immune system receptor activated either by the pathogen itself or by some consequence of its presence. Antibodies can be viewed as a receptor in this context. For example, in individuals with antibodies against a particular pathogen, re-exposure to that pathogen causes first the recognition of the pathogen by the antibody, and then consequent activation of such immune functions as complement activation and Fc-dependent phagocytosis by immune cells.[1]

2.1 Adaptive immunity – receptor repertoire influenced by pathogen exposure

The ability to develop pathogen-specific receptors, such as antibodies, in response to immune challenge developed only in early vertebrates.[2] This system is termed adaptive immunity because an individual's receptor repertoire is adapted to the pathogens previously encountered. However, both plants and those animals that predated the evolution of adaptive immunity can control the deleterious effects of microbial ingress by immune responses in response to infection. Pathogen recognition depends in plants[3] and insects[4] on proteins encoded by germline DNA. The system used is therefore termed innate; it exists in mammals in addition to the adaptive system,[5] providing some immediate defence even in non-immune hosts (Box 8.1).

2.2. Innate immunity – recognition of generic features of pathogens

One mechanism by which pathogen detection by the adaptive immune system occurs has been termed pattern recognition. This model, originally proposed by Medzhitov and Janeway,[5] suggests that germline receptors [pattern recognition receptors (PRR)] for generic features [pathogen-associated molecular patterns (PAMP) present in pathogens allow the discrimination between self and non-self. Numerous PRR have been identified in both vertebrate and invertebrates. Some are soluble and these tend to be multimeric proteins. Mammalian examples are shown in Table 8.1. In the case of some PRR, such as the mannose-binding lectin,[6–9] surfactant protein A[10,11] and the macrophage scavenger receptor,[12] study of the effects of naturally occurring loss of function mutations, or targeted deletions, has confirmed an *in vivo* role for these molecules in vertebrate immune defence.

2.3 Innate Immunity – alternative theories of operation

A second mechanism of innate immunity has also been suggested but is much more controversial. This is because, in contrast to the pattern recognition theory, the molecular basis by which it could operate is less well established. This danger signal theory proposed that a system devoted to self/non-self discrimination might be unnecessary if systems existed for monitoring the damage caused by pathogens, rather than pathogen presence.[18] According to this model, systems responsible for initiating microbe-control measures would detect signals from host cells, termed danger signals, which are released on pathogen damage.

3. TOLL-LIKE RECEPTORS (TLR)

Despite the identification of numerous PRR in vertebrates, the link between these and the initiation of host responses to infection remained obscure for many years. Recently, the discovery of a family of transmembrane receptors essential for responsiveness to pathogens has

	Superfamily (ref)	Examples (ref)	Ligands	Form
Table 8.1 Examples of mammalian pattern recognition molecules				
Soluble	Ficolins (13)	L-ficolin		
		M-ficolin	Bacterial cell wall	Trimeric
	Collectins	Mannose-binding lectin (14)	Varied	Trimeric
		Surfactant Proteins A and D (15)	Bacteria and viruses	
	Pentraxins	C-reactive protein (16)	Varied, including bacteria	Pentameric
Membrane bound	Scavenger receptor	AI scavenger receptor (12)	*Staphylococcus aureus*, other bacteria	Trimeric
		MARCO (17)	Bacteria, dust	
	Integrins	CR3	Varied (see text)	Heterodimer
Soluble and membrane bound	CD14	CD14	See text	See text

clarified the situation and has suggested the fundamental strategies used by vertebrates in their first contact with pathogens. Remarkably, the innate immune defence strategies of vertebrates and invertebrates all appear to involve the same transmembrane receptor family, the TLR, which are currently the subject of intensive research. TLR structure and specificity are discussed in these chapter, which also further explores the implications of these data for human infectious disease pathogenesis and considers the likely role of TLR as disease susceptibility loci in humans.

The strategies one can use to identify a molecule as a component of an immune response are relevant to the interpretation of the experimental data on TLR. There are only a few basic methods, discussed in detail in Box 8.2 but which are also outlined below:

- delete or mutate a gene in an animal and look for phenotypic changes, either by:

  random mutagenesis: the whole genome is mutagenized, and those mutations producing interesting effects are studied further; or

  targeted mutagenesis: the gene of interest is known and is knocked out specifically;

- ectopic expression – the gene is expressed somewhere it is not normally expressed;
- use of a drug or antibody specific to a molecule to investigate the molecule's physiological role.

4. ROLE OF TOLL-LIKE RECEPTORS (TLR) IN *DROSOPHILA* IMMUNE DEFENCE

4.1 *Drosophila* as a model animal

Ease of husbandry, rapid life cycle and powerful techniques for genetic manipulation have made the fruit fly *Drosophila* an important experimental animal in the study of immune function. *Drosophila* is attractive in the study of innate immune function because, unlike the situation

---

Box 8.2 Strategies for identification of immune system components

---

(1) *Delete or mutate an animal and study phenotypic changes*

(a) *Whole animal mutagenesis*

A screening test is used to identify the phenotype of interest. Mutagenesis, either with a chemical mutagen or with a genetic element such as a transposon, is then used on large numbers of animals. Those mutagenized animals with the phenotype of interest are studied further. This technique has been extensively applied to flies[19] and bacteria;[135] similar techniques have also been applied to vertebrates, including mice[136] and fish.[137] The advantage of the technique is that no assumptions need be made about the nature of the genes involved. Multiple alleles of one gene are sometimes recovered, and these may display both gain and lack of function. The major disadvantages are that the gene may be lethal and never recovered; additionally, with most strategies, the gene mutated must be identified as a subsequent exercise, e.g. by positional cloning.[55,56] Additionally, if several genes exist which subserve the same function, neither is likely to be detectable because the probability of mutating both genes in one animal is very low.

Typically, multiple genes producing a similar phenotype are isolated from saturation mutagenesis experiments. This occurs because a series of interacting proteins forms a pathway producing the phenotype of interest. Using classical genetic means, the genes isolated can be ordered, giving rise to the concept of upstream and downstream genes. The order of the genes reflects the order in which the gene products (proteins) interact in the pathway.

(b) *Targeted deletion*

If the gene of interest is known, it can be deleted (knock-out) or replaced with a marker gene (knock-in).

The marker gene, which will be readily detectable, will then be expressed in the same places as the native gene. This is a method of monitoring gene expression *in vivo*.

(2) *Ectopic expression*

If the function of a gene is, for example, a receptor for lipopolysaccharide (LPS), then expression of the gene in cells which are not LPS responsive may cause them to become so. This is referred to as ectopic expression. This has advantages in that the experiment is rapid to perform and fairly well controlled, and DNA for the receptor of interest, and mutants of it, can be introduced, e.g. by transfection. This may be a short-term phenomenon (transient transfection) or permanent (stable transfection). The disadvantages are that the levels of protein expression may differ from those found physiologically, which may be relevant to the observed phenotypic changes. Additionally, even when the gene of interest is essential for a function *in vivo*, if other unknown genes are absolutely required for the function of the receptor, and they are not expressed in the cell transfected, then no phenotypic changes will be evident.

(3) *Block a physiological function using a specific receptor blocker*

If a specific receptor blocker, such as a pharmaceutical compound or monoclonal antibody, is available, then it may be possible to demonstrate a role for the receptor using the blocker, either *in vitro* or *in vivo*. The approach depends on an appropriate level of specificity and potency of the blocker used. The advantage is that modification of the cell of interest is not necessary for the experiment; the disadvantages are that such reagents are time consuming, expensive, difficult and sometimes impossible to generate.

in vertebrates, innate immunity is responsible for all protection of the fly against pathogens. Recent analysis of innate immune function in *Drosophila* have relied on techniques (see Box 8.2 for discussion) including whole animal chemical mutagenesis,[19] transposon-based genome analysis,[20] the construction of animals containing mosaics,[21] and reporter transgenes.[22] Additionally, use has been made of the *Drosophila* cell lines in which transfection experiments can be performed.[23] A summary of the current understanding of innate defence in *Drosophila* is provided in Box 8.3.

4.2 Antimicrobial peptides in *Drosophila*

Natural pathogens of fruit flies include both bacteria and fungi. In response to infection, local responses occur at epithelia.[22,24] Additionally, a systemic response occurs. This involves haemocytes (immune cells present in the haemolymph) which phagocytose and encapsulate invading bacteria. In a reaction which may be enhanced by,[25] but does not absolutely depend on, haemocytes,[26] the fat body (a liver-like organ) produces large quantities of antimicrobial peptides. Antimicrobial peptides are present in both plants, insects and mammals (reviewed in Hancock and Diamond[27]). At least 10 different antimicrobial peptides have been identified in *Drosophila*. These have differing specificities: some such as attacins and diptericin are antibacterial, while drosomycin is antifungal.[23,28,29]

4.3 Specific antimicrobial responses are elicited by specific pathogens

Drosophila can distinguish between systemic infection with fungal and bacterial pathogens, since following infection the fat body produces antimicrobial peptides with specificity appropriate to the invading organism.[30] This process is essential for the survival of the fly on microbial challenge. The *Drosophila* Toll receptor, and other related receptors, are a crucial part of this system.[31–33] The antifungal defence pathway in flies remains the best characterized of all the Toll-signalling systems. This is largely because the Toll pathway is used by the fly for two

---

Box 8.3 Study of the antimicrobial defence in *Drosophila*

Drosophila is a good model for the study of the innate immune function

Ability to make mutants and transgenic animals exceeds mammalian systems

Natural pathogens including fungi and bacteria have been studied

Both local (epithelial) and systemic responses occur, and their control differs

Drosophila has different systems for responding to fungi and bacteria

Different but related pathways mediate pathogen-specific responses

Toll-like receptors are key components of *Drosophila* immune defence

Responses to some pathogens require more than one Toll receptor

Systemic infection produces a response from the fat body, a liver-like organ

Fungal infection is the best understood event

Fungi are important pathogens in *Drosophila*

The antifungal response is initiated in the haemolymph

A cytokine-like molecule is generated by proteolysis by unknown proteins

The cell-surface receptor Toll is not directly involved in fungus recognition

The antibacterial response involves genes other than Toll

Local infection produces a response locally and is poorly understood

Much work remains to be done, since:

> *Drosophila* contains nine Toll-related receptors, and seven have no known function

> At least 30 genes are involved in the antibacterial response in *Drosophila*

purposes: the control of axis formation in the embryo and for antimicrobial defence; the composition of the Toll-dependent pathway used in the establishment of the dorsoventral axis of the fly embryo had been intensively investigated,[34] prior to the discovery of the immune role of Toll.[33–35]

4.4 Antifungal response of *Drosophila*

As illustrated in Fig. 8.1, *Drosophila* Toll is just one component of the antifungal defence system in flies. The recognition of fungi occurs in the haemolymph and Toll does not appear directly involved in this event.[36] The proteins recognizing the fungus are unknown but are presumably pattern recognition receptors of some sort. Although not yet identified in *Drosophila*, fungus-binding PRR which activate serine proteases have been identified in other insects.[37,38] A proteolytic event follows fungal recognition, controlled by a protease inhibitor protein called a serpin.[36] The consequence of the

proteolysis is the activation of a cytokine-like dimeric protein, Spätzle.[39] This event results in activation of the transmembrane receptor Toll. Spätzle is believed to bind to Toll and activate it. Evidence for this is the Spätzle-dependent nature of Toll activation,[23,40,41] that Spätzle protein cannot be isolated from *Drosophila* which have a functional Toll receptor,[41,42] and a recent biochemical study.[43]

Following Toll activation, a signal is transmitted into the cell. Multiple intermediate proteins are involved in this process, which culminates in the activation of transcription factors and the induction of target genes, such as those encoding antifungal peptides. One class of transcription factors activated by Toll proteins is the Rel family, multiple members of which have been shown to be involved in immune function. The details are beyond the scope of this discussion but have been comprehensively reviewed by Karin and Ben-Neriah.[44]

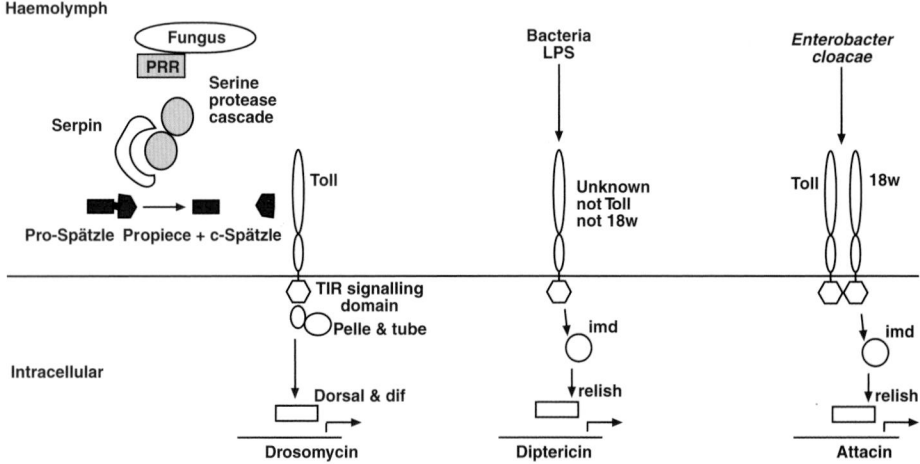

Anti-fungal response Anti-bacterial response

Fig. 8.1 In the antimicrobial defence of the fly, three systems have been identified two of which are illustrated. The one mediating antifungal responses depends on soluble fungus-detection protein(s) triggering a proteolytic cascade which then activates the Toll receptor. The antibacterial defence system includes a system responding to lipopolysaccharide (LPS), which is not as well characterized as the antifungal system. Some responses to Gram-negative bacteria appear to require both Toll and a second Toll receptor, 18-wheeler (18w). (See text for references.)

4.5 Antibacterial response of *Drosophila*

Just as with fungal infections, *Drosophila* responds to bacterial infection by antimicrobial gene induction.[19,20,25] The mechanism by which this occurs is less well understood than the antifungal response. It is not known whether, as with the antifungal response, genes upstream of Toll receptors are required for bacterial recognition. Although a Toll receptor, 18-wheeler (18w), is responsible for induction of some antimicrobial peptides in response to bacterial infection,[28,29,32] other responses do not depend on 18w. This suggests that additional components, which probably include other Toll receptors, are involved. One of these receptors is Toll itself. This is illustrated on the right of Fig. 8.1, showing the response to *Enterobacter cloacae*.[28] In this response, studies of double mutant flies revealed that both 18w and Toll expression is required for some responses.[28] This result is compatible with ectopic expression experiments in the *Drosophila* cell line S2.[23] One explanation for this is that Tolls work together in complexes, as will be discussed later.

4.6 Additional complexities in *Drosophila* antimicrobial defence

Whole genome sequencing of *Drosophila* has shown that there are at least nine Tolls.[23] Of these nine Tolls, the function of two, Toll and 18w, is known. One additional Toll receptor, designated Toll-5, appears to signal by a Toll-like pathway, but no function has been assigned to the other six.[23] Some or all of these molecules are probably involved in immune function but their precise role is obscure at present. Additionally, the signalling pathways downstream of the Tolls are not well characterized. The pathways used by antifungal and antibacterial responses (Fig. 8.1) differ in their dependence on the intracellular tube and pelle proteins,[23] in the protein complexes involved in activation of Rel family members,[45,46] and in use of Rel family members (reviewed by Imler and Hoffman[4]). However the separation of the two signalling pathways is not complete. Thus, flies with a mutation in the *relish* gene, a Rel family member required for antimicrobial gene synthesis, also have decreased antifungal responses. This may be because of the physiological state of the Rel family member involved in drosomycin synthesis is a heterodimer consisting of *relish* and *dif*, another Rel family member.[31]

5. ROLE OF TOLL-LIKE RECEPTORS (TLR) IN VERTEBRATE IMMUNE DEFENCE

The crucial role of Tolls in *Drosophila* caused interest in similar molecules found in vertebrates, which are termed TLR (Box 8.4). To date, ten human TLR have been described in published literature.[47–49] It is possible that analysis of the recently published human genome sequence will reveal further family members.

Targeted deletion of several genes, produces striking phenotypes (see Table 8.2). Each of the TLR is essential for the response of the mice to specific, ubiquitous components of bacteria, as judged by the severe attenuation of these responses in mutant animals. By contrast with the morphogenic role of *Drosophila* Toll and 18w, no developmental abnormality is evident in mice with targeted deletions of Toll-like receptors (see Table 11.2).[50–52]

Therefore, several different molecular systems mediate responses to specific bacterial components. Other uncharacterized pathways, which are probably also TLR dependent, may be responsible for signalling in response to other bacteria, such as *Streptococcus agalactiae*.[59] The relative contribution to stimulation of the

---

Box 8.4 Toll-like receptors (TLR) in vertebrate immune defence

Mammals contain a system for detecting conserved microbial components

Three systems have been identified, each critically dependent on a different TLR

The components detected include bacterial lipoproteins, lipopolysaccharide and DNA

TLR-containing detection systems mediate the earliest responses to microbial invasion

Table 8.2 Effect Toll-like receptors (TLR) – TLR2, TLR4 and TLR9 – evidence from mutant mice

TLR	Activating ligand(s) (ref)	Pathogen susceptibility in knockout mice (ref)
TLR1	Lipoproteins (99)	Hyporesponse to *Borrelia burgdorferi* vaccine (99)
TLR2	Lipoproteins (53) Peptidoglycan (50)	*S. aureus* (54)
TLR3	Double stranded RNA (138)	—
TLR4	Lipopolysaccharide (51,55,56); see also text	*N. meningitides* (57) *Salmonella* (58)
TLR5	Flagellin (148)	—
TLR6	Lipoproteins (100,101)	—
TLR7 and 8	Phsiological ligand unknown; small anti-viral molecules (139)	—
TLR9	Bacterial DNA (52,147); Herpes virus DNA (146)	Herpes simplex virus (146)

— indicates that, at the time of writing, an altered response to an intact microorganism had not been described *in vivo*.

immune system made by the various components of different bacteria, such as lipoproteins, lipopolysaccharide (LPS) and bacterial DNA, differ between bacteria. For example, a recent genetic study of *Neisseria meningitidis*[60] has confirmed that LPS is a crucial immune activator in this Gram-negative organism, but showed that other, non-LPS immune activators are also present. Protective responses to *N meningitidis* depend on TLR4, at least in mice.[57] By contrast,

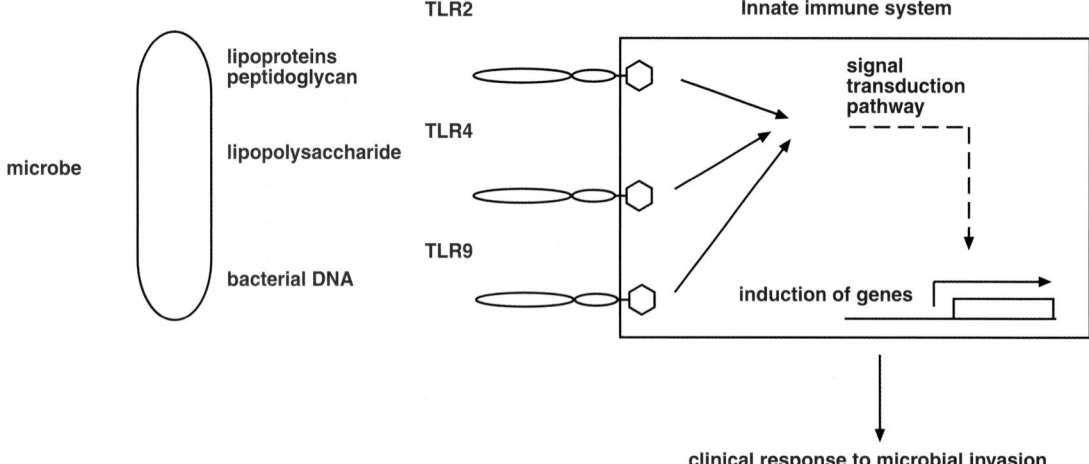

Fig. 8.2 Different Toll-like receptors (TLR) mediate signalling by different microbial components. Multiple TLRs exist, and are transmembrane molecules. Individual TLR have individual specificities. The structures recognized are ubiquitous, and often essential, microbial components. Activation of the TLR activates closely related intracellular signal transduction pathways. The result of these pathways is the induction of proinflammatory genes. See text for references.

stimulation by *Mycobacterium tuberculosis* and *Staphylococcus aureus*, which lack LPS, appears to rely on other components of the cell wall (see Table 8.2), and protective responses depend on TLR2.[54,61] These data suggest that in mammals, as in *Drosophila* (see above), engagement of different TLR will trigger different protective responses to specific bacterial pathogens.

Thus, we suggest that TLR can be viewed as comprising part of a sensory organ, detecting the molecular signatures of invading bacteria. Just as the animal's first image of an external threat is an integration of the signals from the rods and cones of the eye, so the first image of the pathogen within is the integration of the signals from various TLR pathways which detect different parts of the microbial invader. The integration event, which takes place within vertebrate cells stimulated by the pathogen, determines which genes are induced.

At present there is evidence that the magnitude of induction of individual vertebrate immune response genes depends on pathogen[62] and on activation of individual TLR by specific microbial structures.[60,62] Differential induction of patterns of mammalian response genes by microbial signals stimulating different TLR, as occurs in *Drosophila*,[30] is predicted by the above model. This has been demonstrated in the case of TLR2 and TLR4 signalling, as recently reviewed.[63].

5.1 TLR – transmembrane proteins with a common structure

As shown in Fig. 8.3, TLR have a common structure, consisting of an extracellular domain, a transmembrane portion and an intracellular domain. The extracellular domain consists of a series of repeats termed leucine-rich repeats (LRR).[64] By contrast, the intracellular domain is shorter and is required for signalling.[65] This domain does not itself contain known catalytic activity, but instead serves to recruit other signalling molecules that are required for signalling.[66] The intracellular domain, the three-dimensional structure of which has been determined,[67] is termed Toll and interleukin-1 related (TIR), because it is found not only in Toll proteins but also in interleukin-1 receptor family members. It is a structure of great antiquity,

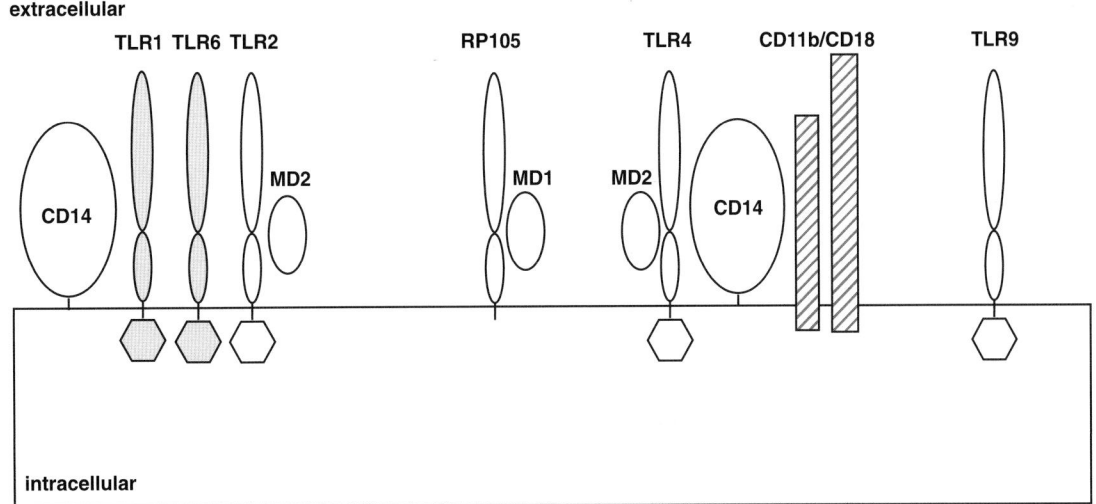

Fig. 8.3 Vertebrate Toll-like receptor (TLR) exist in complexes. TLR are transmembrane molecules with intracellular TIR signalling domains, with the exception of one Toll-like molecule, RP105 which lacks the TIR domain found in other Tolls. RP105 and TLR4 have been shown to cooperate in B-cell lipopolysaccharide (LPS) responsiveness.[69] They respectively bind to two small molecules, MD1[70] and MD2.[71] CD14 is a pattern recognition receptor (PRS)[72] which exists in both soluble and membrane-bound forms, which increases the sensitivity of TLR-dependent signalling,[73–75] as does the integrin CD11b/CD18.[76]

Box 8.5 Vertebrate Toll-like receptors (TLR)

Vertebrate Toll-like receptors:

    are transmembrane proteins

    function as part of a complex with other molecules

    determine specificity of the immune response

    transmit the signal into the cell

The TLR extracellular domain consists mostly of leucine rich repeats (LRR)

The TLR intracellular domain:

    is an ancient signalling domain widely distributed in biology

    is also found in interleukin-1 receptors, hence the name TIR (Toll and interleukin-1 related) domain

    lacks catalytic activity

    recruits other proteins to the complex, initiating signalling

---

found in some plant defence proteins as well as some intracellular vertebrate proteins.[68] The mechanism by which the TIR domain transduces signals into the cell has been comprehensively reviewed.[66] TIR domains are present in all TLR, except for one protein, RP105,[69] which lacks a TIR domain while retaining an immune function.

5.2 TLR operate in cooperation with other molecules

The phenotypes of mice with natural mutations in, or targeted deletions of, TLR[50–55] confirm the essential role of TLR in responses to conserved microbial components. It now is clear, however, that although the TLR are essential, they are not sufficient by themselves and that other molecules are required to mediate physiological responsiveness. These molecules form two classes: adapter proteins which bind to TLR, and TLR which increase, or alter, sensitivity of other TLR to microbial structures.

5.3 MD2 and RP105: components of the TLR complex

The role of TLR4 in LPS signalling was defined by the identification of TLR4 as the product of the mouse *lps* gene, which is essential for LPS responsiveness.[55,56] However, transfection of most cells with TLR4 does not confer LPS responsiveness, suggesting that other proteins are also required.[77–79] A small protein, MD2, sequence analysis of which suggests it to be a secreted protein,[71] binds to TLR4 and is required for TLR4-mediated LPS responsiveness.[71,80] TLR2 can also associate with MD2 and this association increases the responsiveness of TLR2 to a range of microbial products.[81] One possibility, therefore, is that MD2 acts as an adapter molecule, linking different TLR together, either by oligomerization or by interacting with a third, as yet unknown, structure. Two other proteins have also been shown to influence TLR4-dependent LPS responsiveness in B-lymphocytes. These are the protein RP105 and its cofactor MD1.[69,70,82] RP105 is a Toll-like molecule, although it lacks the intracellular signalling domain found in other TLR.[70]

5.4 Interaction between pattern recognition receptor and TLR

CD14 is a PRR[83] which binds to components of many bacteria, including the LPS of Gram-negative organisms, peptidoglycan and lipoteichoic acids of Gram-positive organisms, and the lipoproteins of mycobacteria and spirochaetes.[72,84] CD14 exists in both membrane-bound and soluble forms; animal data suggest it is an important determinant of the extent of some inflammatory processes *in vivo*.[85,86]

Co-transfection experiments suggest that enhanced signalling via TLR, triggered by agonists bound to CD14, is the consequence of PAMP binding to CD14. Probably, this occurs because CD14, by immobilizing the ligand at high local concentration, increases TLR signalling in response to it.[87] Biochemical data support the ligand-induced co-localization of TLR4 and CD14;[88] presumably a similar phenomenon occurs with TLR2, with which CD14 can also cooperate.[75,77,87] The agonists to which CD14 can increase signalling, at least using *in vitro* systems, are diverse and include lipoproteins,[89] lipoteichoic acid, peptidoglycan, whole *S aureus*[73,74] and LPS;[78] however, the *in vivo* relevance of some of these phenomena is not clear.[90,91]

The integrin CD11b/CD18 can also bind,[92] and mediate increased signalling in response to LPS.[93] Studies of macrophages from mice deficient in combinations of CD14 and CD11b/CD18 demonstrate that both may contribute to LPS signalling *in vivo*.[76] Their relative importance depends on the physical state of the agonist.[94] Careful cotransfection experiments, using TLR of different species, confirm that species-specific differences in response to LPS structure, and to related agonists, are due to differences in TLR4 and/or MD2 between species, not to differences in CD11b/CD18 or CD14.[95–98]

5.5 A combinatorial model of TLR function

It is also becoming apparent that combinations of TLR are important for initiating signalling and for determining ligand specificity.[99–101] Using cell lines transfected with TLR and TLR mutants, it has been found that formation of a complex between TLR2 and TLR6 is required for responses to some Gram-positive components.[101] Using different experimental systems, cooperation between TLR2 and TLR1 has also been described in responses to some LPS preparations and to lipoproteins.[99,100] Both of these studies observed a requirement for TLR combinations in the response to specific microbial products, suggesting that combinations of TLR may determine specificity rather than individual proteins. Until it is established which TLR can cooperate with each other, and whether heterodimers or combinations of three or more TLR, constitute the signalling unit, the total number of combinations possible will be unclear.

A combinatorial model of TLR function may explain the observed synergistic stimulatory action on macrophages of combinations of Gram-negative[102] and Gram-positive[103] bacterial components. The basis of the requirement for cooperation between different TLR in initiating signalling may be a need for TIR domains of different types[67] to associate,[101] since heterodimerization of TIR-containing proteins is also necessary for signalling in the interleukin-1 superfamily.[104–106]

5.6 Discrepancies between vertebrate and invertebrate TLR function

An implication of the combinatorial model of TLR function, which is supported by genetic data,[97,98,107] is that some direct interaction between the TLR extracellular domain and the components of microbial pathogen occurs in vertebrate TLR signalling. The cellular location at which this occurs is uncertain; in addition to the cell surface, on which TLR are expressed,[71,108–110] the phagolysosome[111] and intracellular compartments[112] have all been suggested. Irrespective of the location of interaction, the vertebrate system appears to differ in a fundamental way from that used in the *Drosophila* antifungal defence system.[36] One possibility is that two systems exist for activating TLR: some microbial agonists activate TLR by direct interaction, whereas others generate an activating Spätzle-like molecule to produce their effect. This latter mechanism has not been described in vertebrates at the time of writing, although recent data from the frog embryo suggest that mediators similar to the Toll-activating cytokine of the *Drosophila* antifungal response, i.e. Spätzle, must exist in vertebrates.[113,114] One could speculate that the obligate TLR4 cofactor MD2 does, in fact, have a role homologous to that of Spätzle, in that it acts as a secreted molecule with a role in increasing the sensitivity of the TLR2 and TLR4 expressed on other cells. Although evidence that it is secreted is absent at the moment, it is of note that message analysis of monocyte-derived intermediate dendritic cells upregulate MD2 and downregulate TLR2 and TLR4 expression[109] during their differentiation pathway. This suggests that MD2 produced by the intermediate dendritic cells, which are a key regulators of the immune response, is in fact secreted rather than binding to TLR inside the dendritic cell itself.

5.7 Non-bacterial TLR agonists

A more detailed understanding of the mechanism of TLR activation may help to explain the recent discovery of several non-bacterial agonists that activate TLR. These reports all contain controls which appear to exclude endotoxin contamination of protein preparations as an explanation for the observations. Respiratory syncytial virus F glycoprotein stimulates immune cells, and induces a protective response, in a TLR4- and CD14-dependent manner.[115] Additionally, a domain of fibronectin, a connective tissue protein, is reported to act as a TLR4 agonist.[116] A third class of proteins which appear to act as TLR agonists are heat shock proteins (HSP). Recombinant human HSP60, which is a potent adjuvant,[117] stimulates monocytes to produce tumour necrosis factor-alpha (TNF-α). The activity mediated by a recombinant HSP60 preparation is heat labile and resistant to polymyxin B, features which discriminate it from LPS.[118,119] CD14 is required for HSP60 signalling by human monocytes,[120] as is a wild-type *lps* gene.[121] Similar results have been reported with *Chlamydia* HSP60.[118] By contrast to these reports, a report using purified *Escherichia coli* GroEL (HSP60), from which copurification of other proteins was excluded, found that the activity of this protein was heat stable, protease resistant and unaffected by blocking anti-CD14 antibodies.[122] The available data, however, would be compatible with a mechanism of TLR4 activation in which an HSP60–TLR4 interaction was required for TLR4 function. Such an interaction might occur either following release of HSP60[18] at sites of injury[123] or in the Golgi apparatus, a site to which extracellular LPS is transported in a TLR4-dependent fashion.[112,124] More work is clearly needed to understand exactly how agonists as disparate as bacterial LPS, a respiratory virus, fibronectin and HSP all stimulate the same receptor.

Some TLR are also involved in antiviral defence. TLR3 is a receptor for double stranded RNA, an intermediate produced by the reproduction of some viruses.[138] Additionally, TLRs 7 and 8 also induce anti-viral defence. The physiological ligands for TLR7 and TLR8 are unknown, but they can be activated by small antiviral compounds, including imiquimod.[139] Recent data suggests that TLR9, which recognizes double stranded DNA, has a role in defence against herpes simplex virus.[146] Some viruses have systems for activating antiviral TLR.[140]

6. TOLL-LIKE RECEPTOR (TLR) RELEVANCE TO HUMAN MICROBIAL DISEASE SUSCEPTIBILITY

Polymorphisms in crucial immune components are a possible explanation for the varying disease susceptibility of individuals. A strong case can be made for the evaluation of TLR as disease susceptibility genes. This is because, as discussed above:

- TLR are activated by many human pathogens;
- studies with knockout mice support a crucial role for TLR in antimicrobial defence;
- a similar role in humans is supported by studies with human cell lines, in which TLR-blocking antibodies modify inflammatory responses;[59,125]
- differentiation of dendritic cells, driven by TLR-dependent signals, influences the nature of the adaptive immune response;[109,126,127]
- disease susceptibility genes exist that control cytokine secretion and disease susceptibility, e.g. in meningococcaemia.[128] These genes appear to lie upstream of the cytokine gene TNF-α, and TLR are possible candidates.
- cell-surface expression of TLR is positively correlated, at least in the case of LPS and TLR4, with responsiveness;[80,129,130]
- there is marked heterogeneity in expression of TLR between individuals;[109]
- TLR are polymorphic, with polymorphisms in both TLR2[131] and TLR4[132] described. TLR2 polymorphisms are implicated in leprosy pathogenesis in Korean patients.[141,142] Certain TLR4 polymorphisms are associated with responsiveness to endotoxin in the Caucasian population,[132] with rate of progression of atherogenesis,[143] Gram negative septic shock,[144] and with probability of death from meningococcaemia.[145]

7. FURTHER DIRECTIONS

Many crucial issues remain unresolved in the field of TLR signalling. The first concerns how many microbial structures the vertebrate microbial sensory organ, of which TLR are a crucial part, actually detects. Molecular study of those TLR of currently unknown function should address this. The second issue concerns the mechanism and location of the microbe detection event in vertebrates; whether, as in *Drosophila*, some of the detection occurs upstream of the TLR, mediated by specialist detector proteins, or whether, as currently appears to be the case, direct interaction of the microbial structure with the TLR is essential. A better understanding of this may explain the role in TLR activation of some of the non-microbial agonists recently described, such as fibronectin and HSP. Further, the nature of the process by which differential signalling by TLR is integrated into a physiological response, i.e. a pattern of induced genes, is unclear, as is whether the situation in flies, in which responses are tailored to destruction of the invading microbe, also applies to vertebrates. This crucial question awaits experimental investigation. Preliminary data show that at least some TLR are polymorphic and that these polymorphisms may be functional. The extent to which these are relevant to disease susceptibility will be a major challenge in the next few years, which awaits experimental investigation. Finally, in the field of therapeutics, although TLR, being critical components in an important signal transduction system, are clearly candidates for drug development, whether drugs based on TLR modulation will be clinically useful remains to be determined. However, results with recently described anti-TLR2 and anti-TLR4 monoclonal antibodies, which reduce cellular responses to lipoproteins and LPS,[59,125] respectively, combined with a demonstration that LPS chelation alters outcome in meningo-coccaemia,[133] indicate that modulation of TLR function may offer a new means of modulation of the sepsis syndrome, the mortality of which remains high.[134]

GLOSSARY

Adaptive immunity	A system of immunity, found in vertebrates, in which receptors are generated by mutation of germline DNA, driven by antigen exposure.
Complementation	The performance of a function normally subserved by one gene by another such that there is no phenotypic change.
Ectopic expression	Expression of a gene somewhere it is not normally expressed.
Expression	Refers to the process by which the gene is transcribed.
Induction	Causing the expression of a gene.
Innate immunity	A system of immunity which relies only on proteins encoded by the germline (cf. Adaptive immunity).
Leucine-rich repeat (LRR)	A 24–28 amino acid repeat, found in many proteins, including Toll-like receptors (TLR).
Lipopolysaccharide (LPS)	A complex lipid and polysaccharide which is the major lipid of the outer membrane of Gram-negative bacteria.
Lipoprotein	A chemical structure, found in bacteria, by which a protein is conjugated with a lipid.
Microarray	A large collection of DNA fragments, immobilized on a surface so that

hybridization experiments can be carried out on many substrates at once.

Mosaic An organism consisting of two or more populations of cells having different DNA.

Pathogen-associated molecular patterns (PAMP) Repetitive structures, widely distributed among microbes.

Pattern recognition receptors (PRR) A host receptor capable of detecting PAMP and differentiating them from host tissues.

Peptidoglycan A component of bacterial cells walls, both Gram-positive and Gram-negative.

Saturation mutagenesis Mutagenesis of a group of organisms such that every gene present would be expected to be affected by the procedure.

Serpin Serine protease inhibitor. A soluble, naturally occurring protein which inhibits serine protease activity.

Targeted deletion Also known as knock-out, a process by which the natural copy of a gene is destroyed.

Toll and interleukin-1 related (TIR) domain A c. 200 amino acid domain of great antiquity which initiates signalling by those proteins containing it

Transcription factor A protein which, by binding to the promoter (regulatory region) of a gene, regulates gene expression.

Transfection The process of introduction of a gene into a cell, without using an infectious device (such as a virus).

Transgene A gene introduced into an organism artificially.

ACKNOWLEDGEMENTS

The authors wish to thank Dr A Visintin (National Institutes of Health, Bethesda, MD) and Dr S Segal (Wellcome Centre for Human Genetics, Oxford, UK) for helpful comments.

REFERENCES

Further reading

Aderem, A, Ulevitch RJ. Toll-like receptors in the induction of the innate immune response. *Nature* 2000; **406**: 782–7.

Hoffman J, Kafatos F, Janeway C, Ezekowitz R. Phylogenetic perspectives in innate immunity. *Science* 1999; **284**: 1313–18.

Medzhitov R, Janeway Jr C. Innate immune recognition: mechanisms and pathways *Immunol Rev* 2000; **173**: 89–97.

WEBSITES

- http://www.ncbi.nlm.nih.gov/pubmed
  Medline, with links to genomic resources.
- http://www.ncbi.nlm.nih.gov/omim
  Reviews of human genetics, with emphasis on inherited disease.
- http://www.fruitfly.org
  Drosophila genome project.
- http://www.stke.org
  Science's Signal Transduction web resource.

Scientific papers

1. Roitt I. *Roitt's Essential Immunology*, 9th edn. Oxford: Blackwell Science, 1997.
2. Agrawal A, Eastman QM, Schatz DG. Transposition mediated by RAG1 and RAG2 and its implications for the evolution of the immune system. *Nature* 1998; **394**: 744.
3. Bonas U, Ackerveken G. Gene-for-gene interactions: bacterial avirulence proteins specify plant disease resistance. *Curr Opin Microbiol* 1999; **2**: 94.

4. Imler JL, Hoffmann JA. Signaling mechanisms in the antimicrobial host defense of *Drosophila. Curr Opin Microbiol* 2000; **3**: 16.

5. Medzhitov R, Janeway C. Innate immunity: impact on the adaptive immune response. *Curr Opin Immunol* 1997; **9**: 4.

6. Gabolde M, Guilloud-Bataille M, Feingold J, Besmond C. Association of variant alleles of mannnose binding lectin with severity of pulmonary disease in cystic fibrosis: cohort study *Br Med J* 1999; **319**: 1166.

7. Garred P, Madsen HO, Balslev U et al. Susceptibility to HIV infection and progression of AIDS in relation to variant alleles of mannose-binding lectin. *Lancet* 1997; **349**: 236.

8. Hibberd ML, Sumiya M, Summerfield JA et al. Assocation of variants of the gene for mannose-binding lectin with susceptibility to meningococcal disease. Meningococcal Research Group. *Lancet* 1999; **353**: 1049.

9. Wallis R, Cheng JY. Molecular defects in variant forms of mannose-binding protein associated with immunodeficiency. *J Immunol* 1999; **163**: 4953.

10. LeVine AM, Kurak KE, Bruno MD et al. Surfactant protein-A-deficient mice are susceptible to *Pseudomonas aeruginosa* infection. *Am J Respir Cell Molec Biol* 1998; **19**: 700.

11. LeVine AM, Bruno MD, Huelsman KM et al. Surfactant protein A-deficient mice are susceptible to group B streptococcal infection. *J Immunol* 1997; **158**: 4336.

12. Thomas C, Li Y, Kodama T et al. Protection from lethal Gram-positive infection by macrophase scavenger receptor-dependent phagocytosis. *J Exp Med* 2000; **191**: 147.

13. Lu J, Le Y. Ficolins and the fibrinogen-like domain. *Immunobiology* 1998; **199**: 190.

14. Turner MW. Mannose-binding lectin (MBL) in health and disease. *Immunobiology* 1998; **199**: 327.

15. Clark HW, Reid KB, Sim RB. Collectins and innate immunity in the lung. *Microbes Infect* 2000; **2**: 273.

16. Du Clos TW. Function of C-reactive protein. *Ann Med* 2000; **32**: 274.

17. Palecanda A, Paulauskis J, Al-Mutairi E et al. Role of the scavenger receptor MARCO in alveolar macrophage binding of unopsonized environmental particles. *J Exp Med* 1999; **189**: 1497.

18. Matzinger P. Tolerance, danger, and the extended family. *Annu Rev Immunol* 1994; **12**: 991.

19. Wu LP, Anderson KV. Regulated nuclear import of Rel proteins in the *Drosophila* immune response. *Nature* 1998; **392**: 93.

20. Eldon E, Kooyer S, D'Evelyn D et al. The *Drosophila* 18 wheeler is required for morphogenesis and has striking similarities to Toll. *Development* 1994; **120**: 885.

21. Manfruelli P, Reichhart JM, Steward R et al. A mosaic analysis in *Drosophila* fat body cells of the control of antimicrobial peptide genes by the Rel proteins Dorsal and DIF. *Eur Molec Biol Org J* 1999; **18**: 3380.

22. Tzou P, Ohresser S, Ferrandon D et al. Tissue-specific inducible expression of antimicrobial peptide genes in *Drosophila* surface epithelia. *Immunity* 2000; **13**: 737.

23. Tauszig S, Jouanguy E, Hoffmann JA, Imler JL. Toll-related receptors and the control of antimicrobial peptide expression in *Drosophila. Proc Natl Acad Sci USA* 2000; **97**: 10,520.

24. Ferrandon D, Jung AC, Criqui M et al. A drosomycin-GFP reporter transgene reveals a local immune response in *Drosophila* that is not dependent on the Toll pathway. *Eur Molec Biol Org J* 1998; **17**: 1217.

25. Basset A, Khush RS, Braun A et al. The phytopathogenic bacteria *Erwinia carotovora* infects *Drosophila* and activates and immune response. *Proc Natl Acad Sci USA* 2000; **97**: 3376.

26. Braun A, Hoffmann JA, Meister M. Analysis of the *Drosophila* host defense in domino mutant larvae, which are devoid of hemocytes. *Proc Natl Acad Sci USA* 1998; **95**: 14,337.

27. Hancock RE, Diamond G. The role of cationic antimicrobial peptides in innate host defences. *Trends Microbiol* 2000; **8**: 402.

28. Hedengren M, Borge K, Hultmark D. Expression and evolution of the *Drosophila* attacin/diptericin gene family [in process citation]. *Biochem Biophys Res Commun* 2000; **279**: 574.

29. Dushay MS, Roethele JB, Chaverri JM et al. Two attacin antibacterial genes of *Drosophila melanogaster. Gene* 2000; **246**: 49.

30. Lemaitre B, Reichhart JM, Hoffmann JA. *Drosophila* host defense: differential induction of antimicrobial peptide genes after infection by various classes of microorganisms. *Proc Natl Acad Sci USA* 1997; **94**: 14,614.

31. Hedengren M, Asling B, Dushay MS et al. Relish, a central factor in the control of humoral but not cellular immunity in *Drosophila. Molec Cell* 1999; **4**: 827.

32. Williams MJ, Rodriguez A, Kimbrell DA, Eldon ED. The 18-wheeler mutation reveals complex antibacterial gene regulation in *Drosophila* host defense. *Eur Molec Biol Org J* 1997; **16**: 6120.

33. Lemaitre B, Nicolas E, Michaut L et al. The dorsoventral regulatory gene cassette Spatzle/Toll/cactus controls the potent antifungal response in *Drosophila* adults. *Cell* 1996; **86**: 973.

34. Anderson KV. Pinning down positional information: dorsal-ventral polarity in the *Drosophila* embryo. *Cell* 1998; **95**: 439.

35. Levashina EA, Ohresser S, Lemaitre B, Imler JL. Two distinct pathways can control expression of the gene encoding the *Drosophila* antimicrobial peptide metchnikowin. *J Molec Biol* 1998; **278**: 515.

36. Levashina EA, Langley E, Green C et al. Constitutive activation of toll-mediated antifungal defense in serpin-deficienct *Drosophila*. *Science* 1999; **285**: 1917.

37. Satoh D, Horii A, Ochiai M, Ashida M. Prophenoloxidase-activating enzyme of the silkworm, *Bombyx mori*. Purification, characterization, and cDNA cloning. *J Biol Chem* 1999; **274**: 7441.

38. Lee SY, Cho MY, Hyun JH et al. Molecular cloning of cDNA for pro-phenol-oxidase-activating factor I, a serine protease is induced by lipopolysaccharide or 1,3-beta-glucan in coleopteran insect, *Holotrichia diomphalia* larvae. *Eur J Biochem* 1998; **257**: 615.

39. DeLotto Y, DeLotto R. Proteolytic processing of the *Drosophila* Spatzle protein by easter generates a dimeric NGF-like molecule with ventralising activity. *Mech Dev* 1998; **72**: 141.

40. Schneider DS, Jin Y, Morisato D, Anderson KV. A processed form of the Spatzle protein defines dorsal-ventral polarity in the *Drosophila* embryo. *Development* 1994; **120**: 1243.

41. Stein D, Nusslein-Volhard C. Multiple extracellular activities in *Drosophila* egg perivitelline fluid are required for establishment of embryonic dorsal-ventral polarity. *Cell* 1992; **68**: 429.

42. Morisato D, Anderson KV. The spatzle gene encodes a component of the extracellular signaling pathway establishing the dorsal-ventral pattern of the *Drosophila* embryo. *Cell* 1994; **76**: 677.

43. Weber AN, Tauszig-Delamasure S, Hoffman JA et al. Binding of the *Drosophilia* cytokine. Spatzle to Toll is direct and establishes signaling. *Nat Immunol* 2003; **4**: 794.

44. Karin M, Ben-Neriah Y. Phosphorylation meets ubiquitination: the control of NF-κB activity. *Annu Rev Immunol* 2000; **18**: 621.

45. Lu Y, Wu LP, Anderson KV. The antibacterial arm of the *Drosophila* innate immune response requires an IkappaB kinase. *Genes Dev* 2001; **15**: 104.

46. Silverman N, Zhou R, Stoven S et al. A *Drosophila* IkappaB kinase complex required for relish cleavage and antibacterial immunity. *Genes Dev* 2000; **14**: 2461.

47. Rock FL, Hardiman G, Timans JC et al. A family of human receptors structurally related to *Drosophila* Toll. *Proc Natl Acad Sci USA* 1998; **95**: 588.

48. Du X, Poltorak A, Wei Y, Beutler B. Three novel mammalian toll-like receptors: gene structure, expression, and evolution. *Eur Cytokine Netw* 2000; **11**: 362.

49. Chuang TH, Ulevitch RJ. Cloning and characterization of a sub-family of human toll-like receptors: hTLR7, hTLR8 and hTLR9. *Eur Cytokine Netw* 2000; **11**: 372.

50. Takeuchi O, Hoshino K, Kawai T et al. Differential roles of TLR2 and TLR4 in recognition of gram-negative and gram-positive bacterial cell wall components. *Immunity* 1999; **11**: 443.

51. Hoshino K, Takeuchi O, Kawai T et al. Toll-like receptor 4 (TLR4)-deficient mice are hyporesponsive to lipopolysaccharide: evidence for TLR4 as the Lps gene product. *J Immunol* 1999; **162**: 3749.

52. Hemmi H, Takeuchi O, Kawai T et al. A Toll-like receptor recognizes bacterial DNA. *Nature* 2000; **408**: 740.

53. Takeuchi O, Kaufmann A, Grote K et al. Preferentially the R-stereoisomer of the mycoplasmal lipopeptide macrophage-activating lipopeptide-2 activates immune cells through a Toll-like receptor 2- and MyD88-dependent signaling pathway. *J Imunol* 2000; **164**: 554.

54. Takeuchi O, Hoshino K, Akira S. TLR2-deficient and MyD88-deficient mice are highly susceptible to *Staphylococcus aureus* infection. *J Immunol* 2000; **165**: 5392.

55. Poltorak A, Smirnova I et al. Defective LPS signaling in C3H/HeJ and C57BL/10ScCr mice: mutations in Tlr4 gene. *Science* 1998; **282**: 2085.

56. Qureshi ST, Lariviere L, Leveque G et al. Endotoxin-tolerant mice have mutations in Toll-like receptor 4 (Tlr4). *J Exp Med* 1999; **189**: 615.

57. Woods JP, FrelingerJA, Warrack G, Cannon JG. Mouse genetic locus Lps influences susceptibility to *Neisseria meningitidis* infection. *Infect Immunol* 1988; **56**: 1950.

58. Weinstein DL, Lissner CR, Swanson RN, O'Brien AD. Macrophage defect and inflammatory cell recruitment dysfunction in *Salmonella* susceptible C3H/HeJ mice. *Cell Immunol* 1986; **102**: 68.

59. Flo TH, Halaas E, Lien L et al. Human Toll-like receptor 2 mediates monocyte activation by *Listeria monocytogenes*, but not by group B streptococci or lipopolysaccharide. *J Immunol* 2000; **164**: 2064.

60. Pridmore AC, Wyllie DH, Abdillahi F et al. A lipopolysaccharide-deficient mutant of *Neisseria meningitidis* elicits attenuated cytokine release by human macrophages and signals via Toll-like receptor (TLR) 2 but not via TLR4/MD2. *J Infect Dis* 2001; **183**: 89.

61. Thoma-Uszynski S, Stenger S, Takeuchi O et al. Induction of direct antimicrobial activity through mammalian Toll-like receptors. *Science* 2001; **291**: 1544.

62. Cui W, Morrison DC, Silverstein R. Differential tumor necrosis factor alpha expression and release from peritoneal mouse macrophages *in vitro* in response to proliferating gram-positive versus gram-negative bacteria. *Infect Immunol* 2000; **68**: 4422.

63. Vogel SN, Fenton M. Toll-like receptor 4 signalling: new perspectives on a complex signal-transduction problem. *Biochem Soc Trans* 2003; **31**: 664.

64. Kobe B, Deisenhofer J. The leucine-rich repeat: a versatile binding motif. *Trends Biochem Sci* 1994; **19**: 415.

65. Yang RB, Mark MR, Gurney AL, Godowski PJ. Signaling events induced by lipopolysaccharide-activated toll-like receptor 2. *J Immunol* 1999; **163**: 639.

66. O'Neill LA, Greene C. Signal transduction pathways activated by the IL-1 receptor family: ancient signaling machinery in mammals, insects, and plants. *J Leukoc Biol* 1998; **63**: 650.

67. Xu Y, Tao X, Shen B et al. Structural basis for signal transduction by the Toll/interleukin-1 receptor domains. *Nature* 2000; **408**: 111.

68. Slack J, Schooley K, Bonnert T et al. Identification of two major sites in the type I interleukin-1 receptor cytoplasmic region responsible for coupling to pro-inflammatory signaling pathways. *J Biol Chem* 2000; **275**, 4670.

69. Ogata H, Su I, Miyake K et al. The toll-like receptor protein RP105 regulates lipopolysaccharide signaling in B cells. *J Exp Med* 2000; **192**: 23.

70. Miura Y, Shimazu R, Miyake K et al. RP105 is associated with MD-1 and transmits an activation signal in human B cells. *Blood* 1998; **92**: 2815.

71. Shimazu R, Akashi S, Ogata H et al. Md-2, a molecule that confers lipopolysaccharide responsiveness on Toll-like receptor 4. *J Exp Med* 1999; **189**: 1777.

72. Pugin J, Heumann ID, Tomasz A et al. CD14 is a pattern recognition receptor. *Immunity* 1994; **1**: 509.

73. Schwandner R, Dziarski R, Wesche H et al. Peptidoglycan- and lipoteichoic acid-induced cell activation is mediated by toll-like receptor 2. *J Biol Chem* 1999; **274**: 17,406.

74. Yoshimura A, Lien E, Ingalls RR et al. Recognition of Gram-positive bacterial cell wall components by the innate immune system occurs via Toll-like receptor 2. *J Immunol* 1999; **163**: 1.

75. Means TK, Lien E, Yoshimura A et al. The CD14 ligands lipoarabinomannan and lipopolysaccharide differ in their requirement for Toll-like receptors. *J Immunol* 1999; **163**: 6748.

76. Perera PY, Mayadas TN, Takeuchi O et al. CD11b/CD18 acts in concert with CD14 and toll-like receptor (TLR) 4 to elicit full lipopolysaccharide and taxol-inducible gene expression. *J Immunol* 2001; **166**: 574.

77. Kirschning CJ, Wesche H, Merrill Ayres T, Rothe M. Human toll-like receptor 2 confers responsiveness to bacterial lipopolysaccharide. *J Exp Med* 1998; **188**: 2091.

78. Chow JC, Young DW, Golenbock DT et al. Toll-like receptor-4 mediates lipopolysaccharide-induced signal transduction. *J Biol Chem* 1999; **274**: 10,689.

79. Muzio M, Natoli G, Saccani S et al. The human toll signaling pathway: divergence of nuclear factor kappaB and JNK/SAPK activation upstream of tumor necrosis factor receptor-associated factor 6 (TRAF6). *J Exp Med* 1998; **187**: 2097.

80. Akashi S, Shimazu R, Ogata H et al. Cell surface expression and lipopolysaccharide signaling via the toll-like receptor 4-MD-2 complex on mouse peritoneal macrophages. *J Immunol* 2000; **164**: 3471.

81. Dziarski R, Wang Q, Miyake K et al. MD-2 enables Toll-like receptor 2 (TLR2)-mediated responses to lipopolysaccharide and enhances TLR2-mediated responses to Gram-positive and Gram-negative bacteria and their cell wall components. *J Immunol* 2001; **166**:1938.

82. Miyake K, Shimazu R, Kondo J et al. Mouse MD-1, a molecule that is physically associated with RP105 and positively regulates its expression. *J Immunol* 1998; **161**: 1348.

83. Hoffman J, Kafatos F, Janeway C, Ezekowitz R. Phylogenetic perspectives in innate immunity. *Science* 1999; **284**: 1313.

84. Dziarski R, Tapping R, Tobias P. Binding of bacterial peptidoglycan to CD14. *J Biol Chem* 1999; **273**: 8680.

85. Haziot A, Ferrero E, Kontgen F et al. Resistance to endotoxin shock and reduced dissemination of gram-negative bacteria in CD14-deficient mice. *Immunity* 1996; **4**: 407.

86. Cauwels A, Frei K, Sansano S et al. The origin and function of soluble CD14 in experimental bacterial meningitis. *J Immunol* 1999; **162**: 4762.

87. Yang RB, Mark FR, Gray A et al. Toll-like receptor-2 mediates lipopolysaccharide-induced cellular signalling. *Nature* 1998; **395**: 284.

88. Jiang Q, Akashi S, Miyake K, Petty HR. Lipopolysaccharide induces physical proximity between CD14 and toll-like receptor 4 (TLR4) prior to nuclear translocation of NF-kappaB. *J Immunol* 2000; **165**: 3541.

89. Hirschfeld M, Kirschning CJ, Schwandner R et al. Inflammatory signaling by *Borrelia burgdorferi* lipoproteins is mediated by toll-like receptor 2. *J Immunol* 1999; **163**: 2382.

90. Haziot A, Hijiya N, Gangloff SC et al. Induction of a novel mechanism of accelerated bacterial clearance by lipopolysaccharide in CD14-deficient and Toll-like receptor 4-deficient mice. *J Immunol* 2001; **166**: 1075.

91. Haziot A, Hijiya N, Schultz K et al. CD14 plays no major role in shock induced by *Staphylococcus aureus* but down-regulates TNF-alpha production. *J Immunol* 1999; **162**: 4801.

92. Wright SD, Levin SM, Jong MT et al. Cr3 (CD11b/CD18) expresses one binding site for Arg–Gly–Asp-containing peptides and a second site for bacterial lipopolysaccharide. *J Exp Med* 1989; **169**: 175.

93. Ingalls RR, Golenbock DT. CD11c/CD18, a transmembrane signaling receptor for lipopolysaccharide. *J Exp Med* 1995; **181**: 1473.

94. Flo TH, Ryan L, Kilaas L et al. Involvement of CD14 and beta2-integrins in activating cells with soluble and particulate lipopolysaccharides and mannuronic acid polymers. *Infect Immunol* 2000; **68**: 6770.

95. Ingalls RR, Monks BG, Savedra Jr R et al. CD11/CD18 and CD14 share a common lipid A signaling pathway. *J Immunol* 1998; **161**: 5413.

96. Lien E, Means TK, Heine H et al. Toll-like receptor 4 imparts ligand-specific recognition of bacterial lipopolysaccharide. *J Clin Invest* 2000; **105**: 497.

97. Kawasaki K, Gomi K, Nishijima M. Gln(22) of mouse MD-2 is essential for species-specific lipopolysaccharide mimetic action of taxol. *J Immunol* 2001; **166**: 11.

98. Poltorak A, Ricciardi-Castagnoli P, Citterio S, Beutler B. Physical contact between lipopolysaccharide and toll-like receptor 4 revealed by genetic complementation. *Proc Natl Acad Sci USA* 2000; **97**: 2163.

99. Alexopoulou L, Thomas V et al. Hyporesponsiveness to vaccination with *Borrelia burgdorferi* OspA in humans and in TLR1- and TLR2-deficient mice. *Nat Med* 2002; **8**: 878.

100. Wyllie DH, Kiss-Toth E, Visintin A et al. Evidence for an accessory protein function for toll-like receptor 1 in anti-bacterial responses. *J Immunol* 2000; **165**: 7125.

101. Ozinsky A, Underhill DM, Fontenot JD et al. The repertoire for pattern recognition of pathogens by the innate immune system is defined by cooperation between toll-like receptors. *Proc Natl Acad Sci USA* 2000; **97**: 13,766.

102. Manthey CL, Perera PY, Henricson BE et al. Endotoxin-induced early gene expression in C3H/HeJ (Lpsd) macrophages. *J Immunol* 1994; **153**: 2653.

103. Kengatharan KM, De Kimipe S, Robson C et al. Mechanism of gram-positive shock: identification of peptidoglycan and lipoteichoic acid moieties essential in the induction of nitric oxide synthase, shock, and multiple organ failure. *J Exp Med* 1998; **188**: 305.

104. Born TL, Thomassen E, Bird TA, Sims JE. Cloning of a novel receptor subunit, AcPL, required for interleukin-18 signaling. *J Biol Chem* 1998; **273**: 29,445.

105. Greenfeder SA, Nunes P, Kwee L et al. Molecular cloning and characterization of a second subunit of the interleukin 1 receptor complex. *J Biol Chem* 1995; **270**: 13,757.

106. Hoshino K, Tsutsui H, Kawai T et al. Generation of IL-18 receptor-deficient mice: evidence for IL-1 receptor-related protein as an essential IL-18 binding receptor. *J Immunol* 1999; **162**: 5041.

107. Lien E, Chow JC, Hawkins LD et al. A novel synthetic acyclic lipid A-like agonist activates cells via the lipopolysaccharide/Toll-like receptor 4 signaling pathway. *J Biol Chem* 2001; **276**: 1873–80.

108. Lien E, Sellati TJ, Yoshimura A et al. Toll-like receptor 2 functions as pattern recognition receptor for diverse bacterial products. *J Biol Chem* 1999; **274**: 33,419.

109. Visintin A, Mazzoni A, Spitzer JH et al. Regulation of toll-like receptors in human monocytes and dendritic cells. *J Immunol* 2001; **166**: 249.

110. Aliprantis AO, Yang RB, Weiss DS et al. The apoptotic signaling pathway activated by Toll-like receptor-2. *Euro Molec Biol Org* 2000; **19**: 3325.

111. Underhill DM, Ozinsky A, Hajjar AM et al. The toll-like receptor 2 is recruited to macrophage phagosomes and discriminates between pathogens. *Nature* 1999; **401**: 811.

112. Thieblemont N, Wright SD. Transport of bacterial lipopolysaccharide to the golgi apparatus. *J Exp Med* 1999; **190**: 523.

113. Armstrong NJ, Steinbeisser H, Prothmann C et al. Conserved Spatzle/Toll signaling in dorsoventral patterning of *Xenopus* embryos. *Mech Dev* 1998; **71**: 99.

114. Prothmann C, Armstrong NJ, Rupp RA. The Toll/IL-1 receptor binding protein MyD88 is required for xenopus axis formation. *Mech Dev* 2000; **97**: 85.

115. Kurt-Jones EA, Popova L, Kwinn L et al. Pattern recognition receptors TLR4 and CD14 mediate response to respiratory syncytial virus. *Nature Immunol* 2000; **1**: 398.

116. Okamura Y, Watari M, Jerud ES et al. The EDA domain of fibronectin activates toll-like receptor 4. *J Biol Chem* 2001; **276**: 10,229–33.

117. Konen-Waisman S, Cohen A, Fridkin M, Cohen R. Self heat-shock protein (hsp60) peptide serves in a conjugate vaccine against a lethal pneumococcal infection. *J Infect Dis* 1999; **179**: 403.

118. Kol A, Bourcier T, Lichtman A, Libby P. Chlamydial and human heat shock protein 60s activate human vascular endothelium, smooth muscle cells, and macrophages. *J Clin Invest* 1999; **103**: 571.

119. Chen W, Syldath U, Bellmann K et al. Human 60-kDa heat-shock protein: a danger signal to the innate imune system. *J Immunol* 1999; **162**: 3212.

120. Kol A, Lichtman AH, Finberg RN et al. Heat shock protein (HSP) 60 activates the innate immune response: CD14 is an essential receptor for HSP60 activation of mononuclear cells. *J Immunol* 2000; **164**: 13.

121. Ohashi K, Burkart V, Floh S, Kolb H. Heat shock protein 60 is a putative endogenous ligand of the Toll-like receptor-4 complex. *J Immunol* 2000; **164**: 558.

122. Tabona P, Reddi K, Khan S et al. Homogeneous *Escherichia coli* chaperonin 60 induces IL-1 beta and IL-6 gene expression in human monocytes by a mechanism independent of protein conformation. *J Immunol* 1998; **161**: 1414.

123. Frantz S, Kobzik L, Kim YD et al. Toll4 (TLR4) expression in cardiac myocytes in normal and failing myocardium. *J Clin Invest* 1999; **104**: 271.

124. Thieblemont N, Wright SD. Mice genetically hyporesponsive to lipopolysaccharide (LPS) exhibit a defect in endocytic uptake of LPS and ceramide. *J Exp Med* 1997; **185**: 2095.

125. Aliprantis A, Yang R, Mark M et al. Cell activation and apoptosis by bacterial lipoproteins through toll-like receptor-2. *Science* 1999; **285**: 736.

126. Hertz CJ, Kiertscher SM, Godowski PJ et al. Microbial lipopeptides stimulate dendritic cell maturation via Toll-like receptor 2. *J Immunol* 2001; **166**: 2444.

127. Langenkamp A, Messi M, Lanzavecchia A, Sallusto F. Kinetics of dendritic cell activation: impact on priming of TH1, TH2 and nonpolarised T cells. *Nature Immunol* 2000; **1**: 311.

128. Westendorp RG, Langermans JA, Huizinga TN et al. Genetic influence on cytokine production and fatal meningococcal disase. *Lancet* 1997; **349**: 170.

129. Medvedev AE, Kopydlowski KM, Vogel SN. Inhibition of lipopolysaccharide-induced signal transduction in endotoxin-tolerized mouse macrophages: dysregulation of cytokine, chemokine, and toll-like receptor 2 and 4 gene expression. *J Immunol* 2000; **164**: 5564.

130. Nomura F, Akashi S, Sakao Y et al. Endotoxin tolerance in mouse peritoneal macrophages correlates with down-regulation of surface toll-like receptor 4 expression. *J Immunol* 2000; **164**: 3476.

131. Lorenz E, Mira JP, Cornish KL et al. A novel polymorphism in the toll-like receptor 2 gene and its potential associaton wiht staphylococcal infection. *Infect Immunol* 2000; **68**: 6398.

132. Arbour NC, Lorenz E, Schutte BC et al. TLR4 mutations are associated with entodoxin hyporesponsiveness in humans. *Nature Genet* 2000; **25**: 187.

133. Levin M, Quint PA, Goldstein B et al. Recombinant bactericidal/permeability-increasing protein (rBPI21) as adjunctive treament for children with severe meningococcal sepsis: a randomised trial. rBPI21 Meningococcal Sepsis Study Group. *Lancet* 2000; **356**: 961.

134. Astiz ME, Rackow EC. Septic shock. *Lancet* 1998; **351**: 1501.

135. Sun YH, Bakshi S, Chalmers R, Tang CM. Functional genomics of *Neisseria meningitidis* pathogenesis. *Nat Med* 2000; **6**: 1269.

136. Nolan PM, Peters J, Strivens M et al. A systematic, genome-wide, phenotype-driven mutagenesis programme for gene function studies in the mouse. *Nature Genet* 2000; **25**: 440.

137. Ingham PW. Zebrafish genetics and its implications for understanding vertebrate development. *Hum Molec Genet* 1999; **6**: 1755.

138. Alexopoulou L, Holt AC, Medzhitov R et al. Recognition of double-stranded RNA and activation of NF-kappaB by Toll-like receptor 3. *Nature* 2001; **413**: 732.

139. Hemmi H, Kaisho T, Takeuchi O et al. Small anti-viral compounds activate immune cells via the TLR7 MyD88-dependent signaling pathway. *Nat Immonol* 2002; **3**: 106.

140. Harte MT, Haga IR, Maloney G et al. The poxvirus protein A52R targets Toll-like receptor signaling complexes to suppress host defense. *J Exp Med* 2003; **197**: 343.

141. Kang TJ, Chae GT. Detection of Toll-like receptor 2 (TLR2) mutation in the lepromatous leprosy patients. *FEMS Immunol Med Microbiol* 2001; **31**: 53.

142. Kang TJ, Lee SB, Chae GT. A polymorphism in the Toll-like receptor 2 is associated with IL-12 production from monocyte in lepromatous leprosy. *Cytokine* 2002; **20**: 56.

143. Kiechl S, Lorenz E, Reindl M et al. Toll-like receptor 4 polymorphisms and atherogenesis. *N Engl J Med* 2002; **347**: 185.

144. Lorenz E, Mira JP, Frees KL et al. Relevance of mutations in the TLR4 receptor in patients with gram-negative septic shock. *Arch Intern Med* 2002; **162**: 1028.

145. Smirnova I, Mann N, Dols A et al. Assay of locus-specific genetic load implicates rare Toll-like receptor 4 mutations in menigococcal susceptibility. *Proc Natl Acad Sci USA* 2003; **100**: 6075.

146. Lund J, Sato A, Akira S et al. Toll-like receptor 9-mediated recognition of Herpes simplex virus-2 by plasmacytoid dendritic cells. *J Exp Med* 2003; **198**: 513.

147. Bauer S, Kirschning CJ, Hacker H et al. Human TLR9 confers responsiveness to bacterial DNA via species-specific CpG motif recognition. *Pro Natl Acad Sci USA* 2001; **98**: 9237.

148. Hayashi F, Smith KD, Ozinsky A et al. The innate immune response to bacterial flagellin is mediated by Toll-like receptor 5. *Nature* 2002; **410**: 1099.

9

Matrix metalloproteinases and infectious diseases

Nicholas M Price, Jon S Friedland

OBJECTIVES

(1) To briefly review the biology of matrix metalloproteinases (MMP).
(2) To consider the potential roles of MMP in the host response in central nervous system infection and in tuberculosis.

OVERVIEW

Matrix metalloproteinases (MMP) are a family of zinc-containing proteolytic enzymes which have physiological roles in tissue remodelling and development. In terms of immunity to infection, MMP are involved in leucocyte recruitment to sites of invasion by pathogens. However, secreted in excess, MMP have the potential to contribute to tissue destruction and clinical pathology in infectious diseases. In view of their potential harmful effects, MMP secretion is tightly regulated at the level of gene transcription, by secretion as pro-forms requiring enzymatic activation and by specific tissue inhibitors of MMP (TIMP). In the first part of

this chapter, the basic mechanisms of action of MMP and ways in which their tissue levels may be regulated are reviewed. The second part then considers the potential role of MMP in central nervous system infections and in tuberculosis, which has been the focus of our own interest.

1. MATRIX METALLOPROTEINASES: STRUCTURE AND CLASSIFICATION

MMP, or matrixins, are a structurally related family of zinc-containing proteases that degrade specific components of extracellular matrix (ECM).[1] MMP play a major role in normal connective tissue remodelling, such as during embryonic growth or wound repair. In addition, important immunological functions, such as leucocyte recruitment, have also been identified over the past decade. However, despite these physiological roles, excessive MMP activity has been implicated in the immunopathology of a variety of inflammatory diseases such as rheumatoid arthritis and multiple sclerosis. The regulation and specialized immune functions of leucocyte-derived MMP, together with their potential to cause host tissue injury during the host response to infectious diseases, are the central themes of this chapter.

Twenty-three MMP have been identified to date, which may be classified according to their structure and substrate specificity (Table 9.1). However, MMP nomenclature is confusing since some enzymes were named before the full

Table 9.1 Some members of the matrix metalloproteinase (MMP) family

MMP no.	Trivial name	Molecular weight (kDa)	Cellular source	Matrix substrate
Collagenases				
1	Interstitial collagenase	52	Monocytic cells, connective tissue	Collagens I, II, III, X; gelatin; proteoglycans
8	Neutrophil collagenase	75	Neutrophils	Collagens I, II, III; gelatin; proteoglycans
13	Collagenase-3	54	Tumour cells	Unknown
Stromelysins				
3	Stromelysin-1	57	Macrophages, connective tissue	Collagens III, IV, V, IX; proteoglycans; gelatin; fibronectin; laminin; (*activates MMP-1, -8, -9*)
10	Stromelysin-2	53	Macrophages, keratinocytes, tumour cells	As MMP-3 but lower activity
11	Stromelysin-3	55	Tumour stroma	Proteoglycans; fibronectin; gelatin; laminin; collagen IV
Gelatinases				
2	Gelatinase-A	72	Monocytic cells, lymphocytes, connective tissue, tumour cells	Collagens IV, V, VII, IX, XI; gelatin; fibronectin; elastin
9	Gelatinase-B	92	Monocytic cells, lymphocytes, neutrophils, connective tissue, tumour cells	Collagens IV, V, VII, IX, XI; gelatin; elastin
Others				
7	PUMP-1, Matrilysin	28	Monocytic cells, tumour cells	Collagen IV; proteoglycans; gelatin; fibronectin; laminin
12	Metalloelastase	57	Macrophages	Elastin; fibronectin
14–17	Membrane-type MMP e.g. MT1-MMP	66	Lung tissue, tumour cells	(*Activates MMP-2, -13*)

spectrum of their activity was identified. All MMP share several common domain motifs (Fig. 9.1) and are synthesized as inactive pro-enzymes and require proteolytic cleavage of the pro-peptide domain (approximately 80 amino acids long) for functional activation. The cysteine residue (the so-called cysteine switch), within a conserved PRCG(V/N)PD motif, ligates the catalytic zinc and is thought responsible for maintaining this latency. The catalytic domain (approximately 170 amino acids) contains a zinc-binding motif and a conserved methionine, which forms a unique Met-turn structure. The backbone structures within this domain (a five-stranded β-sheet, three α-helices, bridging loops and Met-turn) are similar to those found in three other distinct metallo-proteinase subfamilies (astacins, reprolysins or ADAM, and serralysins), which together with matrixins constitute the metazincins. In addition to another structural zinc ion, the catalytic domain also contains two to three calcium ions that are required for enzymatic activity. The C-terminal, hemopexin-like domain (about 210 amino acids) is involved in determining substrate specificity and has an

ellipsoidal disc shape with a four-bladed β-propeller structure (each blade consists of four antiparallel β-strands and an α-helix). Whilst most MMP are secreted, membrane-bound (-type) MMP (MT-MMP) have been identified which contain a transmembrane domain to anchor these enzymes to the cell surface.

2. MATRIX METALLOPROTEINASE (MMP) EXPRESSION BY LEUCOCYTES AND SPECIALIZED IMMUNE FUNCTIONS

A wide range of cell types responsible for maintenance of connective tissue secrete MMP. In addition, all types of leucocyte produce MMP, although the quantity and range of MMP expressed depends upon the particular cellular subset. For example, macrophages secrete MMP-1, -2, -3 and -9,[2] in addition to matrilysin (MT4-MMP or MMP-17)[3] and the elastase MMP-12.[4] MMP-9 is the quantitatively predominant MMP secreted by human mononuclear phagocytes, whilst only stimulated alveolar macrophages produce MMP-3 and these cells also secrete approximately 20-fold greater amounts of MMP-1 compared with peripheral blood monocytes.[5,6] Thus, the distinct pattern of basal and stimulated MMP expressed by mononuclear phagocytes also depends upon the stage of cellular differentiation or maturation.[2,7] In comparison, T-cells secrete smaller concentrations of only MMP-2 and MMP-9, and neutrophils (PMN) release both MMP-9 and a specific collagenase (MMP-8) from pre-formed granules.[8]

Since ECM maintenance is not a primary function of leucocytes, what is the purpose of MMP secretion by these cells? The role of MMP in cell migration through host tissues to sites of infection is possibly the most important. In particular, MMP-9 facilitates leucocyte extravasation from blood into surrounding connective tissue by degrading type IV collagen, a major component of vascular basement membrane surrounding endothelial cells. In addition, MMP may up- or downregulate the activity of disease-modifying cytokines. For example, active tumour necrosis factor-alpha (TNF-α) is released from its membrane-bound precursor by TNF-α-converting enzyme (TACE), which is a closely related

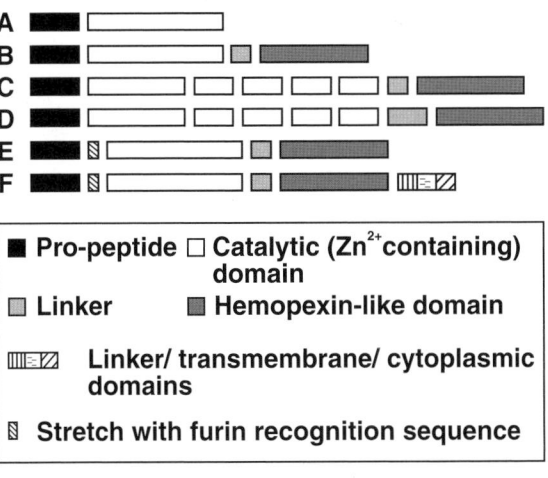

■ **Pro-peptide** □ **Catalytic (Zn²⁺containing) domain**

▨ **Linker** ▨ **Hemopexin-like domain**

▨ **Linker/ transmembrane/ cytoplasmic domains**

▨ **Stretch with furin recognition sequence**

Fig. 9.1 Domain arrangements of matrix metallo-proteinases (MMP). A, Matrilysin (MMP-7); B, intersti-tial collagenase (MMP-1), stromelysin-1 (MMP-3), stromelysin-2 (MMP-10), metalloelastase (MMP-12); C, gelatinase A (MMP-2); D, gelatinase B (MMP-9); E, stromelysin-3 (MMP-11); F, MT-MMP.

zinc-binding metalloproteinase belonging to the adamalysin family.[9] Furthermore, metalloenzymatic cleavage of interleukin (IL)-6 or TNF-α receptors may enhance or antagonize their respective proinflammatory ligands.[10] Finally, in addition to their activity at the cell surface, MMP may release growth factors such as TGF-β$_1$ from bound stores in the ECM or increase the bioavailability of insulin-like growth factor (IGF) by degradation of inhibitory IGF-binding proteins.[11–14]

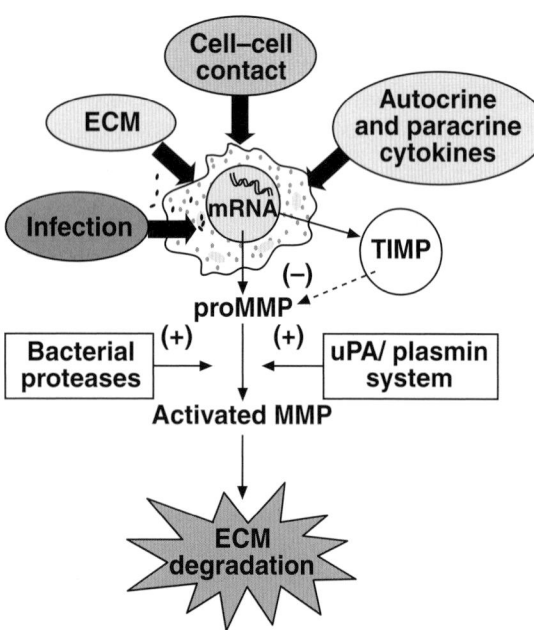

Fig. 9.2 Factors determining monocyte-derived matrix metalloproteinase (MMP) activity during the immune response to infectious diseases. MMP gene expression may be affected by a number of factors including direct contact between cells or with extracellular matrix (ECM), up- and downregulatory cytokines and interaction with the pathogen itself. After secretion, MMP activity is restricted by the presence of protease inhibitors, including specific tissue inhibitors of MMP (TIMP), or increased by proteolytic activation of proMMP. In addition to degrading ECM, activated MMP may increase tissue injury by releasing proinflammatory cytokines from membrane-bound stores. (uPA, urokinase-type plasminogen activator.)

3. REGULATION OF MATRIX METALLOPROTEINASE (MMP) ACTIVITY

Due to the potential harmful effects of excessive proteolytic activity during immune responses, MMP are stringently regulated on three main levels (Fig. 9.2). Firstly, there is tight control at the level of gene transcription. Cytokines and cell adhesion influence the expression of MMP activity at this level. The presence of specific transcriptional regulator protein binding sites, such as for AP-1, in MMP promoter sequences is responsible for controlling MMP gene expression. Secondly, after secretion from the cell, MMP activity is controlled by proteolytic activation of latent proenzymes. Finally, interaction with antiproteases and specific TIMP is critical.

3.1 Regulation of MMP activity by cytokines

The balance between type 1 helper T-cells (Th1) [e.g. TNF-α, and interferon-gamma (IFN-γ)] and Th2 (e.g. IL-4, -10, -13) derived cytokines is thought to be critical in regulating whether the immune response to a wide variety of infectious diseases is protective or destructive. Cytokines have important effects on MMP activity but these are complex. The effect of cytokines on monocytic cell-derived MMP activity is summarized in Table 9.2, although this list is not exhaustive and responses may vary with certain stimuli. TNF-α and IL-1β are important proinflammatory mediators, and induce gene expression and secretion of MMP-9 but not MMP-1 or MMP-3 in human monocyte-derived macrophages.[15] However, granulocyte–macrophage colony-stimulating factor (GM-CSF), when added to either IL-1β or TNF-α, induced MMP-1 and synergistically enhanced MMP-9 synthesis.[16] Interestingly, TNF-α, or IL-1β-induced MMP-9 production was suppressed by the third major cytokine found at inflammatory sites, IFN-γ.[15] In addition, IFN-γ has also been shown to inhibit MMP-1 and MMP-3 secretion by lipopolysaccharide (LPS)-stimulated human macrophages at a pre-translational level.[17]

The Th2-derived cytokines, IL-4 and IL-10, inhibited MMP-1 and MMP-9 secretion by human monocytes and macrophages stimulated with LPS, or killed *Staphylococcus aureus*.[18]

Table 9.2 Effects of cytokines and other mediators on monocytic cell-derived matrix metalloproteinase (MMP) activity

Mediator	Collagenase MMP-1	Stromelysin MMP-3	Gelatinase MMP-9	Inhibitor TIMP-1	Refs
Proinflammatory					
TNF-α	⇔	⇔	⇑	⇑	1
IL-1β	⇔	⇔	⇑	⇑	1
IFN-γ	⇓	⇓	⇓	⇔ ⇓	1–3
GM-CSF	⇑*		⇑	⇑	4
Anti-inflammatory					
IL-4	⇓ ⇑		⇓	⇔	2, 5, 6
IL-6			⇔	⇑	7
IL-10	⇓		⇓	⇑	7
Dexamethasone	⇓	⇓	⇓	⇓	8

GM-CSF, Granulocyte–macrophage colony-stimulating factor; IL, interleukin; INF-γ, interferon-gamma; TIMP, tissue inhibitors of MMP; TNF-α, tumour necrosis factor-alpha.

*GM-CSF in combination with either TNF-α and/or IL-1β.

However, IL-10 had an additional effect since it also stimulated gene expression and secretion of TIMP-1, thereby inhibiting MMP activity by a dual mechanism. Previous studies have shown the importance of a prostaglandin E_2 (PGE_2)-cAMP mediated pathway in MMP secretion by human monocytes stimulated with LPS or concanavalin-A (Con-A).[3,19] This mechanism has been demonstrated by blocking MMP synthesis with indomethacin and reversal of suppression by exogenous PGE_2 or dibutyryl cAMP; the inhibitory effects of IL-4, -10 and IFN-γ may largely be a result of blockade of this pathway.[19–21]

3.2 Regulation of MMP activity by chemokines

Chemokines are chemotactic cytokines, pivotal in leucocyte recruitment to sites of infection, the majority of which can be divided into two subgroups on the basis of structural motifs.[22] In the α or CXC subfamily [e.g. IL-8, IP-10, stromal cell-derived factor (SDF)-1] an intervening amino acid residue separates the first two cysteines. In the β or CC subfamily [e.g. MCP-1, regulated upon activation, normal T expressed and secreted (RANTES), macrophage inflammatory protein (MIP)-1α] these cysteines are adjacent. Chemokines exert their actions by binding to specific cell-surface receptors, which are members of the rhodopsin superfamily of seven-transmembrane G-protein-linked molecules.[23] G-proteins serve to mediate signal transduction events by coupling such surface receptors to intracellular effectors.

Evidence obtained using G-protein ADP-ribosylating agents, cholera and pertussis toxins indicates that G-proteins affect the eicosanoid–cAMP-dependent pathway that results in monocyte-MMP secretion.[24] Cholera toxin enhanced the production of cAMP, prostaglandin H synthase-2, PGE_2 and secretion of MMP-1 and -9 in Con A-stimulated human monocytes and reversed indomethacin-mediated suppression of MMP secretion. In contrast, pertussis toxin, which inhibits intrinsic

G-protein function, reduced the secretion of these MMP in addition to decreasing the production of cAMP, prostaglandin H synthase-2 and PGE2.

However, whilst β-chemokines (MIP-1α, MIP-1β, and RANTES) stimulate proMMP-9 secretion of all human lymphocyte subsets,[25] the functional effect of this in terms of facilitating cell migration is unclear. In order to investigate this in greater detail, T-cell migration across a model basement membrane (BM), made from filters coated with Matrigel (made from BM constituents), have been studied in an *in vitro* chemotaxis system called a modified Boyden chamber.[26–28] Stimulation with RANTES and MIP-1α induced MMP-9 secretion, chemotactic migration and degradation of type IV collagen (a major BM component and an MMP-9 substrate). However, suppression of MMP activity with a hydroxamate-dipeptide inhibitor, GM6001, failed to block migration across BM induced by RANTES and MIP-1α, but not other chemotactic stimuli. One possible explanation for this is that certain chemokines may activate the secretion of proteases that enable BM transmigration. However, MMP-9 secretion and BM invasion by monocytic U937 cells stimulated by TPA or TNF-α was suppressed by physiological MMP inhibitors (TIMP-1 and α$_2$-macroglobulin) but not by blockade of proteinases that are not metalloenzymes (e.g. cathepsin G and leucocyte elastase).[29]

MMP may also directly modify the activity of chemokines and a positive feedback loop was recently demonstrated between MMP-9 secreted by PMN and IL-8, the prototypic CXC chemokine which is active on these leucocytes.[30] Amino terminal truncation of IL-8 (1-77) into IL-8 (7-77) by human PMN MMP-9 resulted in a 10- to 27-fold increased potency in PMN activation, measured by elevated intracellular calcium concentration, chemotaxis and MMP-9 secretion. Interestingly, there is evidence that MMP may also alter the cellular response to chemokines by cleaving their specific receptors from the surface of leucocytes. For example, in TNF-α or LPS-stimulated PMN, proteolytic removal of receptors that bind IL-8, CXCR1 and CXCR2 was blocked by metalloproteinase inhibition.[31]

3.3 Regulation of MMP expression by cell–matrix and cell–cell interactions

Cellular contact with the ECM is also an important stimulus to MMP secretion. Human alveolar macrophages cultured on types I and III collagen induced MMP-1 (but not MMP-9) gene transcription and a 25-fold increase in secretion, via a PGE$_2$-dependent mechanism.[32] In addition, interaction between extravasating leucocytes and endothelial cells,[33] and close contact with other immune cells (see below), may enhance MMP secretion at sites of infection.[34]

3.4 Pro-MMP

Apart from the membrane-bound MMP, most MMP are secreted as inactive zymogens. *In vitro*, these proenzymes can be activated by a variety of proteolytic and non-proteolytic agents (e.g. trypsin, organomercurials, reactive oxygen species, denaturants and SH-active agents). In all of these, the removal of the inhibitory propeptide follows disruption of the Cys–Zn^{2+} 'switch' in a stepwise fashion.[35] *In vivo*, the urokinase-type plasminogen activator (uPA)/plasminogen system, is thought to be particularly important in proMMP activation.[36] This cascade involves conversion of cell-bound plasminogen to plasmin and, once activated, some MMP are capable of activating one another.[37] It has also been discovered that MT-MMP can activate proMMPs at the cell surface. ProMMP-2 activation by MT1-MMP also requires TIMP-2, which forms a receptor complex with MT1-MMP on the cell surface and acts as a concentration mechanism to increase efficiency of activation by co-localizing both active MT1-MMP and zymogen.[38] Interestingly, proteases secreted by some bacteria (e.g. *Pseudomonas* elastase and *Vibrio cholerae* protease) or free radicals generated in infection and inflammation can also activate human proMMP.[39]

3.5 Anti-proteases and TIMP

The major physiologic MMP inhibitors are α2-macroglobulin, present in serum, and a family of specific inhibitors called TIMP (21–32 kDa). Since α2-macroglobulin (780 kDa) is thought to be restricted in its sites of action due to its large size, TIMP are the major MMP regulators in tissue. Four TIMP (TIMP-1–4), which exhibit 41–52% sequence homology, have been identified to date and are secreted by many cells including those of connective tissue.[40] Macrophages secrete both TIMP-1 and -2 constitutively: TIMP-1 is a 32 kDa glycoprotein and quantitatively predominant, whereas TIMP-2 is unglycosylated. TIMP form tight 1:1 stoichiometric complexes with MMP and the balance between the relative local concentrations of MMP and TIMP determines net proteolytic activity. All of the TIMP are potentially capable of inhibiting any MMP,[41] except for the weak, non-inhibitory interaction between TIMP-2 and MT1-MMP (described above), which functions as a membrane-bound receptor for proMMP-2 activation.[42] The N-terminal region of the TIMP appears to be the critical portion of the molecule for inhibition[43] and investigations into the crystal structure of the TIMP-1/MMP-3 complex has revealed that TIMP-1 acts a zinc chelator. TIMP-1 is a wedge-shaped molecule that occupies the entire length of the active-site cleft and the central disulphide-linked segments (Cys 1–Thr 2–Cys 3–Val 4 and Ser 68–Val 69) bidentately chelate the catalytic zinc ion.[44,45] TIMP activity may be restricted by site of secretion. Thus, TIMP-3 is matrix bound and TIMP-4 is principally found in cardiac tissue.

4. MATRIX METALLOPROTEINASES (MMP) AND CENTRAL NERVOUS SYSTEM (CNS) INFECTIONS

Despite the extensive mechanisms in place to regulate MMP activity, there is increasing evidence that these proteases may be involved in the pathogenesis of a wide range of bacterial, viral and fungal infections of the CNS. The potential mechanisms of brain tissue injury by MMP are manifold. There is substantial evidence that elevated MMP activity leads to a breakdown of the blood–brain barrier, a major pathological feature in meningitis, which is responsible for vasogenic oedema and raised intracranial pressure.[46] For example, stereotactic injection of highly-purified activated MMP-7, -8 or -9 into rat brain parenchyma, provoked blood–brain barrier disruption and leucocyte infiltration.[47] Cleavage of myelin proteins,[48] activation of disease-modifying cytokine and direct damage to resident CNS cells are other possible pathological effects of MMP.

In humans, most work has focused on MMP-9 and bacterial meningitis. However, MMP-9 is usually undetectable in normal subjects but was raised in cerebrospinal fluid (CSF) samples from patients with viral[49] and cryptococcal meningitis,[50,51] Lyme disease,[52] human T-cell lymphotrophic virus-1-associated myelopathy[53] and human immunodeficiency virus (HIV) infection.[54] We have found MMP-9 to be raised in Peruvian patients with the parasitic disease neurocyticercosis (unpublished data). Clinical studies reporting an association between cerebral injury and elevated CSF MMP-9 activity suggest that this may have pathological relevance. For example, MMP-9 is raised in 40% of patients with HIV infection and was more commonly elevated in cases with neurological deficit.[54] In addition, both MMP-9 and MMP-8 (but not MMP-2 and -3) were increased in CSF from children with bacterial meningitis, but only CSF MMP-9 concentrations were higher in those who developed hearing impairment or secondary epilepsy.[55] Moreover, recovery from bacterial meningitis is associated with a fall in CSF MMP-9 concentrations.[56]

The most direct evidence for the destructive effect of MMP in CNS infections has come from animal models. For example, intracisternal injection of heat-killed meningococci produced blood–brain barrier disruption, raised intracranial pressure and leucocyte infiltration in rats, paralleled by increased CSF MMP-9 activity 6 hours after meningococcal challenge.[56] The MMP inhibitor batimastat (BB-94), given either before or 3 hours after injection, reduced blood–brain barrier disruption and intracranial pressure but did not inhibit leucocyte influx. In a similar model, increased MMP-9, -3 and -13 mRNA levels were found in brain specimens from meningococcus-injected rats after 6 hours, but MMP-2, -7, -10 remained unchanged.[57] Invading leucocytes are believed to be the most important source of MMP-9 in meningitis and consistent with this was the observation that immunohistochemical staining for MMP-9 was localized to areas of leucocyte infiltration. In contrast, although astrocytes,[58] microglia[59] and endothelial cells[60] secrete MMP-9 in vitro, there was no evidence of significant MMP-9 production by such resident CNS cells in vivo. More recently, mRNA encoding MMP-3, -7, -8, -9 and TNF-α were elevated in cerebral tissue in a rat model of pneumococcal meningitis, and MMP-9 and TNF-α concentrations in CSF were also significantly increased and closely correlated.[61] Interestingly, treatment with GM6001 reduced both CSF MMP-9 and TNF-α, in addition to neuronal injury. It was proposed that such broad inhibition of both TACE and MMP-9 might prevent proteolytic injury by breaking a self-perpetuating cycle of activation and induction by TNF-α and MMP. There are no current data using MMP knockout mice in bacterial meningitis models; however, MMP-9 knockout mice were resistant to cerebral damage from encephalomyelitis induced by heat-killed *Mycobacterium tuberculosis* injected into the hind footpads of mice.[62]

5. MATRIX METALLOPROTEINASES (MMP) AND HOST TISSUE DESTRUCTION IN HUMAN TUBERCULOSIS (TB)

We have investigated MMP secreted by monocytic cells, pivotal in antimycobacterial immunity, in TB. The most common clinical manifestation of TB is interstitial tissue destruction, which classically presents as pulmonary cavitation. However, *M tuberculosis* is also an important cause of a chronic destructive meningo-encephalitis that is fatal if untreated and leaves up to 50% of survivors with residual cerebral damage.[63] However, little is understood about the host immune-derived factors that cause tissue injury in TB.

We recently reported the development of a matrix-degrading phenotype *in vitro* that was related to cerebral injury in patients with tuberculous meningitis.[64] In a cellular model of TB, gene expression and secretion of MMP-9 and TIMP-1 by human monocytic THP-1 cells, pivotal in antimycobacterial immunity and the

predominant leucocyte subset recruited in tuberculous meningitis, was studied. Infection with live, virulent *M tuberculosis* was a potent stimulus for *de novo* MMP-9 mRNA synthesis and resulted in a 10-fold increase in MMP-9 production by monocytic cells compared to controls. Furthermore, phagocytosis of viable, intact, bacilli are not required to stimulate MMP-9 secretion since heat-killed *M tuberculosis* had a similar effect to live organisms and exposure to cell-wall-derived lipoarabinomannan stimulate MMP-9 and MMP-1 secretion by human monocytes.[65] In comparison to MMP-9, there was constitutive TIMP-1 gene expression and secretion by monocytic cells, but the increase in secretion production following infection was delayed and more modest. A similar disproportionate increase in MMP-9 relative to TIMP-1 has been reported in macrophages stimulated by LPS.[5,7]

As an *in vivo* clinical correlate, we studied the secretion of MMP-9 and TIMP-1 in CSF specimens from Vietnamese patients with tuberculous meningitis. MMP-9 activity levels were significantly greater raised in the tuberculous meningitis patient group compared to cases with bacterial and viral meningitis; however, we expected that the levels were likely to reflect both the number and predominant leucocyte subsets recruited in each case. A PMN predominance was found in bacterial meningitis specimens, which is a characteristic clinical feature of this condition, whereas mononuclear cell infiltrates are typical in tuberculous meningitis. Since similar numbers of leucocytes were found in all groups, this suggests that PMN release less MMP-9 than mononuclear cells. Indeed, PMN are shorter lived and release proteases from preformed cytoplasmic granules, rather than synthesizing MMP-9 *de novo* like monocytes.[14,66] Moreover, since tuberculous meninigitis is a meningo-encephalitis, the wide distribution of leucocytes throughout the brain parenchyma may be potentially more harmful than in bacterial meningitis where the inflammatory infiltrate and secretion of MMP-9 is confined to the meninges.[67] In contrast, viral meningitis is characteristically a self-limiting, non-fatal disease. As in our study, other workers in Vietnam found that CSF MMP-9 concentrations in patients with viral meningoencephalitis were similar to controls and only significantly elevated in samples from patients with tuberculous and bacterial meningitis.[51]

In contrast to MMP-9 but similar to our *in vitro* observations, CSF TIMP-1 levels in tuberculous meningitis were similar to the constitutive levels of secretion form non-infected control subjects. A possible consequence of such unrestricted MMP-9 activity is cerebral damage. Importantly, elevated MMP-9 activity but not TIMP-1 levels were related to fatal outcome and signs of local tissue injury (unconsciousness, confusion, neurological deficit), but were not systemic features of generalized infection. Such data are consistent with the findings of another small clinical study in a mixed patient population (including tuberculous and fungal meningitis) who were compared with non-inflammatory CNS disease.[50]

In order to investigate the secretion of MMP-9 *in vivo* in greater detail we have recently examined tissue sections from patients with tuberculous lymphadenitis by immunohistochemistry.[68] A striking finding was that MMP-9 staining strongly localized to monocytic cells, including multinucleate giant cells at the centre of granuloma and adjacent to caseous necrosis. In contrast, there was sparse staining for TIMP-1, again suggesting that monocytic cells develop an unrestricted matrix-degrading phenotype in TB. The histological hallmark of TB is granuloma formation and caseous necrosis. Granulomas, surrounded by T-cells and centred with monocytic and multinucleate giant cells, provide a framework whereby monocytic cells (which become activated to a mycobacteriostatic state) are brought in close apposition with T-cells (secreting cytokines). TNF-α (secreted predominantly by monocytes) and IFN-γ [secreted primarily by lymphocytes and natural killer (NK) cells] are critical for the organization of granuloma and mononuclear cell recruitment, activation and mycobacterial killing.[69] However, granuloma may also displace and destroy host tissue in TB, and a fine balance between Th1 and Th2 cytokines controls whether the granulomatous response is protective or destructive.

Interestingly, nearly all of the monocytic cells within granuloma stained strongly for MMP-9, despite the fact that the proportion of cells infected with tubercle bacilli is characteristically very small. Since secretion of MMP-1 and -9 by monocytes is induced by direct contact with activated lymphocytes, it is possible that similar cell–cell interactions within tissue granuloma stimulate MMP secretion in TB.[34] In a cellular model, we have shown that TNF-α, released by infected monocytic cells, may amplify proteolytic activity by stimulating neighbouring uninfected monocytes to secrete MMP-9. TNF-α is therefore a pivotal mediator of MMP-induced tissue injury in TB. This concept is consistent with recent work suggesting that TNF-α determines the extent of tissue pathology and disease progression during mycobacterial CNS infection in animal models.[70] Interestingly, IL-1 did not have a similar paracrine effect but, paradoxically, IFN-γ, inhibited MMP-9 gene expression and secretion by *M tuberculosis* infected THP-1 monocytic cells.[71] IFN-γ has a critical role in host defence and patients with rare IFN-γ receptor defects have increased susceptibility to mycobacterial infection and are unable to form granuloma.[69] One possible interpretation is that IFN-γ may have a unexpected protective role by preventing excessive MMP-mediated tissue injury in TB, antagonizing the effects of TNF-α.

Finally, although most work has focused on MMP-9 in the immunopathology of TB, *M tuberculosis* also stimulates secretion of 52 kDa interstitial collagenase (MMP-1) by human monocytic cells. Although secretion is delayed and at a lower level, MMP-1 has a significant destructive potential since its specific substrates are the major structural collagens present within lung tissue (collagens type I–IV). In addition, MMP-1 inhibits the activity of the major lung antiproteinase, α_1-antitrypsin, which might potentially lead to unrestricted elastolytic activity causing cavity formation.[72] The role played by MMP-1 and other macrophage-derived MMP, such as MMP-12 implicated in empysema,[73] has not yet been fully dissected in pulmonary TB.

6. PROSPECTS FOR THE FUTURE: A NOVEL APPROACH TO TREATING INFECTION?

There is increasing evidence that MMP play an important role in the immunopathology of TB and other infectious diseases, particularly those affecting the CNS. However, in addition to reducing cerebral injury in rodent models of bacterial meningitis, hydroxamic acid MMP inhibitors have been shown to protect against lethal doses of endotoxin in animal models of septic shock.[74] However, although synthetic MMP inhibitors appear to have a tolerably good side-effect profile in oncology patients, the effectiveness of such strategies in the treatment of infectious diseases has yet to be evaluated in humans. Such an approach recognizes that tissue injury in many infectious diseases results from host- rather than pathogen-derived factors. For example, adjunctive corticosteroid treatment has been used for many years in order to reduce inflammatory tissue injury whilst antituberculous chemotherapy takes effect. Since corticosteroids inhibit MMP synthesis by monocytic cells, MMP inhibitors may provide a more selective way of reducing inflammatory tissue injury without limiting the host's effectiveness at killing pathogens.[74]

REFERENCES

Scientific papers

1. Woessner JF. Matrix metalloproteinases and their inhibitors in connective tissue remodeling. *FASEB J* 1991; **5**: 2145–54.
2. Welgus HG, Campbell EJ, Cury JD et al. Neutral metalloproteinases produced by human mononuclear phagocytes. Enzyme profile, regulation, and expression during cellular development. *J Clin Invest* 1990; **86**: 1496–502.
3. Busiek DF, Baragi V, Nehring LC et al. Matrilysin expression by human mononuclear phagocytes and its regulation by cytokines and hormones. *J Immunol* 1995; **154**: 6484–91.
4. Shapiro SD, Kobayashi DK, Ley TJ. Cloning and characterization of a unique elastolytic metalloproteinase produced by human alveolar macrophages. *J Biol Chem* 1993; **268**: 23,824–9.
5. Welgus HG, Campbell EJ, Bar-Shavit Z et al. *Teitelbaum. 1985.* Human alveolar macrophages produce a fibroblast-like collagenase and collagenase inhibitor. *J Clin Invest* 1985; **76**: 219–24.
6. Campbell EJ, Cury JD, Lazarus CJ, Welgus HG. Monocyte procollagenase and tissue inhibitor of metalloproteinases. Identification, characterization, and regulation of secretion. *J Biol Chem* 1987; **262**: 15,862–8.
7. Campbell EJ, Cury JD, Shapiro SD et al. Neutral proteinases of human mononuclear phagocytes. Cellular differentiation markedly alters cell phenotype for serine proteinases, metalloproteinases, and tissue inhibitor of metalloproteinases. *J Immunol* 1991; **146**: 1286–93.
8. Masure S, Proost P, Van Damme J, Opdenakker G. Purification and identification of 91-kDa neutrophil gelatinase. Release by the activating peptide interleukin-8. *Eur J Biochem* 1991; **198**: 391–8.
9. Black RA, Rauch CT, Kozlosky CJ et al. A metalloproteinase disintegrin that releases tumour-necrosis factor-alpha from cells. *Nature* 1997; **385**: 729–33.
10. Gallea-Robache S, Morand V, Millet S et al. A metalloproteinase inhibitor blocks the shedding of soluble cytokine receptors and processing of transmembrane cytokine precursors in human monocytic cells. *Cytokine* 1997; **9**: 340–6.
11. Fowlkes JL, Enghild JJ, Suzuki K, Nagase H. Matrix metalloproteinases degrade insulin-like growth factor-binding protein-3 in dermal fibroblast cultures. *J Biol Chem* 1994; **269**: 25,742–6.
12. Taipale J, Keski-Oja J. Growth factors in the extracellular matrix. *FASEB J* 1997; **11**: 51–9.
13. Taipale J, Lohi J, Saarinen J et al. Human mast cell chymase and leukocyte elastase release latent transforming growth factor-beta 1 from the extracellular matrix of cultured human epithelial and endothelial cells. *J Biol Chem* 1995; **270**: 4689–96.
14. Hibbs MS, Bainton DF. Human neutrophil gelatinase is a component of specific granules. *J Clin Invest* 1989; **84**: 1395–402.
15. Saren P, Welgus HG, Kovanen PT. TNF-alpha and IL-1beta selectively induce expression of 92-kDa gelatinase by human macrophages. *J Immunol* 1996; **157**: 4159–65.
16. Zhang Y, McCluskey K, Fujii K, Wahl LM. Differential regulation of monocyte matrix metalloproteinase and TIMP-1 production by TNF-alpha, granulocyte–macrophage CSF, and IL-1 beta through prostaglandin-dependent and -independent mechanisms. *J Immunol* 1998; **161**: 3071–6.
17. Shapiro SD, Campbell EJ, Kobayashi DK, Welgus HG. Immune modulation of metalloproteinase production in human macrophages. Selective pretranslational suppression of interstitial

collagenase and stromelysin biosynthesis by interferon-gamma. *J Clin Invest* 1990; **86**: 1204–10.

18. Lacraz S, Nicod LP, Chicheportiche R et al. IL-10 inhibits metalloproteinase and stimulates TIMP-1 production in human mononuclear phagocytes. *J Clin Invest* 1995; **96**: 2304–10.

19. Corcoran ML, Stetler-Stevenson WG, Brown PD, Wahl LM. Interleukin 4 inhibition of prostaglandin E2 synthesis blocks interstitial collagenase and 92-kDa type IV collagenase/gelatinase production by human monocytes. *J Biol Chem* 1992; **267**: 515–19.

20. Wahl LM, Corcoran ME, Mergenhagen SE, Finbloom DS. Inhibition of phospholipase activity in human monocytes by IFN-gamma blocks endogenous prostaglandin E2-dependent collagenase production. *J Immunol* 1990; **144**: 3518–22.

21. Mertz PM, DeWitt DL, Stetler-Stevenson WG, Wahl LM. Interleukin 10 suppression of monocyte prostaglandin H synthase-2. Mechanism of inhibition of prostaglandin-dependent matrix metalloproteinase production. *J Biol Chem* 1994; **269**: 21, 322–9.

22. Adams DH, Lloyd AR. Chemokines: leucocyte recruitment and activation cytokines. *Lancet* 1997; **349**: 490–5.

23. Ben Baruch A, Michiel DF, Oppenheim JJ. Signals and receptors involved in recruitment of inflammatory cells. *J Biol Chem* 1995; **270**: 11,703–6.

24. Corcoran ML, Stetler-Stevenson WG, DeWitt DL, Wahl LM. Effect of cholera toxin and pertussis toxin on prostaglandin H synthase-2, prostaglandin E2, and matrix metalloproteinase production by human monocytes. *Arch Biochem Biophys* 1994; **310**: 481–8.

25. Johnatty RN, Taub DD, Reeder SP et al. Cytokine and chemokine regulation of proMMP-9 and TIMP-1 production by human peripheral blood lymphocytes. *J Immunol* 1997; **158**: 2327–33.

26. Leppert DE, Waubant E, Galardy R et al. T cell gelatinases mediate basement membrane transmigration in vitro. *J Immunol* 1995; **154**: 4379–89.

27. Leppert D, Hauser SL, Kishiyama JL et al. Stimulation of matrix metalloproteinase-dependent migration of T cells by eicosanoids. *FASEB J* 1995; **9**: 1473–81.

28. Xia M, Leppert D, Hauser SL et al. Stimulus specificity of matrix metalloproteinase dependence of human T cell migration through a model basement membrane. *J Immunol* 1996; **156**: 160–7.

29. Watanabe H, Nakanishi I, Yamashita K et al. Matrix metalloproteinase-9 (92 kDa gelatinase/type IV collagenase) from U937 monoblastoid cells: correlation with cellular invasion. *J Cell Sci* 1993; **104**: 991–9.

30. Van den Steen PE, Proost P, Wuyts A et al. Neutrophil gelatinase B potentiates interleukin-8 tenfold by aminoterminal processing, whereas it degrades CTAP-III, PF-4, and GRO- alpha and leaves RANTES and MCP-2 intact. *Blood* 2000; **96**: 2673–81.

31. Khandaker MH, Mitchell G, Xu L et al. Metalloproteinases are involved in lipopolysaccha. *Blood* 1999; **93**: 2173–85.

32. Shapiro SD, Kobayashi DK, Pentland AP, Welgus HG. Induction of macrophage metalloproteinases by extracellular matrix. Evidence for enzyme and substrate-specific responses involving prostaglandin-dependent mechanisms. *J Biol Chem* 1993; **268**: 8170–5.

33. Amorino GP, Hoover RL. Interactions of monocytic cells with human endothelial cells stimulate monocytic metalloproteinase production. *Am J Pathol* 1998; **152**: 199–207.

34. Lacraz S, Isler P, Vey E et al. Direct contact between T lymphocytes and monocytes is a major pathway for induction of metalloproteinase expression. *J Biol Chem* 1994; **269**: 22,027–33.

35. Nagase, H. Activation mechanisms of matrix metalloproteinases. *Biol Chem* 1997; **378**: 151–60.

36. Carmeliet P, Moons L, Lijnen R et al. Urokinase-generated plasmin activates matrix metalloproteinases during aneurysm formation. *Nature Genet* 1997; **17**: 439–44.

37. Murphy G, Docherty AJ. The matrix metalloproteinases and their inhibitors. *Am J Respir Cell Molec Biol* 1992; **7**: 120–5.

38. Strongin AY, Collier I, Bannikov G et al. Mechanism of cell surface activation of 72-kDa type IV collagenase. Isolation of the activated form of the membrane metalloprotease. *J Biol Chem* 1995; **270**: 5331–8.

39. Maeda H, Okamoto T, Akaike T. Human matrix metalloprotease activation by insults of bacterial infection involving proteases and free radicals. *Biol Chem* 1998; **379**: 193–200.

40. Gomez DE, Alonso DF, Yoshiji H, Thorgeirsson UP. Tissue inhibitors of metalloproteinases: structure, regulation and biological functions. *Eur J Cell Biol* 1997; **74**: 111–22.

41. Woessner JF, Jr. Matrix metalloproteinase inhibition. From the Jurassic to the third millennium. *Ann NY Acad Sci* 1999; **878**: 388–403.

42. Strongin AY, Marmer BL, Grant GA, Goldberg GI. Plasma membrane-dependent activation of the 72-kDa type IV collagenase is prevented by complex formation with TIMP-2. *J Biol Chem* 1993; **268**: 14,033–9.

43. Murphy G, Houbrechts A, Cockett MI et al. The N-terminal domain of tissue inhibitor of metalloproteinases retains metalloproteinase inhibitory activity. *Biochemistry* 1991; **30**: 8097–102.

44. Gomis-Ruth FX, Maskos K, Betz M et al. Mechanism of inhibition of the human matrix metalloproteinase stromelysin-1 by TIMP-1. *Nature* 1997; **389**: 77–81.

45. Arumugam S, Hemme CL, Yoshida N et al. TIMP-1 contact sites and perturbations of stromelysin 1 mapped by NMR and a paramagnetic surface probe. *Biochemistry* 1998; **37**: 9650–7.

46. Quagliarello V, Scheld WM. Bacterial meningitis: pathogenesis, pathophysiology, and progress. *N Engl J Med* 1992; **327**: 864–72.

47. Anthony DC, Miller KM, Fearn S et al. Matrix metalloproteinase expression in an experimentally-induced DTH model of multiple sclerosis in the rat CNS. *J Neuroimmunol* 1998; **87**: 62–72.

48. Gijbels K, Proost P, Masure S et al. Gelatinase B is present in the cerebrospinal fluid during experimental autoimmune encephalomyelitis and cleaves myelin basic protein. *J Neurosci Res* 1993; **36**: 432–40.

49. Kolb SA, Lahrtz F, Paul R et al. Matrix metalloproteinases and tissue inhibitors of metalloproteinases in viral meningitis: upregulation of MMP-9 and TIMP-1 in cerebrospinal fluid. *J Neuroimmunol* 1998; **84**: 143–50.

50. Matsuura EF, Umehara F, Hashiguchi T et al. Marked increase of matrix metalloproteinase 9 in cerebrospinal fluid of patients with fungal or tuberculous meningoencephalitis. *J Neurol Sci* 2000; **173**: 45–52.

51. Brown HC, Chau TT, Mai NT et al. Blood–brain barrier function in cerebral malaria and CNS infections in Vietnam. *Neurology* 2000; **55**: 104–11.

52. Perides G, Charness ME, Tanner LM et al. Matrix metalloproteinases in the cerebrospinal fluid of patients with Lyme neuroborreliosis. *J Infect Dis* 1998; **177**: 401–8.

53. Giraudon P, Buart S, Bernard A et al. Extracellular matrix-remodeling metalloproteinases and infection of the central nervous system with retrovirus human T-lymphotropic virus type I (HTLV-I). *Prog Neurobiol* 1996; **49**: 169–84.

54. Sporer B, Paul R, Koedel U et al. Presence of matrix metalloproteinase-9 activity in the cerebrospinal fluid of human immunodeficiency virus-infected patients. *J Infect Dis* 1998; **178**: 854–7.

55. Leppert D, Leib SL, Grygar C et al. Matrix metalloproteinase (MMP)-8 and MMP-9 in cerebrospinal fluid during bacterial meningitis: association with blood–brain barrier damage and neurological sequelae [in process citation]. *Clin Infect Dis* 2000; **31**:80–4.

56. Paul R, Lorenzl S, Koedel U et al. Matrix metalloproteinases contribute to the blood–brain barrier disruption during bacterial meningitis. *Ann Neurol* 1998; **44**: 592–600.

57. Kieseier BC, Paul R, Koedel U et al. Differential expression of matrix metalloproteinases in bacterial meningitis. *Brain* 1999; **122**: 1579–87.

58. Wells GM, Catlin G, Cossins JA et al. Quantitation of matrix metalloproteinases in cultured rat astrocytes using the polymerase chain reaction with a multi-competitor cDNA standard. *Glia* 1996; **18**: 332–40.

59. Gottschall, PE, Yu X, Bing B. Increased production of gelatinase B (matrix metalloproteinase-9) and interleukin-6 by activated rat microglia in culture. *J Neurosci Res* 1995; **42**: 335–42.

60. Herron GS, Werb Z, Dwyer K, Banda MJ. Secretion of metalloproteinases by stimulated capillary endothelial cells. I. Production of procollagenase and prostromelysin exceeds expression of proteolytic activity. *J Biol Chem* 1986; **261**: 2810–13.

61. Leib SL, Leppert D, Clements J, Tauber MG. Matrix metalloproteinases contribute to brain damage in experimental pneumococcal meningitis. *Infect Immunol* 2000; **68**: 615–20.

62. Dubois B, Masure S, Hurtenbach U et al. Resistance of young gelatinase B-deficient mice to experimental autoimmune encephalomyelitis and necrotizing tail lesions. *J Clin Invest* 1999; **104**: 1507–15.

63. Zuger A, Lowy FD. Tuberculosis of the brain, meninges and spinal cord. In: Rom WN, Garay SM, eds. *Tuberculosis*. Little, Brown and Co, 1995.

64. Price NM, Farrar J, Chau TT et al. Identification of a matrix-degrading phenotype in human tuberculosis *in vitro* and *in vivo*. *J Immunol* 2001; **166**: 4223–30.

65. Chang JC, Wysocki A, Tchou-Wong KM et al. Effect of *Mycobacterium tuberculosis* and its components on macrophages and the release of matrix metalloproteinases. *Thorax* 1996; **51**: 306–11.

66. Hibbs MS, Hoidal JR, Kang AH. Expression of a metalloproteinase that degrades native type V collagen and denatured collagens by cultured human alveolar macrophages. *J Clin Invest* 1987; **80**: 1644–50.

67. Adams JH, Graham DI. The nervous systems: infections of the central nervous system. In: MacSween RNM, Whaley K, eds. *Muir's Textbook*

of Pathology. London: Edward Arnold, 1992.

68. Price NM, Friedland JS. TNF-α induces matrix metalloproteinase-9 gene expression and secretion by *Mycobacterium tuberculosis*-infected human monocytic cells. *European Cytokine Network 11* (Special issue ICS/ISICR) 2000; 185.

69. Saunders BM, Cooper AM. Restraining mycobacteria: role of granulomas in mycobacterial infections. *Immunol Cell Biol* 2000; **78**: 334–41.

70. Tsenova L, Bergtold A, Freedman VH et al. Tumor necrosis factor alpha is a determinant of pathogenesis and disease progression in mycobacterial infection in the central nervous system. *Proc Natl Acad Sci USA* 1999; **96**: 5657–62.

71. Gomes JMPF, Price NM, Friedland JS. Interferon-γ and interleukin-10 inhibit matrix metallo-proteinase-9 secretion from *Mycobacterium tuberculosis*-infected human monocytic cells. *European Cytokine Network 11* (Special issue ICS/ISICR) 2000; 191.

72. Desrochers PE, Jeffrey JJ, Weiss SJ. Interstitial collagenase (matrix metalloproteinase-1) expresses serpinase activity. *J Clin Invest* 1991; **87**: 2258–65.

73. Hautamaki RD, Kobayashi DK, Senior RM, Shapiro SD. Requirement for macrophage elastase for cigarette smoke-induced emphysema in mice. *Science* 1997; **277**: 2002–4.

74. Mohler KM, Sleath PR, Fitzner JN et al. Protection against a lethal dose of endotoxin by an inhibitor of tumour necrosis factor processing. *Nature* 1994; **370**: 218–20.

10

HIV and its manipulation of chemokine receptors

Sunil Shaunak

Objectives • Summary • Introduction • A new HIV classification system for HIV-1 • Clinical relevance of chemokine co-receptors • What are chemokines? • Current antiretroviral therapy • Conclusions – new drugs for the future • References

OBJECTIVES

(1) The identification of the mechanism of viral entry into cells and chemokine co-receptor based classification of viral isolates of HIV-1.

(2) The clinical relevance of β-chemokines and chemokine co-receptors in AIDS, and in inflammation.

(3) The influence of wild type chemokine co-receptor gene mutations on susceptibility to infection by HIV-1 and on subsequent disease progression.

(4) New chemokine co-receptor based therapies for HIV-1 infection.

SUMMARY

Laboratory and patient-based studies of the mechanisms by which HIV gains entry into cells have opened up new fields of chemokine and chemokine receptor biology in many areas of medicine. We are only just coming to recognize the seminal role of these molecules in local immunoregulatory pathways in different body compartments and their seminal role in initiating, promoting and maintaining inflammation.

These new insights into acute inflammation and into chronic inflammation should lead to the discovery and the development of important new classes of therapeutic drugs in the forseeable future.

1. INTRODUCTION

The human immunodeficiency virus (HIV) is the infectious agent that leads to the development of the acquired immunodeficiency syndrome (AIDS).[1] Globally, HIV is now predominantly transmitted by heterosexual contact. It has already claimed some 12 million lives. The total number of people living with HIV/AIDS is estimated to be approximately 33.6 million.[2] In reality, the disease is fatal in all but a minority of cases.

1.1 Seroconversion

Acute HIV-1 infection is a transient, symptomatic illness that is associated with high-titre HIV-1 replication, and a robust and expansive immunological response to the invading pathogen. It is often undiagnosed or misdiagnosed. The most common mode of transmission is via genital mucosa. Studies in rhesus monkeys with simian immunodeficiency virus (SIV) suggest that the first cellular targets of the virus are Langerhans cells.[3] These are tissue dendritic cells that are found in the lamina propria of cervicovaginal epithelium. They fuse with CD4+ T-lymphocytes which then migrate to the lymphatic circulation. Within a couple of days, virus can be detected in the draining internal iliac lymph nodes.[4] Shortly thereafter, systemic dissemination occurs and HIV can be cultured from plasma. Breaks in the mucosal barrier and increased inflammation due to genital ulcer disease, urethritis or cervicitis, significantly increase the risk of acquiring HIV infection. Studies of individuals undergoing a seroconversion illness suggested that infection usually occurs with distinct variants of the virus. The subsequent emergence and expansion of viruses with different phenotypes in patients with AIDS triggered a search for new cell-surface molecules that could influence the evolution of the virus and select for the transmission of only some viral phenotypes.

1.2 Reservoirs of HIV-1 replication

The virus infects and replicates in CD4+ positive cells within the lymphatic circulation. Lymphocytes and macrophages account for >98% of all viral replication.[5,6] The acute, high level, cytopathic infection of CD4+ T-lymphocytes reduces the half-life of these cells to about 1.6 days. A second, slower phase, with a half-life in the order of 16 days, has been attributed to the infection of macrophages.[7,8] The hope that highly active antiretroviral therapy (HAART) would lead to the eradication of the virus from the body within a few years has failed to materialize. The re-emergence of virus within 2 weeks of stopping antiretroviral therapy, even in those patients whose plasma HIV RNA had been suppressed to below the limit of detection for several years,[9] suggested that long-lived 'reservoirs' of HIV-1-infected cells exist and persist.[10,11] We have confirmed the existence of these reservoirs of ongoing viral replication by demonstrating episomal HIV-1 DNA in the

peripheral blood of patients with plasma HIV RNA levels <50 copies/ml; their presence is indicative of new, acute infection events occurring despite potent drug therapy.[12]

The precise anatomical location of these reservoirs of ongoing viral replication remains to be defined. Long-lived CD4+ memory T-cells that have been infected by HIV-1 and which have survived cytopathic cell death, constitute one population of cells that is currently under investigation.[13,14] Long-lived tissue-based macrophages are another important focus of current research because they can produce infectious virus for long periods of time without undergoing cell death (Fig 10.1).[15–17]

1.3 Viral entry into cells

Current antiretroviral therapeutic approaches target several viral enzymes. Their failure to stop viral replication throughout the body stimulated new research into the mechanisms by which HIV-1 gains entry into cells. It was hoped that the generation of virus fusion inhibitors would lead to an important new class of drugs that could

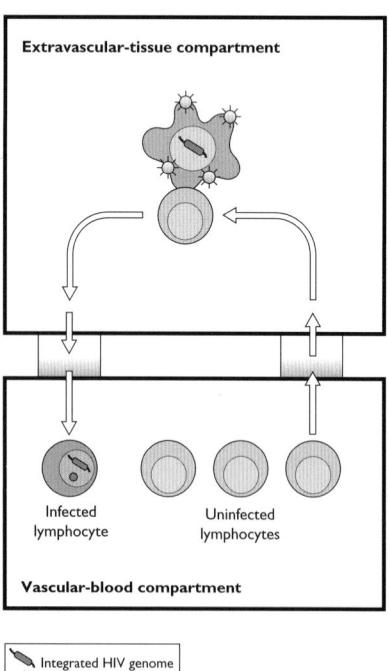

Fig. 10.1

effectively block new rounds of infection in reservoirs of ongoing viral replication. Our recent understanding of the mechanisms by which the virus gains entry into cells has led to the discovery of new chemokines, new chemokine receptors and to a recognition of their seminal role in local immunoregulatory pathways.

The entry of HIV-1 into lymphocytes and macrophages is initiated by the binding of the viral envelope glycoprotein (gp)120 to cell-surface CD4.[18,19] Because three gp120 molecules associate non-covalently with the gp41 trimer to form the viral envelope oligomer, multiple CD4 molecules can bind to the same envelope oligomer with an affinity of 10^{-9} M. This interaction leads to a conformational change in gp120 that exposes a cryptic surface on gp120 within the gp120–CD4 complex; this briefly exposed surface can then bind to a second cell-surface molecule. These co-receptors were discovered to belong to the family of chemokine receptors. Bringing the virion into close apposition to the cell surface allows the viral fusion protein gp41 to insert into the target cell membrane.[20,21] Fusion of the virus with the cell then occurs. The most physiologically relevant and widely used of these chemokine co-receptors are CCR5 and CXCR4; the former mediates the entry of R5 isolates and the latter the entry of X4 isolates of HIV-1. Dual tropic R5X4 isolates can use both co-receptors (Fig. 10.2).[22]

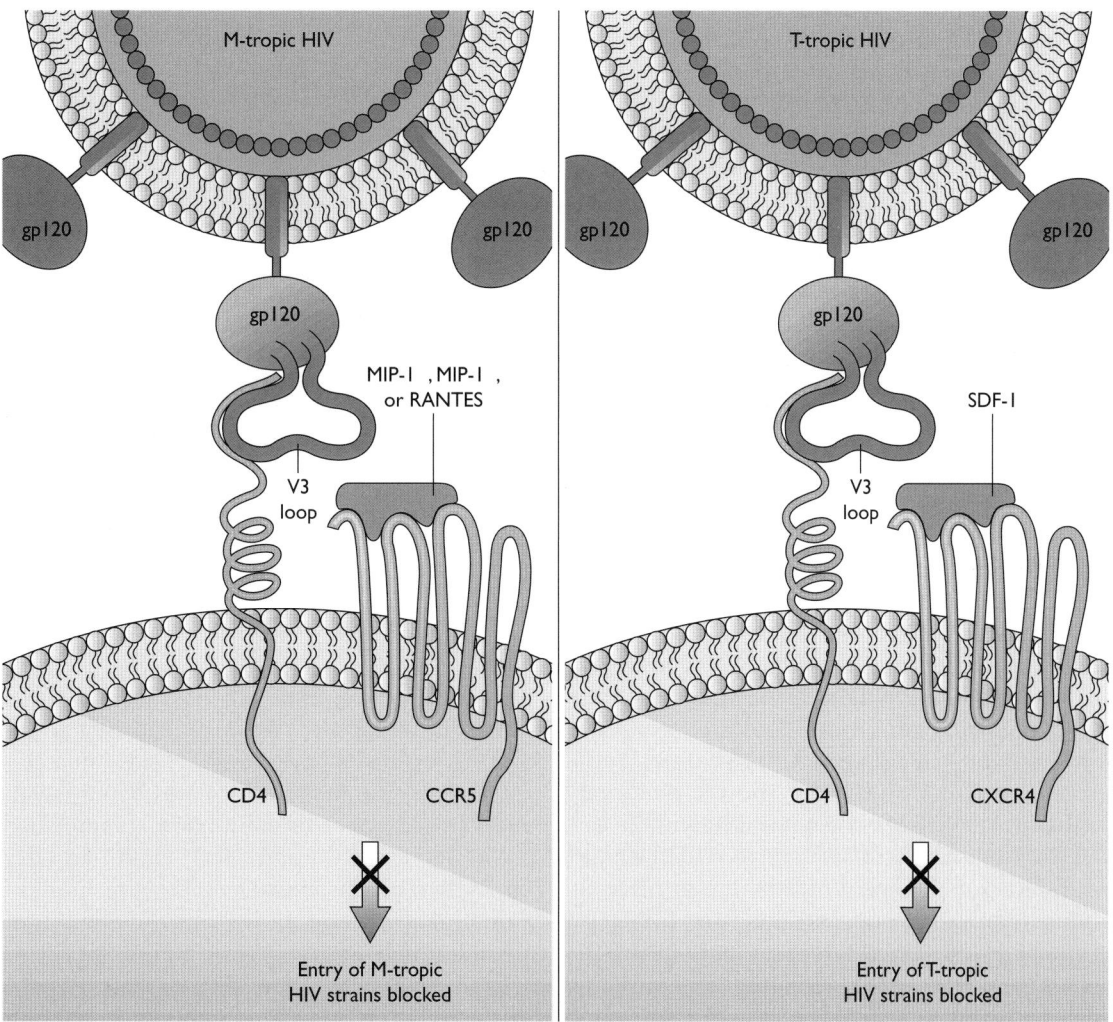

Fig. 10.2

1.4 Syncytium-inducing (SI) and non-syncytium-inducing (NSI) isolates of HIV-1

Around the time these studies were in progress, primary viral isolates of HIV-1 were increasingly being recognized to have a cellular tropism that was distinct from that of laboratory-adapted, T-cell tropic strains of HIV-1. The latter consistently infected T-cell lines and lymphocytes, and they produced syncytia in MT-2 cells. They were termed SI viruses, and did not infect macrophages. Only later were strains of HIV-1 identified that infected macrophages but not T-cell lines, and did not produce syncytia in MT-2 cells. They were termed non-syncytium inducing (NSI) viruses. Broder and Berger[23] went on to show that these differences in the tropism of SI and NSI viruses correlated with sequence-specific changes in the V3 loop region of gp120. This suggested, for the first time, that more than one fusion co-receptor was important in mediating the entry of HIV-1 into CD4+ cells.

1.5 Chemokine co-receptors for HIV-1

Feng et al[24] used a novel functional complementary DNA (cDNA) cloning strategy to identify the first fusion co-receptor for HIV-1. The protein, named fusin, was a G protein-coupled receptor with seven transmembrane regions. Recombinant fusin enabled CD4-expressing non-human cells to support HIV-1 envelope-mediated cell fusion and HIV-1 infection by SI but not NSI isolates. Following its recognition as a member of the CXC family of chemokines, it was renamed CXCR4.[24] Like many other chemokine receptors that have since been discovered, it was initially an orphan receptor whose natural ligand was not known. Only later was the CXC chemokine, stromal cell-derived factor-1 [SDF-1 (now renamed CXCL12)], identified as its natural ligand.[25]

Shortly before the discovery of CXCR4 as a co-receptor for the entry of HIV-1 into cells, it had been noted that supernatants from CD8+ T-lymphocytes contained large amounts of the β-chemokines, macrophage inflammatory protein (MIP)-1αβ now renamed CCL3), MIP-1β, and regulated-upon-activation, normal T expressed and secreted (RANTES). These supernatants had potent activity against NSI strains of HIV-1.[26] As β-chemokine receptors are also seven-transmembrane G-protein-coupled receptors, it was postulated that chemokine receptors could also be important co-receptors for NSI viruses.[27] Several recombinant viruses based on NSI and SI strains of HIV-1 expressing luciferase as a reporter element were constructed. These viruses were fusion but not replication competent, so they could enter cells but could not propagate in them. A series of elegant experiments showed that cells transformed to express hCD4 and the CC-chemokine receptor 5 (CCR5) supported fusion by NSI viruses but not by SI viruses.[28,29] The natural ligands for this receptor were also shown to be the β-chemokines, RANTES, MIP-1α and MIP-1β.

CXCR4 is mainly expressed on naïve CD4+ cells (CD45RA+), whereas CCR5 is predominantly expressed on memory CD4+ cells (CD45RO+) in healthy individuals.[30] Recent reports have also demonstrated enhanced CXCR4 levels on memory CD4+ lymphocytes.[31]

The discovery that some chemokine receptors played such an important role in the entry of HIV-1 into cells led to an explosion in the number of chemokine receptors being described as having a role in viral entry.[32] They are listed in Table 10.1. This list is unlikely to be comprehensive because new chemokine receptors continue to be discovered. They all belong to the seven-transmembrane G-protein-coupled family of receptors.

2. A NEW HIV CLASSIFICATION SYSTEM FOR HIV-1

This new understanding of the cell-surface receptors being used by HIV and SIV to gain entry into cells meant that the increasing number of primary viral isolates being isolated and studied from different body compartments could now be typed and classified more precisely. The classification system proposed by Berger et al[33] is now in widespread use. Viruses are identified by type (e.g. HIV-1, HIV-2 and SIV) as well as by their chemokine co-receptor tropism. They can be monotropic (use only one chemokine receptor) or multitropic (use

Table 10.1 Summary of the HIV and SIV chemokine co-receptors reported to date (adapted from Loetscher et al[82]			
Chemokine receptor	Ligand type	Ligand	Virus
CXCR4	CXC	SDF-1	X4, R5X4, HIV-2
CCR2	CC	MCP-1, MCP-2, MCP-3	R5X4, HIV-2
CCR3	CC	Eotaxin, eotaxin-2 RANTES, MIP-1α,	R5X4, HIV-2
CCR5	CC	MIP-1α, MIP-1β, RANTES	R5, R5X4, HIV-2, SIV
CCR8	CC	I-309	R5X4, HIV-2, SIV
CX_3CR1	CX_3C	Fractalkine	X4, R5X4, HIV-2
STRL33/BONZO	Unknown	Unknown	R5X4, HIV-2, SIV
BOB/GPR-15	Unknown	Unknown	R5X4, HIV-2, SIV
GPR-1	Unknown	Unknown	SIV
Chem23	Unknown	Unknown	R5X4, SIV
APJ	Unknown	Unknown	R5X4, SIV
US28 (CMV)	CC	RANTES, MIP-1α, MCP-1	R5X4, HIV-2

multiple chemokine receptors). NSI isolates that replicate in macrophages and primary CD4+ T-lymphocytes typically use CCR5. SI isolates that replicate in CD4+ T-lymphocytes typically use CXCR4. Dual (i.e. R5X4) and multitropic (e.g. R5X4R3) viruses are typically found circulating in patients with AIDS.[34]

3. CLINICAL RELEVANCE OF CHEMOKINE CO-RECEPTORS

Early studies suggested that dissemination of HIV-1 from lymphoid organs to non-lymphoid tissues was associated with an expansion in the number of chemokine co-receptors being used by the virus.[34] This reflected the observation that a change in the tropism of the virus from an R5 to an R5X4 phenotype was associated with rapid progression of the disease to AIDS and death. However, it has recently been shown that the only physiologically important co-receptors being used by HIV-1 in patients who are clinically well are CCR5 and CXCR4.[22] Spontaneous and repeated switching of the chemokine co-receptors being used by blood-derived isolates of HIV-1 occurs rarely, if at all, in patients who are clinically well.

The situation appears to be different in patients during major opportunistic infections. It has been shown that HIV-1 co-receptor tropism can widen to include CCR5, CXCR4 and CCR3 in patients with severe *Pneumocystis carinii* pneumonia (PCP). This expansion is transient and does not persist >3 months after the acute illness has resolved. It does not extend to include any of the other chemokine co-receptors described in Table 10.1 that have been implicated in viral entry *in vitro*. No autopsy studies of the chemokine co-receptors being expressed by cells in the lung during PCP have been done. However, a detailed study of the *in vivo* distribution of chemokine co-receptors in rhesus macaques and humans found that the macrophages lining the walls of small blood vessels do express CXCR4 and CCR3.[35] PCP-induced alveolitis could therefore promote the local replication of different phenotypes of HIV-1 in cells that have become permissive to infection by HIV-1 during the proinflammatory phase of the pneumonia. This is supported by the observation that alveolar macrophage-derived virus used the CCR5, CCR3, CCR2b and CCR8 co-receptors, whilst simultaneously derived blood virus used only CCR5, CXCR4 and CCR3 in a patient with PCP.[36]

These observations suggest that the pro-inflammatory environment created by an acute opportunistic infection in a non-lymphoid organ can promote the short-term, local evolution of HIV-1 with an expanded chemokine co-receptor tropism. Cilliers et al[37] have also reported the results of a clinical study whose aim was to determine the chemokine co-receptor tropism of primary viral isolates from South African patients presenting for the first time with late-stage AIDS. Their viral isolates used CCR5 and/or CXCR4, as well as CCR3, CCR2b, CCR1, CCR8, V28 and Bob. However, most of these patients also had a major opportunistic infection from which they died. These observations suggest that a *stable* expansion of the tropism of HIV-1 to include the use of multiple chemokine co-receptors is a pre-terminal event in the course of the disease.

4. WHAT ARE CHEMOKINES?

Chemokines are a heterogeneous group of inducible proinflammatory *chemo*attractive cyto*kines* which are highly basic and have a molecular weight of 8–10 kDa.[38] Over 40 have already been identified. They share 20–70% sequence homology with each other and their biological activities are widely conserved. Functionally and structurally, they have been subdivided on the basis of the position of their cysteine residues.[39] The two most extensively characterized groups are the α- and β-chemokines. They differ in that the first two of four cysteine residues of the α-chemokines are separated by one amino acid residue (CXC chemokines), whereas in β-chemokines the first two cysteines are adjacent to each other (CC chemokines). The α-chemokines are further subdivided into those which contain the glutamic acid–leucine–arginine sequence preceding the CXC sequence. They are principally chemotactic for neutrophils. α-Chemokines that do not contain this sequence are chemotactic for lymphocytes. β-Chemokines act as chemoattractants for monocytes, eosinophils, basophils and lymphocytes.[40] Binding of chemokines to their respective receptors leads to a cascade of cellular activation, including the

generation of inositol triphosphate, the release of intracellular calcium and the activation of protein kinase C.[41] Activation of the guanosine-triphosphate-binding proteins Ras and Rho also occurs. These proteins are involved in membrane ruffling, pseudopod formation and adhesion complex formation.[42] Hence, chemokines activate the cellular mechanisms that control chemotaxis. As such, they play a pivotal role in the recruitment of leucocytes to areas of damage.

4.1 Clinical relevance of β-chemokines in HIV-1 infection

The discovery that chemokine receptors acted as secondary receptors for HIV-1 entry led to an interest in whether high levels of endogenous chemokines slowed the progression of the disease to AIDS. Some reports found no correlation between β-chemokine production and the rate of progression to AIDS,[43,44] but others came to the opposite conclusion. In retrospect, many of these early reports of serum β-chemokine levels were flawed because chemokines:

(1) bind to extracellular carbohydrates;
(2) aggregate at high local concentrations;
(3) are spontaneously released by platelets (e.g. RANTES) when blood is collected and plasma separated.[26,45]

More recent studies have, nevertheless, made some important observations. Saha et al[46] found that although β-chemokine production in CD8+ T-cell clones did not correlate with disease status, production of β-chemokines by CD4+ T-cell clones was higher in those patients whose disease did not progress as compared to those in whom it did. This suggested that the *local* production of β-chemokines within the micro-environment of the lymph node can protect cells from infection by HIV-1, and slow the clinical course of the disease. Several other recent reports have also implicated the high endogenous release of β-chemokines as having a protective role.[47] Sustained suppression of plasma HIV-1 RNA in patients on HAART has also been linked to high endogenous levels of β-chemokines.[48,49]

The difficulty in interpreting these measurements of plasma chemokine levels is that they are a very poor indicator of chemokine levels within the microenvironment of an extravascular body compartment in which their biological effects are mediated.[50] Nevertheless, the overall body of evidence does suggest that high levels of endogenously produced β-chemokines do play a significant role in blocking new rounds of infection of CD4+ cells *in vivo* and can thereby slow the clinical progression of the disease.

4.2 Mucosal inflammation

The gastrointestinal tract has recently come to be recognized as a major reservoir of CD4+ T-lymphocytes.[51] Most of these cells are of a memory phenotype expressing CD69 and CD45RO. They also exhibit functional features of activation. *In vitro* studies have suggested that the differentiation of CD4+ T-lymphocytes to a memory phenotype is associated with an increased susceptibility to infection by HIV-1.[52] This finding supports the growing body of evidence that the HIV-1 burden is considerably higher in gut-associated lymphoid tissue than in peripheral blood. This has been confirmed in humans by the demonstration of HIV in the intestinal mucosa of patients whose plasma viral load is < 50 copies/ml.[53] A profound loss of CD4+ T-lymphocytes in the intestine of SIV-infected macaques has also been demonstrated.[54]

In healthy seronegative individuals, the expression of CCR5 is increased in mucosal mononuclear cells compared to that in peripheral blood mononuclear cells. In contrast, CXCR4 is expressed at similar levels on CD45RO+ T-cells in mucosal mononuclear and peripheral blood mononuclear cells. It has recently been shown that mucosal mononuclear cells are more easily infected with HIV-1 than peripheral blood mononuclear cells and may reflect their increased expression of CCR5 as well as their higher state of activation.

Olsson et al[53] have shown that the expression of CCR5 and CXCR4 is significantly greater in HIV-infected lamina propria compared with that in healthy control tissue samples. The pattern was similar in 'inflammatory control' and HIV-infected tissues. These high expression levels suggest that HIV-1, in line with active inflammatory bowel disease, is associated with a strong inflammatory response in the gut lamina propria. Proinflammatory [tumour necrosis factor-alpha (TNF-α) and interleukin (IL)-12] and type 1 [interferon-gamma (INF-γ) and IL-2] cytokines upregulate HIV-1 co-receptor CCR5 mRNA expression, whereas type 2 cytokines upregulate CXCR4. This suggests that CCR5 and CXCR4 expression is altered by the cytokines present in their microenvironment. Increased CCR5 expression is correlated with inflammatory conditions. In cervical mucosa too, infectious and non-infectious inflammation upregulates CCR5 expression.[55]

The presence of very large numbers of effector CD4+ T-lymphocytes expressing CCR5 in mucosal surfaces helps to explain why SIV and HIV are readily transmitted across mucosal surfaces, and why most primary infections are with R5 viruses. Therefore, high levels of CCR5 expression may have an impact on both the effective transmission of the virus and on the prognosis of HIV-infected patients.

4.3 Defective chemokine co-receptors

Some individuals with multiple, high-risk exposures to HIV-1 remain persistently negative for anti-HIV-1 antibodies. CD4+ T-lymphocytes from these individuals [so-called exposed uninfected (EU) individuals] were found to be resistant to infection by HIV-1 *in vitro*.[56] A 32-base pair deletion in the CCR5 gene was found which resulted in the expression of a truncated, non-functional co-receptor variant termed CCR5(Δ32).[57–59] This mutation is frequent in white people but is not found in people from Africa or Asia. It is thought to have occurred relatively recently in evolutionary history. The frequency of heterozygotes declines from 16% in Finland and northeastern Russia to 4% in southern Europe.[60] Individuals with defective CCR5 receptor expression have normal immune defences, suggesting that other chemokine receptors can compensate for the physiological functions of this receptor (Fig. 10.3).

(a)

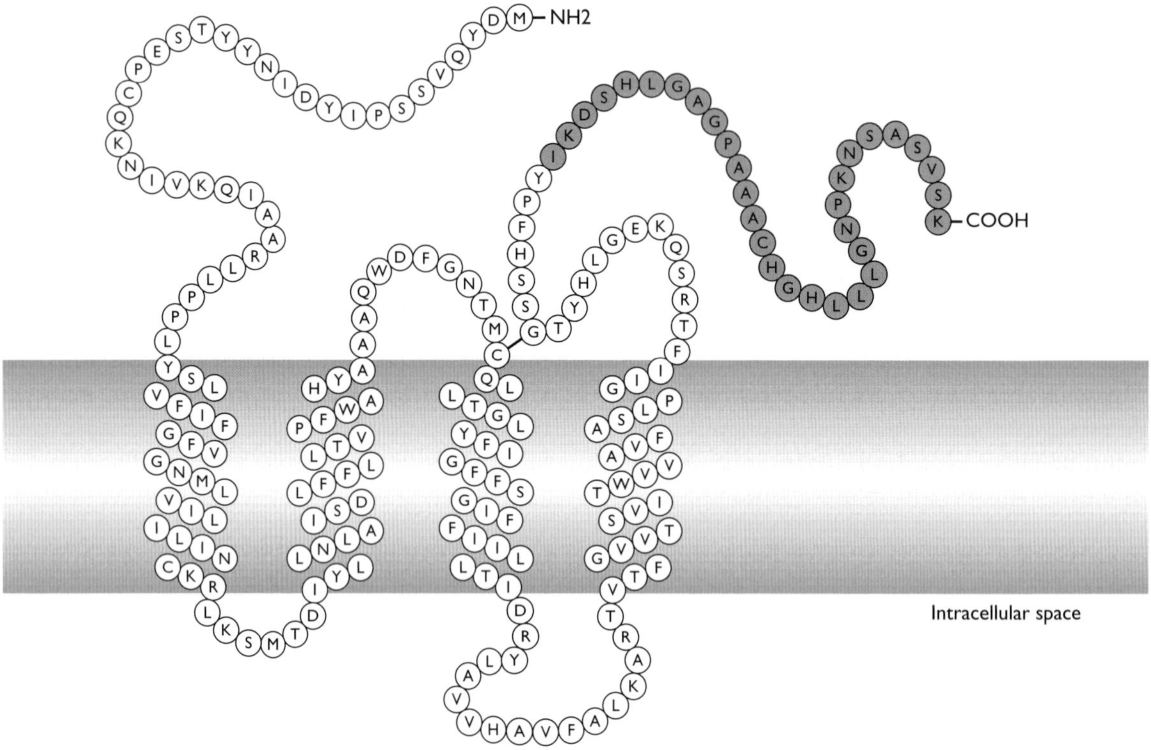

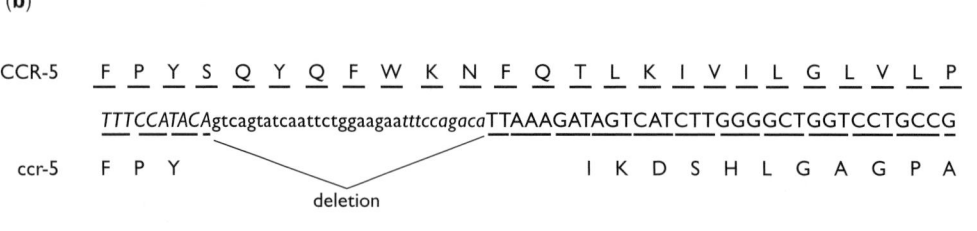

(b)

CCR-5 <u>F</u> <u>P</u> <u>Y</u> <u>S</u> <u>Q</u> <u>Y</u> <u>Q</u> <u>F</u> <u>W</u> <u>K</u> <u>N</u> <u>F</u> <u>Q</u> <u>T</u> <u>L</u> <u>K</u> <u>I</u> <u>V</u> <u>I</u> <u>L</u> <u>G</u> <u>L</u> <u>V</u> <u>L</u> <u>P</u>

*TTTCCATAC*Agtcagtatcaattctggaagaa*tttccagaca*TTAAAGATAGTCATCTTGGGGCTGGTCCTGCCG

ccr-5 F P Y   I K D S H L G A G P A

deletion

CCR-5 <u>L</u> <u>L</u> <u>V</u> <u>M</u> <u>V</u> <u>I</u> <u>C</u> <u>Y</u> <u>S</u> <u>G</u> <u>I</u> <u>L</u> <u>K</u> <u>T</u> <u>L</u> <u>L</u> <u>R</u> <u>C</u> <u>R</u> <u>N</u> <u>E</u> <u>K</u> <u>K</u> <u>R</u>

CTGCTTGTCATGGTCATCTGCTACTCGGGAATCCTAAAAACTCTGCTTCGGTGTCGAAATGAGAAGAAGAGG

ccr-5 A A C H G H L L L G N P K N S A S V S K *

Fig. 10.3

CCR5(Δ32) homozygotes account for 2–4% of all EU subjects, and for as many as 25% of all EU individuals with a prolonged (i.e. >8 years) history of high-risk sexual behaviour.[57–59] These clinical observations emphasize the protective role of the CCR5 defect. Peripheral blood mononuclear cells from individuals homozygous for CCR5(Δ32) cannot be infected with R5 viruses *in vitro*, but can be infected with X4 strains of HIV-1 *in vitro*. Clinically, this resistance to infection by R5 isolates of HIV-1 is reflected by the rarity of HIV+ individuals who are homozygous for CCR5(Δ32); the three cases reported to date were infected by X4 or R5X4 viruses.

Individuals heterozygous for the gene deletion, whilst not protected from acquiring infection, have been found to progress to AIDS more slowly and to have lower viral loads when compared to patients with the wild-type CCR5 gene.[61] In the light of these observations, several groups re-examined their cohorts of HIV-1-infected long-term non-progressors and found that a significant proportion of them had raised serum levels of β-chemokines.[56,62] CD4+ T-cell clones from long-term non-progressors were also found to produce high levels of β-chemokines and they were also less susceptible to infection by R5 viruses *in vitro*.[46]

Several other polymorphisms that can decrease susceptibility to infection by HIV-1 have also been identified. CCR5(m303) carries a T- to A-point mutation in the gene. This introduces a premature stop codon and yields a truncated, non-functional CCR5 protein. It has an allele frequency in white people of <1% and is therefore 10–20 times less frequent than the Δ32 allele.[63] Individuals who are homozygous for this defect have not been identified. However, CCR5(m303) can occur in association with CCR5(Δ32) and mononuclear cells from these individuals [CCR5(Δ32/m303)] are resistant to infection by R5 viruses. A single base mutation in the coding sequence of the CCR2 gene which causes a Val to Ile substitution at position 64 [CCR2(V64I)] has also been reported to correlate with a delay in the onset of AIDS in infected individuals. This defect does not protect against either acquiring HIV infection or change the rate of disease progression.[64,65]

Polymorphisms of the CXCR4 gene have not been reported. Such genotypes may be difficult to find in patients because deletion of the CXCR4 gene is lethal in mice.[66]

One theory for the high frequency of such alleles is that they may have resulted from a positive selection for resistance to infectious pathogens in the recent past. These alleles suppress the proinflammatory effects of these chemokines because they can be deleterious in some circumstances. However, in balanced genetic systems, this type of protective allele can also confer a disadvantage to the host; the HbS allele that confers partial resistance to malaria is a good example. In the case of chemokine receptor polymorphism, the disadvantage is not immediately apparent.

4.4 Other biological functions of CCR5

Having established that CCR5 was an important co-receptor for HIV infection, its normal biological function needed to be defined. CCR5 knockout mice (CCR5–/–) were found to develop normally with no observable histological abnormalities in their organs when compared with wild-type mice. Furthermore, CCR5 knockout mice do not display the major defects in leucocyte recruitment that have been reported for CCR1 and CCR2 knockout mice. Although these initial studies suggested a relatively normal immunological phenotype for the CCR5–/– mouse, more subtle abnormalities are now coming to light in these animals.

The first of these was that CCR5–/– mice display slightly reduced clearance of *Listeria* from the liver but not from spleen. They also have moderately reduced survival after intermediate dose treatment with lipopolysaccharide (LPS).[67] More notable were the studies of intratracheal inoculation with *Cryptococcus neoformans* which demonstrated that:

(1) a cell-mediated immune response to a single pathogen can be differentially regulated at different sites in the body such as the lung and the brain;
(2) CCR5 plays a role in tissue-specific recruitment of leucocytes;

(3) CCR5 is not required for leucocyte recruitment during a type 1 helper T-cell (Th1) response but may play a role in innate recognition of shed microbial products.[68]

CCR5 deficiency prevents mononuclear cell recruitment into the brain but not into the lungs.[68] In contrast, T-cell deficiency inhibits leucocyte recruitment into both the lungs and the brain during *Cryptococcus neoformans* infection. It remains to be established how CCR5 mediates such specific tissue trafficking during a cell-mediated immune response.

The most recent evidence for subtle immune dysregulation was a study that investigated whole blood immunoglobulin (Ig) G concentrations for herpesviruses in 157 normal adult blood donors. Individuals who were CCR5−/− were 9.2 times more likely to be seronegative for varicella-zoster virus than non-carriers. No differences were seen for any of the other herpesviruses.[69] There is little doubt that other subtle immunological abnormalities will be identified in individuals homozygous for the gene deletion as other cohorts of patients with specific diseases are studied.

5. CURRENT ANTIRETROVIRAL THERAPY

The three classes of drugs currently being used to treat HIV-1-positive patients are the nucleoside reverse-transcriptase inhibitors, non-nucleoside reverse-transcriptase inhibitors and the protease inhibitors. Clinical trials have confirmed the superiority of drug combinations over monotherapy and have led to the concept of HAART. Suppression of the viral load to below the detection limit of currently available assays (HIV-1 RNA <50 copies/ml) can now be achieved in 60–90% of patients receiving HAART for the first time. This has had a major impact on the clinical course of the disease and reduced the frequency of opportunistic infections occurring in HIV-positive patients.[70]

Unfortunately, initial optimism about the prognosis of patients with HIV/AIDS receiving HAART has been tempered by long-term experience. In everyday clinical use, only 50% of patients achieve sustained plasma HIV-1 RNA

levels of <50 copies/ml for one of several reasons.[71,72] Complex dosing schedules seriously disrupt lifestyle, patient compliance deteriorates with time and drug toxicity has become a real problem.[73] Complex treatment regimens and the incomplete suppression of viral replication have led to the emergence of resistant viruses, thereby limiting the long-term efficacy of current antiretroviral drugs.

5.1 Co-receptor-based therapies for inflammation

The idea of blocking viral entry into cells as an adjunctive therapy for the treatment of HIV-1 infection is currently a subject of intense study. The initial optimism surrounding chemokine co-receptor antagonists has faded because of the unexpected growth of the chemokine family and because of the considerable redundancy within the system. Nevertheless, the idea of influencing the degree of inflammation rather than abolishing inflammation with chemokine receptor antagonists remains a valid target for new drugs.

The first chemokine antagonist was obtained by truncation of IL-8. Studies with this and other truncated chemokines showed that receptor selectivity is primarily determined by the NH_2-terminal of the molecule. However, despite a large body of *in vitro* data that have shown that these molecules can effectively block chemokine receptors, chemokine mutants which act as antagonists do not make for ideal drugs. As proteins, they pose enormous problems in relation to effective delivery to their point of action and they are unlikely to be orally active.

5.2 Co-receptor-based therapies for HIV-1 infection

These would be highly-targeted drug therapies which would block viral entry into cells. There are two ways in which the entry of HIV into cells could be blocked with receptor antagonists. The first is simply by steric hindrance in which binding of the chemokine to its receptor prevents HIV from interacting with the chemokine receptor. The second is based on the capacity of chemokines to induce endocytosis of their receptors because removal of the chemokine receptor from the cell surface prevents it from acting as an HIV co-receptor. Chemokine inhibition of HIV entry by steric hindrance could be achieved by an agonist or an antagonist as both types of proteins will bind to the receptor. A truncated RANTES protein, 9-68 RANTES, as well as Met-RANTES, did not elicit calcium mobilization or chemotactic responses in primary cells; these proteins are thus functional antagonists. Both are capable of inhibiting HIV infectivity, albeit less potently than RANTES itself.[74] When seven-transmembrane receptors are internalized into endosomes, they can follow one of two pathways: (1) transport to the lysosomal compartment where they are degraded or (2) recycling to the cell surface. These alternative pathways have not yet been extensively studied for chemokine receptors, but evidence exists for both. CXCR2 has been shown to undergo lysosomal degradation, whereas CXCR4 and CCR5 have been shown to recycle to the cell surface. Aminooxypentone (AOP)-RANTES has the capacity to prevent CCR5 recycling, correlating with its higher affinity for CCR5 and for its greater potency in inhibiting infection by HIV than RANTES alone.[75]

5.3 Therapeutic drugs

Current treatments for HIV-1 are all directed at proteins produced by the virus. Targeting chemokine receptors would be a therapy directed at a host protein. The development of small molecular weight ligands for chemokine receptors will not be a trivial task. Intense efforts from the major pharmaceutical companies have, to date, resulted in very few reports of co-receptor specific compounds; however, several have recently been described in the patent and scientific literature and examples include:

(1) *AMD 3100* – a bicyclam that acts as an antagonist of CXCR4, which is in early clinical trials.[76]
(2) *derivatives of RANTES* – some of these are in early clinical trials. *TAK-779* is another small molecule under evaluation; it binds to CCR5 and is able to block the binding of gp120 to CD4.

(3) *T-20* – a synthetic peptide which binds to gp41 *on the virus*, therefore acting after gp120 has bound to CD4 to block fusion of the virus envelope with that of CD4+ cells. Early reports of the *in vivo* anti-HIV-1 activity of this molecule from small clinical trials are promising.[77,78]
(4) *Sulphated dextrins* – dextrin 2-sulphate is a member of a new class of polymer-based drugs that block fusion at a post-gp120–CD4 step. They are currently in early clinical trials as part of a salvage regimen of drugs in patients with AIDS and are also being evaluated as vaginal virucides.[79–81]

6. CONCLUSIONS – NEW DRUGS FOR THE FUTURE

There is now little doubt that detailed study of the mechanisms by which HIV gains entry into cells has opened up the new fields of chemokine and chemokine receptor biology. We are only just beginning to recognize the seminal role of these molecules in local immunoregulatory pathways in different body compartments, as well as their importance in initiating and maintaining inflammation. The new insights into acute and chronic inflammation which will follow in the next few years will lead to important new classes of therapeutic drugs for treating a variety of medical conditions.

REFERENCES

Scientific papers

1. Coffin J, Haase A, Levy JA et al. What to call the AIDS virus? *Nature* 1986; **321**: 10.
2. UNAIDS/WHO. *AIDS epidemic update 1999.* Geneva: Joint United Nations Programme on AIDS and World Health Organization.
3. Spira AI, Marx PA, Patterson BK et al. Cellular targets of infection and route of viral dissemination after an intravaginal inoculation of SIV into rhesus macaques. *J Exp Med* 1996; **183**: 215–25.
4. Schacker T, Little S, Connick E et al. Rapid accumulation of HIV in lymphatic tissue reservoirs during acute and early HIV infection: implications for timing of antiretroviral therapy. *J Infect Dis* 2000; **181**: 354–7.

5. Embretson J, Zupancic M, Ribas JL et al. Massive covert infection of helper T lymphocytes and macrophages by HIV during the incubation period of AIDS. *Nature* 1993; **362**: 359–62.

6. Pantaleo G, Graziosi C, Demarest JF et al. HIV infection is active and progressive in lymphoid tissue during the clinically latent stage of disease. *Nature* 1993; **362**: 355–8.

7. Perelson AS, Neumann AU, Markowitz M et al. HIV-1 dynamics *in vivo*: virion clearance rate, infected cell life-span, and viral generation time. *Science* 1996; **271**: 1582–6.

8. Perelson AS, Essunger P, Cao Y et al. Decay characteristics of HIV-1-infected compartments during combination therapy. *Nature* 1997; **387**: 188–91.

9. Chun TW, Davey-RT J, Engel D et al. Re-emergence of HIV after stopping therapy. *Nature* 1999; **401**: 874–5.

10. Finzi D, Hermankova M, Pierson T et al. Identification of a reservoir for HIV-1 in patients on highly active antiretroviral therapy. *Science* 1997; **278**: 1295–300.

11. Wong JK, Hezareh M, Gunthard HF et al. Recovery of replication-competent HIV despite prolonged suppression of plasma viremia. *Science* 1997; **278**: 1291–5.

12. Sharkey ME, Teo I, Greenough T et al. Persistence of episomal HIV-1 infection intermediates in patients on highly active anti-retroviral therapy. *Nature Med* 2000; **6**: 76–81.

13. Chun TW, Finzi D, Margolick J et al. *In vivo* fate of HIV-1-infected T cells: quantitative analysis of the transition to stable latency. *Nature Med* 1995; **1**: 1284–90.

14. Chun TW, Stuyver L, Mizell SB et al. Presence of an inducible HIV-1 latent reservoir during highly active antiretroviral therapy. *Proc Natl Acad Sci USA* 1997; **94**: 13,193–7.

15. Meltzer MS, Nakamura M, Hansen BD et al. Macrophages as susceptible targets for HIV infection, persistent viral reservoirs in tissue, and key immunoregulatory cells that control levels of virus replication and extent of disease. *AIDS Res Hum Retroviruses* 1990; **6**: 967–71.

16. Teo I, Veryard C, Barnes H et al. Circular forms of unintegrated HIV-1 DNA and high levels of viral protein expression: association with dementia and multinucleated giant cells in the brains of patients with AIDS. *J Virol* 1997; **71**: 2928–33.

17. Lambotte O, Taoufik Y, de Goer MG et al. Detection of infectious HIV in circulating monocytes from patients on prolonged highly active antiretroviral therapy. *J AIDS* 2000; **23**: 114–19.

18. Dalgleish AG, Beverley PC, Clapham PR et al. The CD4 (T4) antigen is an essential component of the receptor for the AIDS retrovirus. *Nature* 1984; **312**: 763–7.

19. Maddon PJ, Dalgleish AG, McDougal JS et al. The T4 gene encodes the AIDS virus receptor and is expressed in the immune system and the brain. *Cell* 1986; **47**: 333–48.

20. Kwong PD, Wyatt R, Robinson J et al. Structure of an HIV gp120 envelope glycoprotein in complex with the CD4 receptor and a neutralizing human antibody. *Nature* 1998; **393**: 648–59.

21. Rizzuto CD, Wyatt R, Hernandez Ramos N et al. A conserved HIV gp120 glycoprotein structure involved in chemokine receptor binding. *Science* 1998; **280**: 1949–53.

22. Veryard C, Javan C, Shaunak S. Repeated and spontaneous switching of the chemokine co-receptors used by HIV-1 is rare *in vivo*. *AIDS* 2000; **14**: 2942–3.

23. Broder CC, Berger EA. Fusogenic selectivity of the envelope glycoprotein is a major determinant of HIV-1 tropism for CD4+ T-cell lines vs. primary macrophages. *Proc Natl Acad Sci USA* 1995; **92**: 9004–8.

24. Feng Y, Broder CC, Kennedy PE et al. HIV-1 entry cofactor: functional cDNA cloning of a seven-transmembrane, G protein-coupled receptor. *Science* 1996; **272**: 872–7.

25. Bleul CC, Farzan M, Choe H et al. The lymphocyte chemoattractant SDF-1 is a ligand for LESTR/fusin and blocks HIV-1 entry. *Nature* 1996; **382**: 829–33.

26. Cocchi F, de Vico AL, Garzino DA et al. Role of β-chemokines in suppressing HIV replication. *Science* 1996; **274**: 1394–5.

27. Alkhatib G, Combadiere C, Broder CC et al. CC CKR5: a RANTES, MIP-1α, MIP-1β receptor as a fusion cofactor for macrophage-tropic HIV-1. *Science* 1996; **272**: 1955–8.

28. Deng H, Liu R, Ellmeier W et al. Identification of a major co-receptor for primary isolates of HIV-1. *Nature* 1996; **381**: 661–6.

29. Dragic T, Litwin V, Allaway GP et al. HIV-1 entry into CD4+ cells is mediated by the chemokine receptor CC-CKR-5. *Nature* 1996; **381**: 667–73.

30. Bleul CC, Wu L, Hoxie JA et al. The HIV coreceptors CXCR4 and CCR5 are differentially expressed and regulated on human T lymphocytes. *Proc Natl Acad Sci USA* 1997; **94**: 1925–30.

31. Anton PA, Elliott J, Poles MA et al. Enhanced levels of functional HIV-1 co-receptors on human mucosal T cells demonstrated using intestinal biopsy tissue. *AIDS* 2000; **14**: 1761–5.

32. Choe H, Farzan M, Sun Y et al. The β-chemokine receptors CCR3 and CCR5 facilitate infection by primary HIV-1 isolates. *Cell* 1996; **85**: 1135–48.

33. Berger EA, Doms RW, Fenyo EM et al. A new classification for HIV-1. *Nature* 1998; **391**: 240.

34. Xiao L, Rudolph DL, Owen SM et al. Adaptation to promiscuous usage of CC and CXC-chemokine coreceptors *in vivo* correlates with HIV-1 disease progression. *AIDS* 1998; **12**: F137–F143.

35. Zhang L, He T, Talal A et al. *In vivo* distribution of the HIV/SIV coreceptors: CXCR4, CCR3, and CCR5. *J Virol* 1998; **72**: 5035–45.

36. Singh A, Besson G, Mobasher A et al. Patterns of chemokine receptor fusion cofactor utilization by human immunodeficiency virus type 1 variants from the lungs and blood. *J Virol* 1999; **73**: 6680–90.

37. Cilliers T, Orlovic D, Morris L. South African HIV-1 subtype C isolates are able to utilize a variety of chemokine receptors. *XIII International AIDS Conference*. Durban, South Africa, July 2000. (MoPeA2019.)

38. Murphy PM. The molecular biology of leukocyte chemoattractant receptors. *Annu Rev Immunol* 1994; **12**: 593–633.

39. Baggiolini M, Dewald B, Moser B. IL-8 and related chemotactic cytokines-CXC and CC chemokines. *Adv Immunol* 1994; **55**: 97–179.

40. Luster AD. Chemokines – chemotactic cytokines that mediate inflammation. *N Engl J Med* 1998; **338**: 436–45.

41. Lodi PJ, Garrett DS, Kuszewski J et al. High-resolution solution structure of the β-chemokine hMIP-1β by multidimensional NMR. *Science* 1994; **263**: 1762–7.

42. Laudanna C, Campbell JJ, Butcher EC. Role of Rho in chemoattractant-activated leukocyte adhesion through integrins. *Science* 1996; **271**: 981–3.

43. Clerici M, Balotta C, Trabattoni D et al. Chemokine production in HIV-seropositive long-term asymptomatic individuals. *AIDS* 1996; **10**: 1432–3.

44. Zanussi S, D'Andrea M, Simonelli C et al. CD8+ cells in HIV infection produce MIP-1α and RANTES: a comparative study in long-term survivors and progressor patients. *Immunol Lett* 1996; **53**: 105–8.

45. Mackewicz CE, Barker E, Levy JA. Role of β-chemokines in suppressing HIV replication. *Science* 1996; **274**: 1393–5.

46. Saha K, Bentsman G, Chess L et al. Endogenous production of β-chemokines by CD4+, but not CD8+, T-cell clones correlates with the clinical state of HIV-1 infected individuals and may be responsible for blocking infection with non-syncytium-inducing HIV-1 *in vitro*. *J Virol* 1998; **72**: 876–81.

47. Blaak H, Ran LJ, Rientsma R et al. Susceptibility of *in vitro* stimulated PBMC to infection with NSI HIV-1 is associated with levels of CCR5 expression and β-chemokine production. *Virology* 2000; **267**: 237–46.

48. Kumar D, Parato K, Kumar A et al. Sustained suppression of plasma HIV RNA is associated with an increase in the production of mitogen-induced MIP-1α and MIP-1β. *AIDS Res Hum Retroviruses* 1999; **15**: 1073–7.

49. Garzino DA, Moss RB, Margolick JB et al. Spontaneous and antigen-induced production of HIV-inhibitory β-chemokines are associated with AIDS-free status. *Proc Natl Acad Sci USA* 1999; **96**: 11,986–91.

50. Andersson J, Andersson U. Characterization of cytokine production in infectious mononucleosis studied at a single-cell level in tonsil and peripheral blood. *Clin Exp Immunol* 1993; **92**: 7–13.

51. Veazey RS, DeMaria M, Chalifoux LV et al. Gastrointestinal tract as a major site of CD4+ T cell depletion and viral replication in SIV infection. *Science* 1998; **280**: 427–31.

52. Zhang Z, Schuler T, Zupancic M et al. Sexual transmission and propogation of SIV and HIV in resting and activated CD4+ T cells. *Science* 1999; **286**: 1353–7.

53. Olsson J, Poles M, Spetz AL et al. HIV-1 infection is associated with significant mucosal inflammation characterised by increased expression of CCR5, CXCR4 and β-chemokines. *J Infect Dis* 2000; **182**: 1625–35.

54. Veazey RS, Tham IC, Mansfield KG et al. Identifying the target cell in primary SIV infection: highly activated memory CD4+ T cells are rapidly eliminated in early SIV infection *in vivo*. *J Virol* 2000; **74**: 57–64.

55. Patterson BK, Landay A, Andersson J et al. Repertoire of chemokine receptor expression in the female genital tract: implications for human immunodeficiency virus transmission. *Am J Pathol* 1998; **153**: 481–90.

56. Paxton WA, Martin SR, Tse D et al. Relative resistance to HIV-1 infection of CD4 lymphocytes from persons who remain uninfected despite multiple high-risk sexual exposure. *Nature Med* 1996; **2**: 412–17.

57. Samson M, Libert F, Doranz BJ et al. Resistance to HIV-1 infection in Caucasian individuals bearing

mutant alleles of the CCR-5 chemokine receptor gene. *Nature* 1996; **382**: 722–5.

58. Liu R, Paxton WA, Choe S et al. Homozygous defect in HIV-1 coreceptor accounts for resistance of some multiply-exposed individuals to HIV-1 infection. *Cell* 1996; **86**: 367–77.

59. Dean M, Carrington M, Winkler C et al. Genetic restriction of HIV-1 infection and progression to AIDS by a deletion allele of the CKR5 structural gene. *Science* 1996; **273**: 1856–62.

60. Libert F, Cochaux P, Beckman G et al. The ΔCCR5 mutation conferring protection against HIV-1 in Caucasian populations has a single and recent origin in Northeastern Europe. *Hum Molec Genet* 1998; **7**: 399–406.

61. Zimmerman PA, Buckler WA, Alkhatib G et al. Inherited resistance to HIV-1 conferred by an inactivating mutation in CC chemokine receptor 5: studies in populations with contrasting clinical phenotypes, defined racial background, and quantified risk. *Molec Med* 1997; **3**: 23–36.

62. Ullum H, Cozzi LA, Victor J et al. Production of β-chemokines in HIV infection: evidence that high levels of MIP-1β are associated with a decreased risk of HIV disease progression. *J Infect Dis* 1998; **177**: 331–6.

63. Quillent C, Oberlin E, Braun J et al. HIV-1-resistance phenotype conferred by combination of two separate inherited mutations of CCR5 gene. *Lancet* 1998; **351**: 14–18.

64. Michael NL, Louie LG, Rohrbaugh AL et al. The role of CCR5 and CCR2 polymorphisms in HIV-1 transmission and disease progression. *Nature Med* 1997; **3**: 1160–2.

65. Mummidi S, Ahuja SS, Gonzalez E et al. Genealogy of the CCR5 locus and chemokine system gene variants associated with altered rates of HIV-1 disease progression. *Nature Med* 1998; **4**: 786–93.

66. Tachibana K, Hirota S, Iizasa H et al. The chemokine receptor CXCR4 is essential for vascularization of the gastrointestinal tract. *Nature* 1998; **393**: 591–4.

67. Zhou Y, Kurihara T, Ryseck RP et al. Impaired macrophage function and enhanced T cell-dependent immune response in mice lacking CCR5, the mouse homologue of the major HIV-1 coreceptor. *J Immunol* 1998; **160**: 4018–25.

68. Huffnagle GB, McNeil LK, McDonald RA et al. Role of CCR5 in organ-specific and innate immunity to *Cryptococcus neoformans*. *J Immunol* 1999; **163**: 4642–6.

69. Wienckle JK, Kelsey KT, Zuo Z et al. Genetic resistance factor for HIV-1 and immune response to varicella-zoster virus. *Lancet* 2001; **357**: 360–1.

70. Hirschel B, Opravil M. The year in review: antiretroviral treatment. *AIDS* 1999; **13 (Suppl A)**: S177–S187.

71. Fatkenheuer G, Theisen A, Rockstroh J et al. Virological treatment failure of protease inhibitor therapy in an unselected cohort of HIV-infected patients. *AIDS* 1997; **11**: F113–F116.

72. Casado JL, Perez-Elias MJ, Antela A et al. Predictors of long-term response to protease inhibitor therapy in a cohort of HIV-infected patients. *AIDS* 1998; **12**: F131–F135.

73. Moyle GJ, Gazzard BG, Cooper DA et al. Antiretroviral therapy for HIV infection. A knowledge based approach to drug selection and use. *Drugs* 1998; **55**: 383–404.

74. Simmons G, Clapham PR, Picard L et al. Potent inhibition of HIV-1 infectivity in macrophages and lymphocytes by a novel CCR5 antagonist. *Science* 1997; **276**: 276–9.

75. Mack M, Luckow B, Nelson PJ et al. Aminooxypentane–RANTES induces CCR5 internalization but inhibits recycling: a novel inhibitory mechanism of HIV infectivity. *J Exp Med* 1998; **187**: 1215–24.

76. De Clercq E. The emerging role of fusion inhibitors in HIV infection. *Drugs* 1999; **2**: 321–31.

77. Kilby JM, Hopkins S, Venetta TM et al. Potent suppression of HIV-1 replication in humans by T-20, a peptide inhibitor of gp41-mediated virus entry. *Nature Med* 1998; **4**: 1302–7.

78. Pilcher CD, Eron-JJ J, Ngo L et al. Prolonged therapy with the fusion inhibitor T-20 in combination with oral antiretroviral agents in an HIV-infected individual. *AIDS* 1999; **13**: 2171–3.

79. Javan CM, Gooderham NJ, Edwards RJ et al. Anti-HIV type 1 activity of sulfated derivatives of dextrin against primary viral isolates of HIV type 1 in lymphocytes and monocyte-derived macrophages. *AIDS Res Hum Retroviruses* 1997; **13**: 875–80.

80. Shaunak S, Gooderham NJ, Edwards RJ et al. Infection by HIV-1 blocked by binding of dextrin 2-sulphate to the cell surface of activated human peripheral blood mononuclear cells and cultured T-cells. *Br J Pharmacol* 1994; **113**: 151–8.

81. Shaunak S, Thornton M, John S et al. Reduction of the viral load of HIV-1 after the intraperitoneal administration of dextrin 2-sulphate in patients with AIDS. *AIDS* 1998; **12**: 399–409.

82. Loetscher P, Moser B, Baggiolini M. Chemokines and their receptors in lymphocyte traffic and HIV infection. *Adv Immunol* 2000; **74**: 127–80.

11

Viral evasion of the immune system

Babak Javid, Paul J Lehner

Objectives • Introduction and overview • Inhibition of major histocompatibility complex class I restricted antigen presentation • Inhibition of major histocompatibility complex class II restricted antigen presentation • Inhibition of apoptosis • Interference with cytokines and chemokines • Inhibition of humoral responses • Complement evasion • Future perspectives and implications • Glossary • References

OBJECTIVES

(1) To review many mechanisms which viruses use to overcome host defence to infection.
(2) To consider the equilibrium between the virus and the human immune system.

1. INTRODUCTION AND OVERVIEW

Viruses are obligate intracellular parasites, and utilize the host cell's organelles and metabolic pathways for their own reproduction. At the most basic level, a virus particle (a virion) consists of a nucleic acid genome packaged within a protein coat. For viral replication to occur the virion must deliver the nucleic acid to the host cell. Viral entry, replication and the measures used by the host to eliminate the virus have been the subject of intense study for many years. More recent is the realization that coexistence with the host requires a virus to deal with the complexities of both the innate and acquired immune system that may be activated from the moment of viral entry.

Viruses exist both as extracellular virion particles and intracellular genomes. Prior to gaining cellular access a virus must successfully breach the host's first-line defences. At the very

least, this involves penetration of the protective external skin or epithelial layer and avoidance of the many arms of the host innate immune system. Once inside a cell, viral safety is only assured if viral genomes are maintained within the host cell by limited gene expression. The moment viral replication is initiated, with consequent expression of viral gene products, the virus can be visualized by the host immune system. Indeed, as we shall discuss, multiple pathways of antigen presentation have evolved to allow the cell to continually 'sample' its different intracellular compartments for the presence of foreign, especially viral, material. Viral proteins can be transported to the cell surface and recognition of a viral fragment by the T-cell immunosurveillance system will result in destruction of the cell. Thus, the innate and adaptive immune system provide a challenge to any incoming pathogen (see Fig. 11.1).

One of the most exciting and productive areas of immunology and virology over the last decade has been an appreciation of the delicate equilibrium between the virus and its host – more specifically, the immune system of the host. To be genetically successful a virus needs

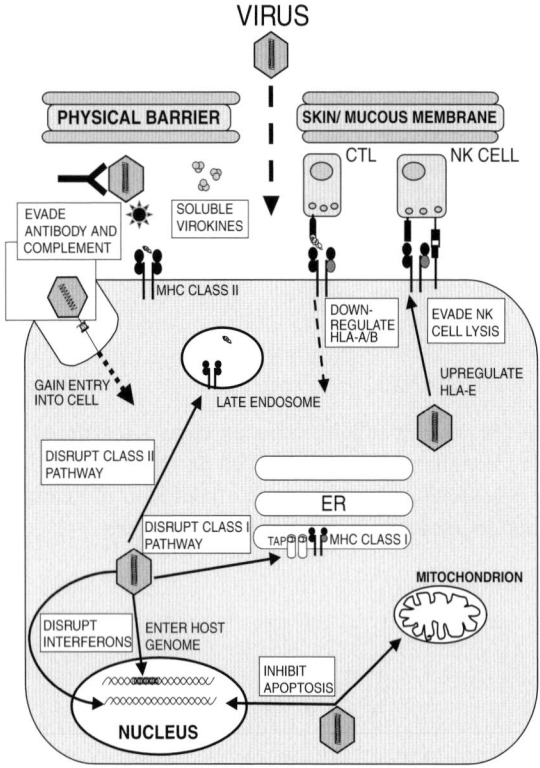

Fig. 11.1 Strategies employed by viruses to evade the host immune response. After breaching a physical barrier to gain access to host tissue, a virus has to avoid antibody and complement before entering a host cell. Inside the cell, a virus has to avoid detection by disrupting antigen-processing pathways, and inhibit apoptosis and cell lysis by natural killer (NK) cells. Viruses also interfere with cell signalling by mimicking interferons and other cytokines. (CTL, cytotoxic T-lymphocytes; ER, endoplasmic reticulum; HLA, human leucocyte antigen; MHC, major histocompatibility complex.)

to overcome the host immune system and at the same time retain a reservoir for infection. Therefore, the rapid elimination of the host by an extremely virulent virus may not necessarily be a useful long-term strategy.

Depending on the constraints of their genome size, different viruses have developed a multitude of strategies that allow them to defend their ecological niche. RNA viruses have smaller genomes than their DNA counterparts due to the higher error rate of RNA polymerase. As such, their proteins are often multifunctional

and adept at rapid mutation, which may be used for avoiding both B- and T-cell epitopes. DNA viruses are not so constrained and have, in some cases, such as the herpes viruses and poxviruses, devoted up to 50% of their genome to immune subversion. Indeed, there is evidence to suggest that different components of the immune system continue to co-evolve with viruses and their subversive tactics – a strategic game of cat and mouse.

Why is the study of viral evasion important? Viruses have spent millions of years learning the cell biology of the immune system in their efforts to avoid immune detection. There are therefore many reasons to study viral evasion of the immune system:

(1) Viral genomes are relatively small and compact, and many of the clinically important viral genomes have been sequenced. In principle, it should be possible to identify the gene products responsible for viral evasion and we have, as a consequence, learnt several basic principles of cell biology and immunology from the study of viruses.
(2) There is the hope and expectation that a further understanding of basic immunological concepts, in particular how a virus avoids immune system detection, will be helpful for improved vaccine strategies.
(3) The identification of viral proteins responsible for immune subversion, in particular the soluble small molecules, may provide potential tools for both antiviral and anti-inflammatory strategies.

Viral immunoevasion gene products fall into two main categories. Viral genes with homology to cellular genes, which are presumed to have been seconded and modified for the benefit of the virus, and those with no known homologues. The latter would suggest either genes which are truly virus specific and have evolved solely for the purpose of viral evasion or genes for which no homologues have yet been described.

In this chapter we will review some of the important means of escape by different viruses. The chapter is in no way exhaustive (comprehensive reviews can be found in Tortorella et al 2000 and Alcami and Koszinowski 2000) but illustrates some general principles of the immune system and the remarkable strategies used by viruses to overcome them.

2. INHIBITION OF MAJOR HISTOCOMPATIBILITY COMPLEX (MHC) CLASS I RESTRICTED ANTIGEN PRESENTATION

2.1 Overview of MHC class I antigen presentation

All nucleated cells express MHC class I molecules. The MHC class I antigen-presentation pathway allows the intracellular protein content of the cell to be displayed at the cell surface, in the form of small peptides (reviewed in Pamer and Cresswell 1998) to cytotoxic T-lymphocytes (CTL). These peptides can be derived from any intracellular protein and may therefore be cellular or viral in origin. Peptides derived from a viral protein will be recognized as foreign and subsequently destroyed by the CTL. The class I presentation pathway is therefore of fundamental importance in defence against viruses.

The presentation of peptide to CTL at the cell surface is the final step in an intracellular process which involves the cytosolic degradation of protein to peptide by the proteasome, the transport of peptide from the cytosol to the endoplasmic reticulum (ER) via the transporters associated with antigen processing (TAP)

Table 11.1 Viral interference with major histocompatibility complex (MHC) class I and natural killer (NK) cells

Virus	Gene/protein	Mechanism
Adenovirus	E3/19k	Retains class I molecules in the ER
EBV	EBNA-1	Resistant to proteasome-mediated proteolysis
HCMV	pp65	Inhibits processing of IE-1 transcription factor
	US2, US11	Relocates MHC class I heavy chains for degradation
	US3	Binds and retains class I molecules in the ER
	US6	Inhibits TAP-mediated peptide transport
	UL18	Class I homologue
	UL40	Upregulates HLA-E (NK cell inhibitory receptor CD94 target)
HIV	Nef	Rapid endocytosis of cell surface MHC class I
	Vpu	Destabilizes newly synthesized class I molecules
HHV-8	K3, K5	Promote endocytosis of class I molecules
HSV	ICP-47	Inhibits TAP-mediated peptide transport
MCMV	m4	Binds MHC class I molecules
	m6	Targets class I molecules for lysosomal degradation
	m144	Class I homologue (inhibits NK cell lysis)
	m152	Retains class I in ER/Golgi intermediate compartment

EBNA, EBV nuclear antigen; EBV, Epstein-Barr virus; ER, endoplasmic reticulum; HCMV, human cytomegalovirus; HHV, human herpesvirus; HIV, human immunodeficiency virus; HLA, human leucocyte antigen; HSV, herpes simplex virus; IE-1, immediate–early-1; MCMV, mouse cytomegalovirus; TAP, transporters associated with antigen processing.

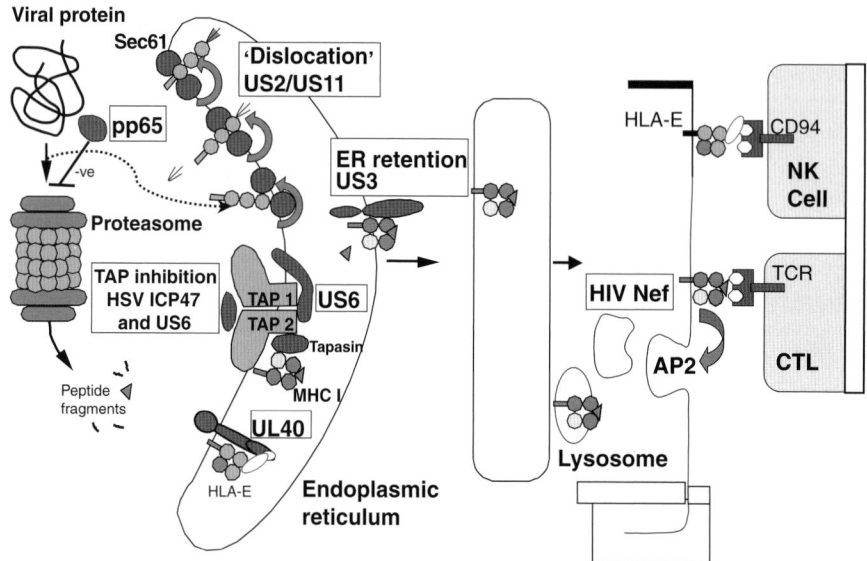

Fig. 11.2 Viral inhibition of major histocompatibility complex (MHC) class I processing and antigen presentation. Examples of how viruses interrupt the MHC class I pathway. Viruses interrupt the pathway at various levels including degradation of viral proteins by the proteasome, inhibition of transporter-associated antigen processing (TAP)-dependent peptide transport, degradation of class I molecules and removal of class I from the cell surface. (AP, Adaptor protein; CTL, cytotoxic T-lymphocyte; ER, endoplasmic reticulum; HIV, human immunodeficiency virus; HLA, human leucocyte antigen; HSV, herpes simplex virus; ICP, infected cell protein; TCR, T-cell receptor; US, unique short.)

molecules, and peptide loading and transport of class I molecules from the ER to the cell surface. Efficient peptide loading requires the formation of a TAP/class I ER protein complex, whose minimal components include TAP1 and TAP2, tapasin, MHC class I heavy chains, β2M, and calreticulin. Many viruses encode gene products which interfere with class I processing and presentation (reviewed in Fruh et al 1999; Table 11.1 and Fig. 11.2). The large double-stranded DNA viruses, in particular, have evolved elaborate strategies to avoid class I antigen presentation. In many of these infections, e.g. human cytomegalovirus (HCMV) infection, it is still possible to detect virus-specific CTL, suggesting that viral deterrence is defective. With human viruses, and in the absence of a good model, this is difficult to test. With murine and other animal viruses there are some examples which suggest that

these viral gene products affecting class I are required for viral success. The effects are not all or nothing but almost certainly affect the intricate balance between the virus and its host, which in the case of herpes viruses in immunocompetent subjects allows for successful, and often lifelong, infection.

2.2 Inhibition of generation of antigenic peptide

Viral proteins expressed in the cytosol are candidates for proteasomal degradation and subsequent loading onto class I molecules. To avoid this process and prevent CTL detection, viruses may inhibit the proteasome and thus prevent self-degradation. During latency, the Epstein-Barr virus (EBV) protein, EBV nuclear antigen-1 (EBNA-1), is expressed in B-cells but no B-cell specific EBNA-1 CTL have been identified. This is due to inhibition of proteasomal processing by EBNA-1,[1] a glycine–alanine–rich phosphoprotein which is thought to prevent degradation of EBNA-1 but not other proteins. The molecular mechanism by which EBNA-1 resists proteolysis is poorly understood.

A second example of a viral gene product which affects proteasomal degradation is HCMV-derived matrix protein phosphoprotein 65 (pp65). Together with the immediate–early-1 (IE-1) protein, pp65 is expressed during the immediate–early phase of HCMV infection and the IE-1-specific CTL response is lost following coexpression of pp65.[2] Since the pp65 protein has kinase activity, it has been suggested that phosphorylation of the viral protein may limit access to the processing machinery with consequent evasion of CTL recognition.

2.3 Inhibition of TAP-mediated peptide translocation

TAP allows cytosolic peptides access to the lumen of the ER for subsequent loading onto class I molecules. As the majority of peptides require TAP transport, it represents a potential bottleneck in class-I-mediated presentation and is therefore a good target for viral inhibition. Two herpesvirus family members, herpes simplex virus (HSV) and HCMV, express well-characterized TAP inhibitors, and other herpesviruses are known to inhibit TAP, though the responsible proteins have not been defined. The HSV immediate–early gene product, infected cell protein 47 (ICP-47), binds TAP on the cytosolic side of the ER membrane and inhibits peptide transport[3] by preventing other peptides from binding to TAP – in effect, it plugs the transporter and prevents further peptide translocation.

In contrast, HCMV has a very different TAP inhibitor. The unique short (US) gene, US6, whose product is expressed both in the early and late phases of infection, binds TAP on the ER lumenal side, the opposite side from ICP-47, and effectively inhibits peptide translocation. US6 does not prevent peptide binding to TAP, but prevents interaction of TAP with its energy source, ATP.[4] In the absence of ATP binding and hydrolysis, TAP is functionally inert and is unable to transport peptide.

2.4 Inhibition of MHC class I trafficking through the secretory pathway

The adenovirus E3/19k protein was the first described viral protein that decreases cell-surface class I expression.[5] It is now known to do this by two independent mechanisms. E3/19k encodes a terminal dilysine motif in its cytoplasmic tail and causes ER retention through an interaction with the retrieval protein COP-I, which prevents protein traffic beyond the Golgi. E3/19k binds peptide-loaded MHC class I molecules via the α1 and α2 regions of the class I heavy chain, and therefore prevents their transport to the cell surface. More recently it was found that independent of its effect on class I molecules, E3/19k can bind TAP and may inhibit tapasin activity, thus preventing efficient peptide loading of MHC class I molecules.[6] Other viral proteins such as the HCMV US3 protein, also retain class I in the secretory pathway, though in the absence of an ER-retention motif, the responsible mechanism is unclear.

Two HCMV encoded proteins, US2[7] and US11, have a remarkable ability to prevent class I expression by promoting the degradation of newly synthesized class I heavy chains in the cytosol. These two viral proteins bind nascent class I heavy chains and return them, via the Sec61p translocon, to the cytosol for deglycosylation and degradation by the proteasome. This process, known as retrograde translocation, is now recognized as an important 'garbage disposal' route for a large number of misfolded ER proteins, an example being the cystic fibrosis transmembrane regulator (CFTR). It is possible that US2 and US11 may promote a normal pathway for removing unwanted ER proteins and confer specificity to their target proteins by direct binding to class I heavy chains.

The murine equivalent of HCMV, the mouse cytomegalovirus (MCMV), encodes several proteins (see Table 11.1) which affect class I presentation.[8] It should be noted that none of these proteins share homology with the gene products from HCMV that inhibit class I. Despite these two viruses sharing 70% sequence homology, they have clearly evolved different gene products for effectively the same purpose, i.e. class I inhibition. Thus, the viruses appear to have co-evolved with their hosts and away from family members.

The MCMV product of the m152 gene retains class I molecules within the ER–Golgi intermediate compartment through a retention signal within its lumenal region. In contrast, the m6 gene product binds and targets class I for degradation in lysosomes through the use of a dileucine, lysosomal signalling motif.

2.5 Removal of class I from the cell surface

Two viruses encode gene products which downregulate expression of mature MHC class I molecules once they have reached the cell surface. The human immunodeficiency virus (HIV) product, Nef, targets human leucocyte antigen (HLA)-A and HLA-B gene products (reviewed in Piguet et al 1999) and accelerates their endocytosis. In the presence of Nef, class I MHC molecules are relocalized from the cell surface to the trans-Golgi network (TGN). Nef-induced downregulation of MHC class I expression, and targeting of class I to the TGN, requires the binding of Nef to PACS-1, a molecule that controls the TGN localization of the cellular protein furin. This interaction is dependent on Nef's cluster of acidic amino acids. The HIV protein Vpu targets only newly synthesized class I molecules, causing their destabilization.

Human herpesvirus 8 (HHV-8), the causative agent of Kaposi's sarcoma, also decreases cell-surface class I expression. HHV-8 encodes two gene products, K3 and K5,[9,10] which promote endocytosis of class I molecules from the cell surface. The molecular mechanism remains unclear, though both of these proteins are members of the 'RING' family of proteins, ubiquitin E3-ligases, which promote internalization through ubiquitination of their target proteins.

2.6 Inhibition of natural killer cell lysis

NK cells are a critical component of the innate immune system. They are directly cytotoxic and secrete proinflammatory cytokines such as interferon-gamma (IFN-γ) (reviewed in Lanier 2000). Their role in viral defence is well illustrated by humans congenitally deficient in NK cells, who suffer overwhelming herpesvirus infections.[11]

NK cells destroy virus-infected and tumour cells, without the need for previous antigen stimulation. NK cells possess killer-activating and killer-inhibitory receptors. In part, target cells are recognized by decreased expression of MHC class I molecules, which normally interact with killer-inhibitory receptors on the NK cell surface. Engagement of the killer-activating receptor issues a 'kill' instruction to the NK cell, which is normally overridden by killer-inhibitory receptors on recognition of class I molecules (Fig. 11.3).

NK cells also express triggering receptors that are specific for non-MHC ligands. The nature of the ligands recognized on target cells is not well defined. NKp46 is one of the main activating receptors for human NK cells[12] and sialylated NKp46 oligosaccharides may bind viral glyco-proteins such as the influenza protein haemagglutinin, leading to activation of the NK cell.

We have described how class I subversion is used by many viruses as a strategy to prevent immune detection. Reduced cell-surface class I expression will make the infected cells targets for NK cell lysis. The class I HLA-A and H-B gene products appear to be predominantly involved with presentation of endogenous peptide to CTL, while the HLA-C, -E and -G gene products inhibit NK-mediated cell lysis. Selective allele-specific class I downregulation, as seen with HIV Nef allows evasion from both CD8+ CTL and NK cells. Similarly, HLA-C and H-G gene products are resistant to degradation by US11 and US2. Some viruses have evolved further strategies to avoid NK cell detection, usually by production of MHC class I homologues, of which the best characterized is m144.

The MCMV gene product m144 binds β_2 microglobulin and is homologous with murine MHC class I.[13] m144-Transfected cells are less susceptible to NK cell lysis than their wild-type counterparts, and m144-deleted MCMV shows a replication deficit which is due to NK cell activity. The ligand for m144 remains to be identified.

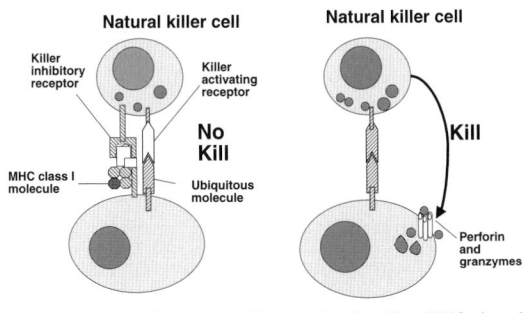

Fig. 11.3 The absence of cell-surface class I molecules promotes natural killer (NK) cell cytolysis. While positive stimulation may be initiated by an array of co-stimulatory receptors found on the surface of normal cells, specificity is provided by inhibitory signals transduced by receptors for major histocompatibility complex (MHC) class I. Cytolysis of the target cell is achieved by release of perforin and granzymes from NK cell granules, which induce apoptosis in the abnormal cell.

The HCMV gene product, UL18, was identified as a class I homologue following the sequencing of the HCMV.[14] However, despite a string of *Nature* papers, the function of this protein remains controversial and UL18 expression has not been seen following HCMV infection. Despite claims to the contrary, UL18 expression appears to be associated with enhanced rather than diminished NK cell activity.[15] The natural ligand for UL18 is a novel immunoglobulin (Ig) superfamily member,[16] leucocyte immunoglobulin-like receptor-1 (LIR-1), and not CD94 as was initially reported. *Molluscum contagiosum* (MCV), a human poxvirus, also encodes a class I homologue, though its function has not been discerned.

The HCMV product UL40 provides a beautiful example of elegance in viral strategy.[17] In wild-type cells, HLA-E binds signal-sequence peptides from HLA-A and -B alleles and traffics them to the cell surface for interaction with the NK cell receptor CD94. Following HCMV infection, these signal peptides are prevented from loading HLA-E due to TAP inhibition by US6.

This would make the cell susceptible to NK cell lysis, as CD94 would be unable to identify its ligand. Remarkably, the signal sequence from UL40 is identical to the HLA-A and -B alleles, and so binds HLA-E in a TAP-independent fashion, thus allowing HLA-E to reach the cell surface and bind CD94.

3. INHIBITION OF MAJOR HISTOCOMPATIBILITY COMPLEX (MHC) CLASS II RESTRICTED ANTIGEN PRESENTATION

3.1 Overview of MHC class II antigen presentation

The class I antigen-presentation pathway samples endogenous proteins, i.e. proteins synthesized within the cell, for presentation as peptides at the cell surface. In contrast, the MHC class II pathway allows the presentation of peptides derived from exogenous proteins, i.e. proteins which reach the cell via the exogenous route (reviewed in Pieters 2000). This route will include pathogens which enter the cell via phagocytosis or receptor-mediated endocytosis.

How do class II molecules reach the endosomal compartments for peptide loading? Mature class II molecules consist of an antigenic peptide bound to an αβ heterodimer. However, in the ER, nascent αβ dimers associate with a third protein, the invariant chain (Ii), which binds the peptide groove of the class II molecule, preventing the binding of endogenous peptide in the ER. A dileucine motif within the Ii directs the αβ/Ii complex from the TGN to endosomal compartments where protease cleavage of the Ii leaves a remnant peptide. Exogenous proteins are degraded to peptides within endosomes and, with help from the class-II-dedicated peptide editor HLA-DM, bind MHC class II molecules. From these compartments, peptide-bound MHC class II molecules traffic to the cell surface and are presented to CD4+ lymphocytes. MHC class II molecules are expressed on B-lymphocytes, dendritic cells and macrophages, and can be induced on other cell types.

CD4+ T-cells are polarized to become type 1 helper T-cells (Th1), as well as being required for CTL activation. The class II presentation pathway is therefore a viable target for viral evasion. It is perhaps surprising that, to date, relatively few viral gene products have been identified which target the class II presentation pathway (see Table 11.2).

3.2 Inhibition of MHC class II expression at the cell surface

In addition to targeting class I molecules for proteasomal degradation, the HCMV gene product US2 also targets the MHC class II HLA-DR and -DM molecules for proteasomal degradation.[18] How US2 interacts with both MHC class I and class II proteins which share little sequence homology is at present unclear.

Viruses also interfere with MHC class II molecule expression at the transcriptional level. Gene products from HCMV[19] and MCMV affect the IFN-γ signalling cascade, which induces transcription of class II genes. The adenovirus E1A product also interferes with transcription factors involved with IFN-α and IFN-γ signalling pathways.

3.3 Interference with the endocytic pathway

Traffic of vesicles both to and from the plasma membrane is a complex and highly regulated process. Both clathrin and non-clathrin coated pits (COP) form vesicles that target different organelles depending on the exact proteins involved.

Bovine (BPV) and human (HPV) papillomaviruses express proteins which interfere with trafficking (see Table 11.2). BPV E6 interacts with the adaptor protein-1 (AP-1) which is involved in the transport of vesicles to early endosomes from the TGN. Both papillomaviruses express E5 which interacts with a subunit of the vacuolar ATPase proton pump and is proposed to collapse the pH gradient necessary for antigen processing.[20]

3.4 Downregulation of CD4

HIV-1 uses CD4 and the chemokine receptors CCR5 and CXCR4 to enter and infect cells (reviewed in Collins and Baltimore 1999). In

Table 11.2 Viral interference with major histocompatibility complex (MHC) class II

Virus	Gene/protein	Mechanism
Adenovirus	E1A	Interferes with MHC class II upregulation (IFN-γ signal transduction cascade)
EBV	BZLF2	Interferes with MHC class II antigen presentation
HCMV	US2	Targets class II HLA-DM and -DR chains for degradation
	IE/E product	Interferes with MHC class II upregulation (IFN-γ signal transduction cascade)
HIV	Nef	Rapid endocytosis of CD4, may interfere with class II processing by acidifying lysosomes
	Vpu	Targets CD4 for degradation
HPV/BPV	E5/E6	Interferes with MHC class II processing. E5 acidification of lysosomes, E6 interaction with AP complex
HSV (KOS)	Unknown	Interferes with MHC class II presentation

AP, adaptor protein; BPV, bovine papillomavirus; EBV, Epstein-Barr virus; HCMV, human cytomegalovirus; HIV, human immunodeficiency virus; HLA, human leucocyte antigen; HPV, human papillomavirus; HSV, herpes simplex virus; IE/E, intermediate–early/early; IFN-γ, interferon-gamma.

addition, intracellular CD4 inhibits virion release by binding gp120 and preventing its incorporation into the virion. HIV decreases cell-surface CD4 expression as well as newly synthesized CD4. HIV Nef is responsible for the decrease in cell-surface CD4 while the HIV product Vpu induces degradation of newly synthesized CD4. Neither of these viral proteins are required for replication but both are essential for pathogenicity. Nef interacts with CD4 at the cell surface and increases CD4 endocytosis, and subsequent transport to lysosomes and the ER Golgi intermediate compartment (ERGIC). Endocytosis is achieved through interaction of Nef with AP-1, through a dileucine motif 20 amino acids proximal to CD4's transmembrane region. Transferring these 20 amino acids to CD8 causes rapid internalization of the chimeric CD8.

Vpu, together with gp160, induces degradation of newly synthesized CD4 by the proteasome. Vpu has a hydrophobic amino terminal, which tethers it to the plasma membrane, and a charged cytoplasmic domain, both of which are essential for its function. CD4 degradation is dependent on potential ubiquitin-binding sites and Vpu appears to connect CD4 with the cytosolic degradation machinery through cellular intermediaries.

4. INHIBITION OF APOPTOSIS

4.1 Triggers of apoptosis and death receptors

Apoptosis, or programmed cell death, may occur following a direct cell insult, such as viral infection, or follow recognition by CTL or NK cells (see Rathmell and Thompson 1999 for review). From a viral perspective, apoptosis is usually an undesirable consequence of infection as it limits the time available for viral replication and virion production, and thus prevents latent infection. However, at later stages of infection, apoptosis could allow release of virions and facilitate viral dissemination.

When an infected cell is attacked by a CTL or NK cell, perforin-induced membrane pores allow granzymes to enter the target cell. These activate the caspase enzymes that mediate apoptosis. Alternatively, Fas ligand (FasL) on the NK cell can bind Fas on the target cell, or NK cells release soluble tumour necrosis factor (TNF) to bind the TNF receptor (TNFR). Both of these events lead to activation of caspases and initiate apoptosis through the death signal.

Therefore, it will come as no surprise that, as seen with the class I antigen-presentation pathway, the cellular proteins responsible for apoptosis are targeted by viral anti-apoptotic mechanisms.[21] This viral strategy of immune evasion must have occurred early as anti-apoptotic mechanisms are seen in organisms which lack an acquired immune system (Fig. 11.4).

Several poxviruses have gene products that manipulate TNF signalling. The TNFR homologue, MT-2, from myxoma virus, has two isoforms.[22] A secreted isoform binds and neutralizes the activity of extracellular TNF-α, and an intracellular isoform protects infected T-cells from apoptosis by an unknown mechanism. Cowpox virus encodes three different TNFR homologues that neutralize TNF and lymphotoxin-α;[27] HCMV encodes the TNFR homologue UL144, though its function is undetermined.

Adenovirus encodes several proteins [E3/10.4k, E3/14.5k or receptor internalization and degradation (RID)], which specifically inhibit Fas-dependent apoptosis but do not affect perforin-mediated killing.[21] These adenoviral proteins cause the internalization and lysosomal destruction of Fas and epidermal growth factor receptor from the cell surface.

Ligation of trimerized TNFR causes assembly of their cytosolic domains with Fas-associated and TNFR-associated death domains (FADD and TRADD, respectively), and activate signals via caspases to trigger apoptosis. FADD and caspases associate through homologous protein interaction motifs with the dramatically named death effector domains (DED). Several herpesviruses [HHV8, herpes virus saimiri (HVS)] and MCV encode gene products, named viral FLICE inhibitory proteins (vFLIP), that encode two DED, which bind Fas and interfere directly with the FADD–caspase interaction to prevent caspase recruitment.

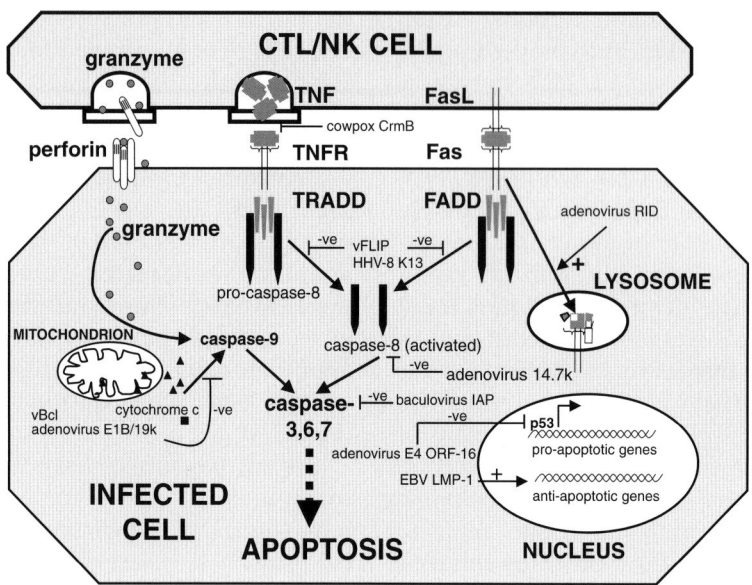

Fig 11.4: Viral inhibition of apoptosis. Some examples of how viruses prevent programmed cell death by interfering with host effectors along multiple pathways. (CrmB, Cytokine response modifier B; CTL, cytotoxic T-lymphocyte; FADD, Fas-associated death domain; FaSL, Fas ligand; HHV, human herpesvirus; LMP, latent membrane protein; NK, natural killer; RID, receptor internalization and degradation; TNF, tumour necrosis factor; TNFR, TNF receptor; TRADD, TNFR-associated death domain; vBcL, viral BcLs; vFLIP, viral FLICE inhibitory proteins)

4.2 Interference with regulators of programmed cell death

4.2.1 Caspase inhibitors

Many apoptotic stimuli converge at the level of caspase activation, the final common pathway of apoptosis. Caspases are aspartate-specific cysteine proteases that coordinate apoptosis by proteolytically activating other caspases and other cellular targets, leading to cell suicide. They therefore represent important targets for viral subversion.

A well-characterized caspase inhibitor is the cytokine response modifier A (CrmA) of cowpox virus.[25] It is a potent inhibitor of caspase-1 and caspase-8. These caspases are involved in the maturation of IL-1β, and CrmA. By blocking caspase-8 and the production of IL-1β, CrmA reduces the IL-1β inflammatory response. Inhibition of caspase-8 prevents the apoptotic signal induced by a wide range of stimuli, including TNF, FasL and granzyme B.

4.2.2 Bcl-2 homologues

The Bcl-2 family are an important family of anti-apoptotic proteins, and like the caspases are critical regulators of apoptosis.[26] Many viruses encode either Bcl homologues (e.g. EBV, HHV-8, HVS; see Table 11.3) or alter Bcl cellular levels. For example, EBV encodes two Bcl homologues, and the gene product LMP-1 increases cellular levels of Bcl-2[27] and other proteins that promote cell survival. Lymphocytes are particularly sensitive to regulation by Bcl, and the lymphotropic herpesviruses encode several Bcl modulatory products. In keeping with the observation that Bcl and Fas coordinate distinct apoptotic pathways, many of these viruses (HHV-8, HVS, bovine herpesvirus) also encode vFLIP.

Table 11.3 Viral inhibitors of apoptosis

Cellular target	Virus	Gene/protein	Mechanism
Fas/TNF	Adenovirus	RID complex	Targets Fas for lysosomal degradation
	Cowpox	CrmB	Neutralizes TNF and lymphotoxin-α
		CrmC	Neutralizes TNF but not lymphotoxin-α
	HCMV	UL144	TNF homologue, function unclear
	Myxoma	MT-2	TNFR homologue. Secreted form blocks TNFα. Intracellular form prevents T-cell apoptosis.
vFLIP	HHV-8	k13	vFLIP contain two DED and prevent activation of caspases by death receptors
	HVS	ORF-71	
Caspases	Adenovirus	14.7k	Inhibits caspases, interacts with caspase-8
	Baculovirus	p35, IAP	Inhibits multiple caspases
	ASFV	A224L	IAP homologue
	Cowpox	CrmA/SPI-2	Serpin, inhibits caspases-1/-8, granzyme B
	Vaccinia	SPI-2/B13R2	Serpin, homologous to CrmA
Bcl-2	Adenovirus	E1B 19k	Bcl-2 homologue
	HHV-8	ORF-16	
	HVS	ORF-16	
	EBV	LMP-1	Upregulates Bcl-2, many other functions
Others	HCMV	IE-1/IE-2	Inhibits TNF-induced apoptosis

ASFV, African swine fever virus; DED, death effector domains; EBV, Epstein-Barr virus; HCMV, human cytomegalovirus; HHV, human herpesvirus; HVS, herpes virus saimiri; IAP, inhibitor of apoptosis; IE, intermediate–early; LMP, latent membrane protein; ORF, open reading frame; RID, receptor internalization and degradation; TNF, tumour necrosis factor; TNFR, TNF receptor; vFLIP, viral FLICE inhibitory proteins.

5. INTERFERENCE WITH CYTOKINES AND CHEMOKINES

5.1 Interference with cytokines and cytokine receptors

Cytokines are secreted polypeptides that play a key role in the initiation and regulation of both the innate and adaptive immune response, while chemokines regulate leucocyte trafficking to sites of infection. Cytokines are produced very early in viral infection and are largely responsible for the symptoms of acute viral illness such as fever (e.g. IL-1β) and myalgia. They are essential in the clearance of virus and their modulation contributes to the pathogenicity of viruses (see Tables 11.4 and 11.5).

Table 11.4 Viral interference with cytokine signalling

Cellular target or homologue	Virus	Gene/protein	Mechanism
TNFR	Cowpox	CrmB	Secreted, binds TNF-α and lymphotoxin-α
		CrmC	Secreted, binds TNF-α
	Myxoma	MT-2	Secreted, binds rabbit TNF
IL-1β	Vaccinia	B15R	Secreted, binds IL-1β, blocks febrile response
		B13R	Inhibits ICE
	Cowpox	CrmA/SPI-2	Inhibits several caspases including ICE
IL-12	Measles	Haemagglutinin	Binds CD46, blocking IL-12 production
Chemokine receptors	Cowpox, variola, vaccinia	p35	Binds CC chemokines
	HCMV	US28	CC chemokine receptor, sequesters and internalizes chemokines
	HHV-6, -7	U12	CC chemokine receptor
	HHV-8	ORF-74	Constitutively activated receptor, binds CC and CXC chemokines. Induces cell proliferation
Viral cytokines	EBV	BCRF-1	IL-10 homologue, antagonizes Th1 response
	HHV-6	U83	CC, CXC agonist. ?Aids viral dissemination
		vIL-6	Angiogenic factor, B-cell growth factor
	HHV-8	vMIP-1	CCR8 agonist. Th2 attractant
		vMIP-II	Chemokine receptor antagonist, Th2 attractant

BCRF, B-cell receptor factor; EBV, Epstein-Barr virus; HCMV, human cytomegalovirus, HHV, human herpesviruses; ICE, IL-1β converting enzyme; IL, interleukin; LT, lymphotoxin; MIP, macrophage inflammatory protein; ORF, open reading frame; Th1/2, type 1/2 helper T-cells; TNF, tumour necrosis factor; TNFR, TNF receptor; v, viral.

Viruses are adept at altering host interactions with cytokines.[28] The large DNA viruses, in particular the herpesviruses and poxviruses, encode a large number of molecules which mimic cytokines (virokines) and cytokine receptors (viroceptors). These viral agents compete with host chemokines and cytokines for binding in their efforts to subvert the immune response.

Cowpox encodes two TNFR homologues, CrmB and CrmC, which bind TNF-α,[29] as does myxoma virus product MT-2, inhibiting the effector functions of TNF, including apoptosis (see Fig. 11.4).

Some poxviruses possess soluble IFN homologues that are species specific whereas others are active across several species, reflecting

Table 11.5 Interference with interferons

Cellular target or homologue	Virus	Gene/protein	Mechanism
IFN-α/β	Adenovirus	E1A	Blocks IFN-induced pathways
	EBV	EBNA-2	Downregulates IFN-induced transcription
	HHV-8	γIRF	Represses IFN-induced transcription
	HSV	$\gamma_1 34.5$	Reverses IFN-induced block on translation
	Hepatitis B	Capsid protein	Blocks IFN signalling
	Vaccinia	B18R	Secreted, IFN-α homologue, inhibits IFN-α
PKR/ RNAseL	EBV	EBER1	Blocks PK activity
	Hepatitis C	E2	Inhibits PKR activation
	HIV	TAR RNA	Recruits cellular PKR inhibitor, TRBP
	HSV	2′-5′(A)	RNA analogue, inhibits RNAseL
	Vaccinia	K3L	eIF2α homologue, blocks PKR
		E3L	Sequesters dsRNA, prevents PKR activation
IFN-γ	Myxoma	MT-7	Secreted, IFN-γR homologue, sequesters IFN-γ and disrupts chemokine gradients
	Vaccinia	B8R	Secreted, IFN-γR homologue, sequesters IFN-γ

EBER1, Epstein-Barr virus small RNA; EBNA, Epstein-Barr virus nuclear antigen; EBV, Epstein-Barr virus; eIF2, a translation initiation factor; HHV, human herpesvirus; HIV, human immunodeficiency virus; HSV, herpes simplex virus; IFN, interferon; PK, protein kinase; PKR, dsRNA-dependent PK; TAR, transactivation response element; TRBP, trans-activation response RNA-binding protein; VIRF, viral interferon regulatory factor.

the pathogenicity pattern of the particular virus. Vaccinia virus infects many species and possesses an IFN-γ homologue active in rats, humans, cows and rabbits. In contrast, myxoma has a similar protein, MT-7, that is active only against rabbit IFN-γ.[30]

Chemokines set up solid phase gradients by which leucocytes can be guided to the site of inflammation. Recruitment is also facilitated by upregulation of leucocyte adhesion molecules. MT-7 adheres to the heparin-binding regions of several chemokine families, thus preventing them from binding to heparin and disrupting the solid-phase chemokine gradient.

Vaccinia encodes for p35,[31] the product of which, although showing no sequence homology to chemokine receptors, binds more avidly to CC chemokines than host receptors, suggesting competitive inhibition.

The γ-herpesviruses HHV-8 and HVS encode a transmembrane chemokine receptor,[32] open reading frame-74 (ORF-74), which has sequence homology to CXCR2, and IL-8 receptor. HHV-8 is the causal agent in Kaposi's sarcoma and ORF-74 is thought to be important in the pathogenesis of vascularized tumours.[33] ORF-74 expression in transgenic mice results in Kaposi's-sarcoma-like lesions. ORF-74 is constitutively active and causes inflammatory-like signal transduction cascades and binds IL-8. Its signalling is blocked by IFN-γ, viral macrophage inflammatory protein (vMIP)-II (see below) and stromal cell-derived factor-1α.

The herpesviruses HHV-6 and HHV-7 infect CD4+ T-cells. They downregulate CXCR4 at the cell surface,[34] causing a decreased response to CXCR4's ligand, stromal cell-derived factor-1. HHV-8 encodes vMIP-II, an inhibitor of CC and CXC receptor antagonists. In the host, CC and CXC chemokines do not share receptors, while virokines have evolved to disable multiple receptor types.

Some virokines have agonistic properties to serve viral replication and spread. The HHV-6 peptide U83 binds to CC or CX3C receptors and may recruit monocytes to aid viral dissemination.

CD4+ lymphocyte subsets express different chemokine receptors important in differentiating a Th1 from a Th2 response. Several viruses shift the balance from Th1 to Th2, presumably allowing a survival advantage. MIP-1 and MIP-II are CCR8 agonists, preferentially expressed by Th2. They also antagonize CCR5 and CXCR3 found on Th1. HHV-8 vMIP-1 and vMIP-II thus recruit Th2 in areas of infection. MCV encodes for viral homologues of IL-18 binding protein. This peptide mops up IL-18.[35] IL-18 is involved in NK cell activation and induction of a Th1 response.

5.2 Interference with intracellular cytokine signalling

Due to their largely intracellular life cycle, viruses can influence cytokine effector function along various steps in their pathways. With regard to type 1 IFN, different viruses target subsequent steps of its signalling pathway.[36] For example, HCMV infection lowers levels of proximal receptor-mediated transducers, as does the adenovirus product E1A. HHV-8 encodes for two proteins that are homologous to and compete with immune regulatory factors that regulate IFN-induced transcription.

Type 1 IFN induces several antiviral agents. dsRNA-dependent protein kinase (PKR) is induced by IFN and arrests protein synthesis by phosphorylating a translation initiation factor,

eIF2. HSV activates a protein phosphatase to dephosphorylate eIF2;[37] whereas hepatitis C virus[38] and vaccinia K3L virus inhibit PKR by production of a competing peptide. Both adenovirus and EBV code for RNA that inhibits PKR activation.

6. INHIBITION OF HUMORAL RESPONSES

For viral dissemination, viruses need to enter and leave the host cell, exposing them to further host defences. While cell-mediated immunity is required to clear virus, antibody and complement are important in preventing infection, especially following initial exposure when protective antibody has been produced.

Antibody can block viral receptors required for cell entry and bind viral coat structures. Antibody-coated virions are phagocytosed by cells expressing IgG Fc receptors (FcR). NK cells also recognize infected cells via FcR and cause antibody-dependent cell lysis.

Virions bound by IgM and IgG can activate the classical complement pathway, and virus particles can directly activate the alternate pathway, causing lysis of enveloped virus. Cells expressing complement receptors (CR) can clear C3- and C4-bound virus. Complement can opsonize virions for phagocytosis by professional antigen-presenting cells, which in turn can present processed antigen to effector cells. Complement degradation products such as C3b attract an inflammatory response, and dendritic cells with Fc CR1 and CR2 can internalize opsonized viral particles for presentation to germinal centre B-cells, allowing specific antibody production.

The low fidelity of RNA polymerase may result in multiple random mutations in RNA viruses. This genetic variation results in epitope escape, allowing evasion of antibody responses, as characterized in both HIV and influenza A.

Many herpesviruses encode FcR (see Table 11.6). Antibody to the virus or infected cell is bound by the Fc region, preventing Fc-dependent immune activation. This strategy may be prevalent in herpesvirus due to their persistence. The herpesvirus life cycle involves latency after primary infection, with periodic reactivation in a host no longer naïve to the pathogen.

Table 11.6 Viral inhibition of humoral and complement responses

Function	Virus	Gene/protein	Mechanism
Inactivation of C3 and C3 convertase	HVS	ORF-4	C4bp, CD46
	Cowpox	IMP	C4bp
	HSV-1/-2	gC-1/2	CR1
Inhibition of membrane-attack complex	HVS	HVS CD59 (ORF15)	CD59 homologue
	Vaccinia, HIV, HCMV	Host CD55, CD59, CD46	Host proteins incorporated into viral envelope
Viral FcγR	HSV-1	gE–gl	Binding of IgG and inhibition of Fc-dependent immune activation
	HSV-2	gE	

FcR, Fc Receptor; HCMV, human cytomegalovirus; HIV, human immunodeficiency virus; HSV, herpes simplex virus; HVS, herpes virus saimiri; Ig, Immunoglobulin; IMP, inflammation modulatory protein; ORF, open reading frame.

7. COMPLEMENT EVASION

Complement is an important component of the innate immune system and activation initiates a rapid amplification cascade (reviewed in Morgan 2000). There are multiple host regulators of complement activation (RCA) which prevent tissue damage. RCA degrade C3 and C5 convertases, allow cleavage of C3b and C4b by factor I and, in the case of CD55 and CD59, protect host cells from membrane attack complexes. Viral RCA homologues manipulate the host's own regulatory machinery to regulate complement attack.

Poxviruses encode homologues of RCAs;[39] the cowpox inflammation modulatory protein (IMP) dampens the inflammatory response to infection by inhibiting C3a and C5a. HVS encodes a CD59 homologue, which anchors in the infected cell membrane, protecting against complement-induced cell lysis.[40] Enveloped viruses (e.g. poxviruses, HIV and HCMV) leave the infected cell cloaked in the host membrane.

This provides camouflage from host humoral defences and allows hijacking of host membrane proteins, including CD55 and CD59. HIV uses host attack by complement and antibody to its advantage. Follicular dendritic cells trap opsonized HIV through complement and FcR without internalization. HIV then 'hitchhikes' on the dendritic cell to lymph nodes where the neutralized but still infectious virus is transmitted to CD4+ lymphocytes.

8. FUTURE PERSPECTIVES AND IMPLICATIONS

Viruses exhibit diverse mechanisms to evade host immune defences. Many viral gene products are homologous to host proteins and have presumably been hijacked and modified for the virus's advantage. In other instances, novel peptides with no similarity in primary sequence to host proteins have co-evolved to mimic host devices.

The larger viruses can express multiple tiers of defence against the host immune system. For example, HCMV has strategies to avoid attack by complement and antibody before entering the cell. HCMV prevents antigen being presented onto MHC class I and surface expression of class I molecules. It subverts MHC class II presentation and prevents NK cell lysis of infected cells. HCMV inhibits apoptosis, and interferes with host cytokine and chemokine signalling and release. Do these multiple mechanisms represent viral redundancy, or does HCMV require different strategies at different points of infection? The answers to these questions will only come from studying the *in vivo* effects of these genes in animal models.

Many viruses have been implicated in oncogenesis. There are parallels between viral and tumour evasion, and some of the principles of viral evasion could equally be applied. Similar to virally infected host cells, tumours need to escape host immune surveillance. Tumour cells also express foreign antigens which can be presented at the cell surface on MHC class I molecules and, like viruses, evolve mechanisms to avoid detection, such as decreased cell-surface class I expression and suppression of cell suicide.

Already, many antiviral agents such as INF are being used in immunotherapy of cancers. A better understanding of virus immunobiology will have therapeutic implications beyond new antiviral drugs and vaccine design. Autoimmune disease also subverts physiological immune responses, such as inhibition of programmed cell death, and anti-inflammatory agents, such as soluble TNFR, are being used in the treatment of autoimmune diseases such as rheumatoid arthritis.

Viruses are arguably the most successful parasites. Further study of how they have co-evolved with their host will have wide-ranging implications in the study and practice of immunology, infectious disease and oncology.

GLOSSARY

ABC transporter	A superfamily of ATP-binding cassette transporters that incorporate a transmembrane sequence and nucleotide-binding domain. Important members include TAP, CFTR (cystic fibrosis transmembrane regulator) and MDR-1 (multiple-drug-resistant transporter-1).
Adaptive immune system	Immunity mediated by lymphocytes and characterized by antigen specificity and memory.
Apoptosis	Programmed cell death or 'cell suicide'. An active process characterized by endonuclease digestion of DNA.
Caspase	A family of cysteine proteases that coordinate apoptosis by proteolytically activating other caspases and cellular targets.
Coated protein (COP)	A type of coated protein, as opposed to clathrin, involved in endocytosis of coated pits.
Cytolytic lymphocyte (CTL)	CD8+ T-cells which recognize foreign antigens presented on MHC class I molecules via their T-cell receptor, and proceed to effector functions such as cell lysis.
Cytokine	Secreted polypeptides that regulate the immune response. A subset, chemokines, are involved in the chemotaxis of specific cell types in inflammation.
Death receptor	A variety of cellular receptors that when ligated initiate apoptosis.
Endosome	An intracellular compartment, i.e. not within the cytosol.

Innate immune system	Immunity characterized by a limited array of, but functionally wide ranging, invariant receptors. It does not vary with repeated exposure to pathogen.	**Sec61 channel**	Channel in the endoplasmic reticulum membrane responsible for both secretory protein import of newly synthesized proteins and export of misfolded proteins back to the cytosol.
Interferon (IFN)	Cytokines that can induce resistance to viral infection. They include type I interferons (IFN-α and IFN-β) and IFN-γ. The latter is important in initiating a Th1 response.	**Secretory pathway**	Pathway taken by newly synthesized proteins to the cell surface and other cellular destinations such as endosomes.
Major histocompatibility complex (MHC)	A cluster of genes on human chromosome 6 that encode MHC molecules. MHC class I molecules present peptides generated in the cytosol to CD8+ CTL. MHC class II molecules present peptides derived from outside of the cell and degraded in endosomes to CD4+ cells. The MHC also encodes for other proteins involved in antigen processing such as TAP.	**Transporter associated with antigen processing, (TAP)**	A heterodimer ABC transporter located in the endoplasmic reticulum (ER) that translocates the majority of peptides loaded onto MHC class I from the cytosol into the ER.
		Tapasin	A TAP-associated protein which bridges TAP and MHC class I, and enables class I molecules to load peptide.
Natural killer (NK) cell	Large granular lymphocytes (non-T, non-B) that cause lysis of target cells by release of perforins and granzymes. They are important mediators of innate immunity against viruses and tumour cells.	**Type 1 helper T-cell (Th1) response**	Inflammatory response from Th1 CD4+ T-lymphocytes that secrete IFN-γ and tumour necrosis factor alpha (TNF-α).
		Type 2 helper T-cell (Th2) response	CD4+ T-lymphocyte secrete interleukin (IL)-4 and IL-5, and help antibody production by B-cells.
Proteasome	The major cytosolic protease. It is a large multimeric complex that degrades cellular proteins that have been tagged by ubiquitination and is responsible for production of peptide ligands for MHC class I molecules.	**Ubiquitin**	A polypeptide that targets a protein for degradation.
		Virion	A viral particle composed of folded genetic material (DNA or RNA) and a protein coat.

REFERENCES

Further reading

Alcami A, Koszinowski UH. Viral mechanisms of immune evasion. *Immunol Today* 2000; **21**; 447–55.

Collins KL, Baltimore D. HIV's evasion of the cellular immune response. *Immunol Rev* 1999; **168**: 65–74.

Fruh K, Gruhler A, Krishna RM, Schoenhals GJ. A comparison of viral immune escape strategies targeting the MHC class I assembly pathway. *Immunol Rev* 1999; **168**: 157–66.

Lanier LL. Turning on natural killer cells. *J Exp Med* 2000; **191**; 1259–62.

Morgan BP. The complement system: an overview. *Methods Molec Biol* 2000; **150**: 1–13.

Pamer E, Cresswell P. Mechanisms of MHC class I-restricted antigen processing. *Annu Rev Immunol* 1998; **16**: 323–58.

Pieters J. MHC class II-restricted antigen processing and presentation. *Adv Immunol* 2000; **75**: 159–208.

Piguet V, Schwartz O, Le Gall S, Trono D. The downregulation of CD4 and MHC-I by primate lentiviruses: a paradigm for the modulation of cell surface receptors. *Immunol Rev* 1999; **168**: 51–63.

Rathmell JC, Thompson CB. The central effectors of cell death in the immune system. *Annu Rev Immunol* 1999; **17**: 781–828.

Tortorella D, Gewurz BE, Furman MH et al. Viral subversion of the immune system. *Annu Rev Immunol* 2000; **18**: 861–926.

Scientific papers

1. Levitskaya J, Coram M, Levitsky V et al. Inhibition of antigen processing by the internal repeat region of the Epstein-Barr virus nuclear antigen-1. *Nature* 1995; **375**: 685–8.
2. Gilbert MJ, Riddell SR, Plachter B, Greenberg PD. Cytomegalovirus selectively blocks antigen processing and presentation of its immediate-early gene product. *Nature* 1996; **383**: 720–2.
3. Hill A, Jugovic P, York I et al. Herpes simplex virus turns off the TAP to evade host immunity. *Nature* 1995; **375**: 411–15.
4. Hewitt EW, Gupta SS, Lehner PJ. The human cytomegalovirus gene product US6 inhibits ATP binding by TAP. *Eur Molec Biol Org J* 2001; **20**: 387–96.
5. Mahr JA, Gooding LR. Immune evasion by adenoviruses. *Immunol Rev* 1999; **168**: 121–30.
6. Bennett EM, Bennink JR, Yewdell JW, Brodsky FM. Cutting edge: adenovirus E19 has two mechanisms for affecting class I MHC expression. *J Immunol* 1999; **162**: 5049–52.

7. Wiertz EJ, Tortorella D, Bogyo M et al. Sec61-mediated transfer of a membrane protein from the endoplasmic reticulum to the proteasome for destruction. *Nature* 1996; **384**: 432–8.
8. Hengel H, Reusch U, Gutermann A et al. Cytomegaloviral control of MHC class I function in the mouse. *Immunol Rev* 1999; **168**: 167–76.
9. Ishido S, Wang C, Lee BS et al. Downregulation of major histocompatibility complex class I molecules by Kaposi's sarcoma-associated herpesvirus K3 and K5 proteins. *J Virol* 2000; **74**: 5300–9.
10. Stevenson PG, Efstathiou S, Doherty PC, Lehner PJ. Inhibition of MHC class I-restricted antigen presentation by gamma 2-herpesviruses. *Proc Natl Acad Sci USA* 2000; **97**: 8455–60.
11. Biron CA, Byron KS, Sullivan JL. Severe herpesvirus infections in an adolescent without natural killer cells. *N Engl J Med* 1989; **320**: 1731–5.
12. Mandelboim O, Lieberman N, Lev M et al. Recognition of haemagglutinins on virus-infected cells by NKp46 activates lysis by human NK cells. *Nature* 2001; **409**: 1055–60.
13. Cretney E, Degli-Esposti MA, Densley EH et al. m144, a murine cytomegalovirus (MCMV)-encoded major histocompatibility complex class I homologue, confers tumor resistance to natural killer cell-mediated rejection. *J Exp Med* 1999; **190**: 435–44.
14. Beck S, Barrell BG. Human cytomegalovirus encodes a glycoprotein homologous to MHC class-I antigens. *Nature* 1988; **331**: 269–72.
15. Leong CC, Chapman TL, Bjorkman PJ et al. Modulation of natural killer cell cytotoxicity in human cytomegalovirus infection: the role of endogenous class I major histocompatibility complex and a viral class I homolog. *J Exp Med* 1998; **187**: 1681–7.
16. Cosman D, Fanger N, Borges L et al. A novel immunoglobulin superfamily receptor for cellular and viral MHC class I molecules. *Immunity* 1997; **7**: 273–82.
17. Tomasec P, Braud VM, Ricards C et al. Surface expression of HLA-E, an inhibitor of natural killer cells, enhanced by human cytomegalovirus gpUL40. *Science* 2000; **287**: 1031.
18. Tomazin R, Boname J, Hegde NR et al. Cytomegalovirus US2 destroys two components of the MHC class II pathway, preventing recognition by CD4+ T cells. *Nature Med* 1999; **5**: 1039–43.
19. Miller DM, Zhang Y, Rahill BM et al. Human cytomegalovirus inhibits IFN-alpha-stimulated

antiviral and immunoregulatory responses by blocking multiple levels of IFN-alpha signal transduction. *J Immunol* 1999; **162**: 6107–13.

20. Andresson T, Sparkowski J, Goldstein DJ, Schlegel R. Vacuolar H(+)-ATPase mutants transform cells and define a binding site for the papillomavirus E5 oncoprotein. *J Biol Chem* 1995; **270**: 6830–7.

21. Hardwick JM. Viral interference with apoptosis. *Semin Cell Dev Biol* 1998; **9**: 339–49.

22. Schreiber M, Sedger L, McFadden G. Distinct domains of M-T2, the myxoma virus tumor necrosis factor (TNF) receptor homolog, mediate extracellular TNF binding and intracellular apoptosis inhibition. *J Virol* 1997; **71**: 2171–81.

23. Loparev VN, Parsons JM, Knight JC et al. A third distinct tumor necrosis factor receptor of orthopoxviruses. *Proc Natl Acad Sci USA* 1998; **95**: 3786–91.

24. Shisler J, Yang C, Walter B et al. The adenovirus E3-10.4K/14.5K complex mediates loss of cell surface Fas (CD95) and resistance to Fas-induced apoptosis. *J Virol* 1997; **71**: 8299–306.

25. Dbaibo GS, Hannun YA. Cytokine response modifier A (CrmA): a strategically deployed viral weapon. *Clin Immunol Immunopathol* 1998; **86**: 134–40.

26. Chao DT, Korsmeyer SJ. BCL-2 family: regulators of cell death. *Annu Rev Immunol* 1998; **16**: 395–419.

27. Henderson S, Rowe M, Gregory C et al. Induction of bcl-2 expression by Epstein-Barr virus latent membrane protein 1 protects infected B cells from programmed cell death. *Cell* 1991; **65**: 1107–15.

28. Alcami A, Koszinowski UH. Viral mechanisms of immune evasion. *Immunol Today* 2000; **21**: 447–55.

29. Hu FQ, Smith CA, Pickup DJ. Cowpox virus contains two copies of an early gene encoding a soluble secreted form of the type II TNF receptor. *Virology* 1994; **204**: 343–56.

30. Mossman K, Upton C, McFadden G. The myxoma virus-soluble interferon-gamma receptor homolog. M-T7, inhibits interferon-gamma in a species-specific manner. *J Biol Chem* 1995; **270**: 3031–8.

31. Smith CA, Smith TD, Smolak PJ et al. Poxvirus genomes encode a secreted, soluble protein that preferentially inhibits beta chemokine activity yet lacks sequence homology to known chemokine receptors. *Virology* 1997; **236**: 316–27.

32. Kledal TN, Rosenkilde MM, Coulin F et al. A broad-spectrum chemokine antagonist encoded by Kaposi's sarcoma-associated herpesvirus. *Science* 1997; **277**: 1656–9.

33. Bais C, Santomasso B, Coso O et al. G-protein-coupled receptor of Kaposi's sarcoma-associated herpesvirus is a viral oncogene and angiogenesis activator. *Nature* 1998; **391**: 86–9.

34. Yasukawa M, Hasegawa A, Sakai I et al. Down-regulation of CXCR4 by human herpesvirus 6 (HHV-6) and HHV-7. *J Immunol* 1999; **162**: 5417–22.

35. Novick D, Kim SH, Fantuzzi G et al. Interleukin-18 binding protein: a novel modulator of the Th1 cytokine response. *Immunity* 1999; **10**: 127–36.

36. Guidotti LG, Chisari FV. Noncytolytic control of viral infections by the innate and adaptive immune response. *Annu Rev Immunol* 2001; **19**: 65–91.

37. He B, Gross M, Roizman B. The gamma(1)34.5 protein of herpes simplex virus 1 complexes with protein phosphatase 1alpha to dephosphorylate the alpha subunit of the eukaryotic translation initiation factor 2 and preclude the shutoff of protein synthesis by double-stranded RNA-activated protein kinase. *Proc Natl Acad Sci USA* 1997; **94**: 843–8.

38. Taylor DR, Shi ST, Romano PR et al. Inhibition of the interferon-inducible protein kinase PKR by HCV E2 protein. *Science* 1999; **285**: 107–10.

39. Kotwal GJ, Isaacs SN, McKenzie R et al. Inhibition of the complement cascade by the major secretory protein of vaccinia virus. *Science* 1990; **250**: 827–30.

40. Rother RP, Rollins SA, Fodor WL et al. Inhibition of complement-mediated cytolysis by the terminal complement inhibitor of herpesvirus saimiri. *J Virol* 1994; **68**: 730–7.

41. Burton GF, Masuda A, Heath SL et al. Follicular dendritic cells (FDC) in retroviral infection: host/pathogen perspectives. *Immunol Rev* 1997; **156**: 185–97.

12

Pathogenicity islands

Kate E Unsworth, David W Holden

OBJECTIVES

(1) To consider the function of pathogenicity islands (PAI) and their role as virulence determinants.
(2) To review the role and regulation of PAI in bacterial infection.

OVERVIEW

Pathogenicity islands are bacterial DNA segments carrying one or more virulence genes that have been acquired *en bloc* from a foreign source. The genome of a pathogen often represents a 'mosaic' of these recently acquired islands scattered along a backbone of relatively ancient DNA. They can frequently be identified by markedly different G+C content to the chromosomal backbone, and other features suggest that their acquisition is mediated by mobile genetic elements such as bacteriophages. Genes for a wide variety of important virulence traits are associated with PAI, and study of these is providing important insights into the biology of bacterial pathogens. The products of PAI may well represent important targets for antimicrobial therapy, vaccines and diagnostic tools of the future.

1. INTRODUCTION

Over the past few decades, it has become apparent that an important driving force in the evolution of bacterial virulence has been the acquisition of large segments of foreign DNA from unrelated sources (horizontal transfer). The significance of horizontal gene transfer in the emergence of new clinical problems was first appreciated in the 1950s, with the rapid global spread of bacterial multidrug resistance.[1] The first pathogenicity island, a horizontally acquired DNA segment whose resident genes are involved in virulence, was described in the early 1980s.[2] It has since been found that PAI encode a broad spectrum of virulence factors and are central players in bacterial pathogenicity. The acquisition of PAI has been instrumental in the recent emergence of clinically significant pathogens, including epidemic *Vibrio cholerae* 0139 and *Escherichia coli* 0157:H7.[3,4]

2. PATHOGENICITY ISLANDS AND EVOLUTION OF BACTERIAL VIRULENCE

2.1 Evolution of bacterial virulence

In most cases, virulence involves expression of a large number of bacterial gene products. These can be grouped into two classes.[5] First are those genes whose products are required for basic physiological processes such as biosynthetic pathways. Many of these factors are obviously necessary for bacterial growth within a host (e.g. synthesis of a cell wall or essential amino acids), but they are also found in the non-virulent relatives of pathogens and are not specific adaptations for a pathogenic lifestyle. These genes cannot be described solely as virulence factors. The second class of virulence-related genes comprises those which are only found in pathogenic organisms and whose products play a specific role in the pathogenic process (Table 12.1). For example, products of genes unique to a pathogen may have roles in determining host and tissue tropism, multiplication within the host (which necessitates evasion, resistance or subversion of host defence mechanisms), cytotoxicity, and dissemination between

hosts.[6] Many pathogens probably evolved from benign relatives by acquiring large units of such genetic information, conferring the ability to colonize new host niches.[5] In many cases, these blocks of DNA are found on plasmids. However, many virulence genes are found on the bacterial chromosome. These genes tend to be found in functionally-related groups which appear to be different from the surrounding chromosome, probably because they have been acquired together from a distant source by horizontal transfer.

Full genome sequence data are becoming available for an increasing number of pathogenic and non-pathogenic bacteria (see Websites). Inspection of these genomes has led to the idea that some microbial chromosomes can be thought of as a backbone into which many horizontally transmitted segments are inserted. For example, although *Salmonella typhimurium* and *Salmonella typhi* are considered members of the same species, 20% of the genome of *S typhimurium* is not present in *S typhi* and vice versa.[7] These so-called islands represent genetic cassettes encoding diverse functions, ranging from biosynthetic pathways

Table 12.1 Classes of virulence-related genes			
Virulence function	**Example**	**Organism**	**Function**
Host tropism	*spv* operon	*Salmonella typhimurium*	Required for murine typhoid, not human typhoid
Tissue tropism	P-related fimbriae	UPEC	Specific adherence to uroepithelial cells
Evasion of host defences	IgA protease	*Neisseria gonorrhoeae*	Cleaves IgA molecules
Specific nutrient acquisition	Yersiniabactin	Many Gram-negative pathogens	Secreted high-affinity iron-binding complex
Cytotoxicity	IpaB	*Shigella* spp.	Macrophage apoptosis
Dissemination	SopB	*Salmonella* spp.	Fluid secretion by intestinal epithelial cells

UPEC, Uropathogenic *Escherichia coli*.

to toxins.[8] An important subset of these genomic islands are those termed PAI, which contain genes whose products are involved in bacterial virulence.

2.2 Characteristics of PAI

The first described PAI was found in uropathogenic *E coli*. (UPEC).[2] As further PAI have been identified in a wide range of bacterial species, a working definition of a PAI has evolved (Box 12.1).[9,10] Most importantly, a PAI is a region of the genome of a pathogenic organism carrying virulence determinants which is absent, or sporadically distributed, in non-pathogenic close relatives. A PAI may harbour only one virulence gene (referred to as a pathogenicity islet), such as the *sifA* islet, that encodes a secreted protein involved in intracellular multiplication of *S typhimurium*,[11] or contain several virulence-associated operons. For instance, *Salmonella* pathogenicity island 1 (SPI-1) of *S typhimurium* encodes both a secretion system involved in host cell invasion and an iron-uptake system required for systemic infection of mice.[12–14] Some PAI are very large, e.g. PAI II of UPEC is around 190 kilobases (kb) in size. Some distinguishing features of PAI are vestiges of their horizontal acquisition and distant origins. The overall nucleotide composition of the island often differs considerably from the average for the recipient, reflecting the different codon usage of the source genome. Genetic signatures of the transfer event may be present, such as direct repeats (which may arise from integration of mobile genetic elements such as transposons or bacteriophages), integrase or transposase genes, or plasmid origins of replication. Some PAI are unstable and have a relatively high rate of spontaneous loss from the chromosome. For example, the PAI encoding toxic shock syndrome toxin 1 (TSST-1) of *Staphylococcus aureus* is excised from the chromosome at high frequencies by staphylococcal bacteriophages.[15] However, as a genome evolves, these distinguishing characteristics of a PAI become obscured through mutation and the boundaries may become more difficult to delineate. This often seems to be the case with PAI of Gram-positive pathogens. For example, the *vir* regulon encoding M-protein, which protects *Streptococcus pyogenes* from phagocytosis, is absent from other streptococcal species but does not contain any other obvious hallmarks of horizontal acquisition.

3. VIRULENCE DETERMINANTS ENCODED BY PATHOGENICITY ISLANDS

Bacterial pathogens have acquired PAI encoding a wide range of virulence determinants. These include mechanisms for resisting the defences of the host, colonization, and nutrient acquisition factors and toxins that specifically modify host cell function. Some of these activities are mediated by specialized bacterial secretion systems.

3.1 Secretion systems

The site of action of most virulence factors is outside the bacterium, either the bacterial cell surface or a more remote location. Therefore, an important property of pathogenic bacteria is their ability to deliver virulence determinants to the correct locality. This may simply involve secretion across the bacterial cell membranes or may require a further step, such as translocation across a eukaryotic membrane. PAI of several Gram-negative pathogens, including *Salmonella*, *E coli*, *Bordetella* and *Pseudomonas*, encode specialized export structures called type III secretion systems (TTSS).[16] Almost all described TTSS are encoded by horizontally transmitted

---

Box 12.1 Common features of pathogenicity islands (adapted from Hacker et al[9])

They contain one or many virulence genes

They are absent in non-pathogenic relatives

Their G+C content differs from genome average

They are flanked by direct repeats/tRNA genes/insertion sequence elements

They contain 'mobility' genes (integrases, transposases, origins of replication)

They are unstable (can be lost by the recipient strain)

elements (Table 12.2) and are highly conserved amongst different bacterial species. These TTSS consist of several proteins which form a molecular syringe, injecting the effector proteins directly across bacterial and eukaryotic cell membranes into the target cell cytoplasm.[16] Sequence analysis supports the hypothesis that TTSS have been independently acquired by a number of Gram-negative pathogens from an unknown source(s).[17] Although the TTSS themselves are highly conserved, the secreted effector proteins are often encoded on separate PAI elsewhere in the genome and are more divergent in sequence and function.[16] Furthermore, the eukaryotic membrane targeted may differ; most TTSS deliver proteins across the plasma membrane, but *Salmonella* and *Chlamydia* reside in membrane-bound vacuoles within host cells and probably translocate proteins across the vacuolar membrane as well (Fig. 12.1). TTSS are an illustration of the flexibility afforded by horizontal transfer, as they appear to have been adopted by many pathogens as a generalized method of targeting toxins into the eukaryotic cell with diverse consequences (Fig. 12.1). Secretion of virulence factors by another specialized virulence-associated secretion system (type IV; TFSS) has recently been demonstrated for several pathogenic species, including the CagA antigen by *Helicobacter pylori* (Table 12.2).[18,19]

Table 12.2 Type III and IV secretion systems of mammalian pathogens

Organism	Description	Function of secreted proteins	Genomic location
Type III secretion systems			
EPEC/EHEC	LEE	Pedestal formation	PAI
Yersinia spp	Yop virulon	Antiphagocytosis	Plasmid
Yersinia spp	*ysa* region	Virulence in mice	Chromosomal
Shigella spp	Entry region	Invasion of epithelial cells, intracellular spread, macrophage apoptosis	Plasmid
Salmonella typhimurium	SPI-1	Invasion of epithelial cells, macrophage apoptosis	PAI
S typhimurium	SPI-2	Survival/multiplication in macrophages	PAI
Chlamydia psittaci		Not determined	Not determined
Pseudomonas aeruginosa		Epithelial cell damage	PAI
Bordetella pertussis	Bpel	Not determined	Not determined
Type IV secretion systems			
Helicobacter pylori	Cag PAI	Induces interleukin-8 secretion by enterocytes	PAI
Brucella spp		Survival/multiplication in macrophages	Not determined
Legionella pneumophilia	*icm/dot* region	Survival/multiplication in macrophages	Chromosomal
B pertussis	Ptl	ADP-ribosylating toxin	Not determined

PAI, Pathogenicity islands.

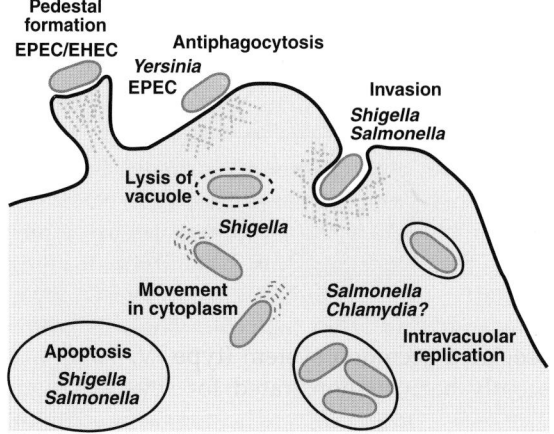

Fig. 12.1 The diverse functions of type III secretion systems (TTSS). TTSS translocate toxins across different host cell membranes. The effects of these translocated toxins are diverse but some common themes are discernible. A target of many TTSS is the host cell actin cytoskeleton (dotted lines), although the effect of cytoskeletal manipulation varies from system to system. The TTSS of *Shigella* and *Salmonella* SPI-1 are very similar, and both are involved in inducing macrophage apoptosis as well as mediating host cell invasion. The TTSS of *Chlamydia* could play a role similar to that of *Salmonella* SPI-2, in generating an intracellular environment suitable for bacterial replication. The TTSS of both *Yersinia* and enteropathogenic *Escherichia coli* (EPEC) paralyse the phagocytic machinery of the host cell. (EHEC, enterohaemorrhagic *E coli*.)

3.2 Avoidance of the immune system

The role of many virulence factors is to prevent destruction of the bacterium by the host immune system. Variation of surface antigens is a common theme in immune avoidance, and rapid acquisition and/or loss of genetic material by horizontal transfer may contribute to this process. For example, a major antigen present on Gram-negative bacterial surfaces is the O lipopolysaccharide antigen. There are many variants of the O antigen, which form the basis for one method of identifying Gram-negative bacterial isolates. It is highly likely that the recent pandemic *V cholerae* strain O139 emerged after the previously prevalent strain O1 El Tor acquired a new PAI. This PAI replaced part of

the O antigen cluster of O1 El Tor,[3] and seems to encode a different set of O antigen and capsule biosynthetic proteins.[20] The lack of effective cross-immunity against O139 strains led to the resurgence of clinical cholera in populations resistant to infection with O1 *V cholerae*.[21]

Further PAI-encoded mechanisms to avoid host immune killing include serum resistance (e.g. the *Shigella flexneri* Pic complement resistance protein, encoded on *Shigella* island 1[22]) and induction of macrophage apoptosis (e.g. SipB, encoded by *Salmonella* SPI-1 and translocated by the SPI-1 TTSS[23,24]).

3.3 Adherence and colonization factors

The ability to adhere to an epithelial surface is essential for the majority of pathogenic or commensal bacteria which interact with a mammalian host. Many pathogens remain at an epithelial surface during infection and replicate in the extracellular milieu. Adherence is usually mediated by molecules which are secreted onto the bacterial cell surface and which bind specific ligands on the host cell surface or extracellular matrix. A great number of adherence factors have been identified, and these are divided into two major groups: fimbriae (pili) and afimbrial adhesins. Fimbrial adhesins are complex rod-shaped structures that project from the bacterial surface and mediate contact between bacteria and host cells. In UPEC, *prf* (P-related fimbriae) pilus genes are located on a PAI that also encodes other uropathogenicity factors, including an α-haemolysin.[25,26]

Deletion of this PAI occurs naturally at a relatively high frequency and results in loss of virulence.[26] An unusual adhesion system is encoded by the locus of enterocyte effacement (LEE), a 35 kb PAI present in enteropathogenic *E coli* (EPEC) and enterohaemorrhagic *E coli* (EHEC), which encodes a TTSS.[27] This injects the Tir (translocated intimin receptor) protein into the membrane of host intestinal epithelial cells, where it acts as a receptor for another LEE-encoded protein, intimin,[28] resulting in tight adherence to epithelial cells. Pathogens often possess a complex array of adhesins, and the range of adhesins expressed by a pathogen may play a significant role in determination of host and tissue tropism and, therefore, pathogenic potential. For example, *E coli* strains possessing PAI encoding S fimbriae, which bind sialic acid receptors found on brain microvascular endothelial cells, can cause sepsis or meningitis.[29,30]

3.4 Modulators of host cell function

Many virulence factors encoded by PAI alter the activities of host cells by interfering with eukaryotic signalling pathways. This can have a variety of effects, including bacterial uptake by normally non-phagocytic cells, inhibition of phagocytosis, diversion of intracellular trafficking pathways and induction of host cell apoptosis.

3.4.1 Invasion

Most pathogens able to induce their uptake by host cells use one of relatively few mechanisms. For example, *Salmonella* and *Shigella* trigger their uptake by injecting proteins into the host cell cytoplasm via TTSS encoded on PAI. These activate host cell signalling cascades, leading to dramatic cytoskeletal rearrangements.[31] Proteins translocated by the TTSS involved in *Salmonella* invasion are encoded both within the PAI encoding the secretion system and on PAI elsewhere in the genome.[32–34] Although their origins appear to be diverse, the secreted proteins act in concert to direct efficient internalization of bacteria (Fig. 12.2).[31,35]

3.4.2 Intracellular survival and multiplication

Survival and replication within host cells is an important stage in the pathogenesis of several bacterial species.[36] Following uptake, bacteria are enclosed within a membrane-bound compartment (phagosome). Normally, this fuses with other compartments that deliver toxins. These include a vacuolar proton pump, which causes the phagosomal pH to fall dramatically, a cocktail of degradative enzymes from lysosomes, and other toxic molecules including highly destructive reactive oxygen and nitrogen intermediates (Fig. 12.3).[36,37] Intracellular pathogens utilize an array of mechanisms to escape from, withstand or prevent the effects of these processes (Fig. 12.3).[36,37] Some *Listeria* spp possess a PAI-like gene cluster encoding a pore-forming toxin (listeriolysin O). This lyses the phagosomal membrane, leaving the bacteria free in the cytoplasm where they are inaccessible to the cell's defences and able to obtain nutrients.[38] Other pathogens, such as *S typhimurium*, *Mycobacterium tuberculosis*, *Chlamydia* spp and *Legionella pneumophilia*, remain within the phagosome. They convert this into a compartment in which they can multiply, by preventing or resisting acidification or delivery of toxic lysosomal contents, and recruiting additional membrane and nutrients. The only bacterial factors whose role in this process have been identified are SpiC and SifA, both of which are translocated by the TTSS encoded on the second pathogenicity

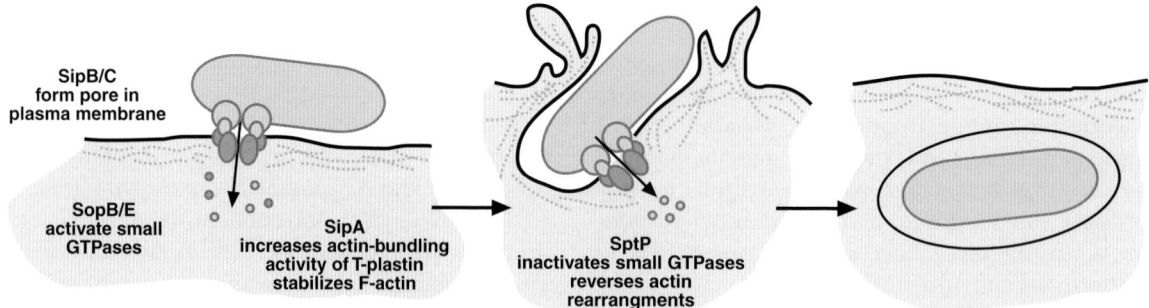

Fig. 12.2 *Salmonella typhimurium* invasion mediated by the SPI-1 type III secretion system (TTSS). The SPI-1 TTSS secretes proteins that work in concert to bring about bacterial uptake. SipB and -C form a pore in the host cell plasma membrane, through which other effectors are translocated. SipA, SopB and SopE induce actin rearrangements which generate extensive membrane ruffling, leading to bacterial internalization. SptP mediates the reversal of these actin rearrangements after bacterial uptake has occurred.

island of *S typhimurium* (SPI-2). SpiC is an inhibitor of macrophage phago-lysosomal fusion;[39] and SifA is required for maintenance of the membrane-bound compartment in which *Salmonella* resides[11] and, although it is secreted by the SPI-2 TTSS, is encoded on a separate pathogenicity islet.

3.5 Nutrient acquisition factors

The ability to compete for nutrients, against host defences and other resident microorganisms, is an essential facet of pathogenesis. One particularly well-studied aspect of this is iron acquisition. Many bacteria secrete low molecular mass iron-binding compounds called siderophores and use cognate siderophore uptake systems to transfer siderophore-bound iron into the bacterial cell. One example of a siderophore is yersiniabactin, which is encoded by the so-called high PAI of *Yersinia* spp and is required for virulence in a mouse model of plague.[40] Further examples of iron transporters encoded by PAI include the siderophore aerobactin, encoded by SHI-2 of *S flexneri*,[41,42] the Sit1 iron transporter encoded by SPI-1 of *S typhimurium*[12,14] and the *pit2* operon of the recently described *Streptococcus pneumoniae* PPI-1 which encodes an ABC transporter required for iron uptake and full virulence of *S pneumoniae*.[43]

4. ROLE OF PAI IN THE EVOLUTION OF BACTERIAL PATHOGENS

4.1 *E coli*

E coli is an excellent illustration of the impact that horizontal transfer of pathogenicity cassettes (both plasmid-encoded and PAI) has had in the evolution of virulence. Most *E coli* strains are non-pathogenic and many are free-living; some reside as commensals in the intestinal tract. However, a number of *E coli* strains are pathogens and can cause a wide range of diseases, ranging from diarrhoea, urinary tract infections (UTI) and haemolytic uraemic syndrome to septic shock, meningitis and pneumonia.[44] In the majority of cases, a particular strain of pathogenic *E coli* is specifically associated with only one disease. This is a

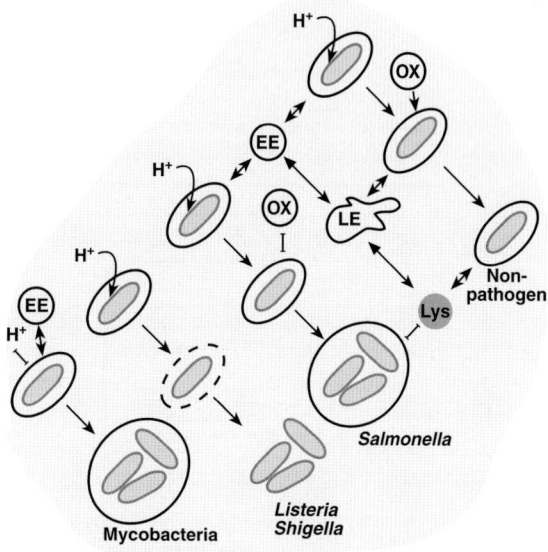

Fig. 12.3 Intracellular pathogens avoid host cell defences by altering the trafficking of their phagosomes, *Listeria* and *Shigella* lyse the phagosomal membrane and replicate in the host cell cytosol. Mycobacteria prevent vacuolar acidification (H⁺) and replicate within an early endosome (EE)-like compartment. *Salmonella* withstand the effects of vacuolar acidification, but prevent interactions with late endosomes (LE) and lysosomes (Lys), and with the effectors of the oxidative burst (OX).

reflection of the pathway by which pathogenic *E coli* are thought to have evolved; different strains arose in parallel from commensal ancestors through the acquisition of distinct sets of horizontally-acquired virulence determinants (Fig 12.4). A recent comparison of the genome sequences of non-pathogenic *E coli* K-12 and EHEC O157:H7 revealed an astonishing 1387 new genes in the pathogenic strain, including nine horizontally-acquired islands > 15 kb encoding putative virulence factors.[45]

A good example of the effect of PAI on the virulence phenotype of *E coli* is the role of PAI I and PAI II of strains that cause UTI. Both PAI encode haemolysins, while PAI II also contains genes for Prf-type fimbriae which are necessary for adherence to uroepithelial cells.[25,46,47] If these

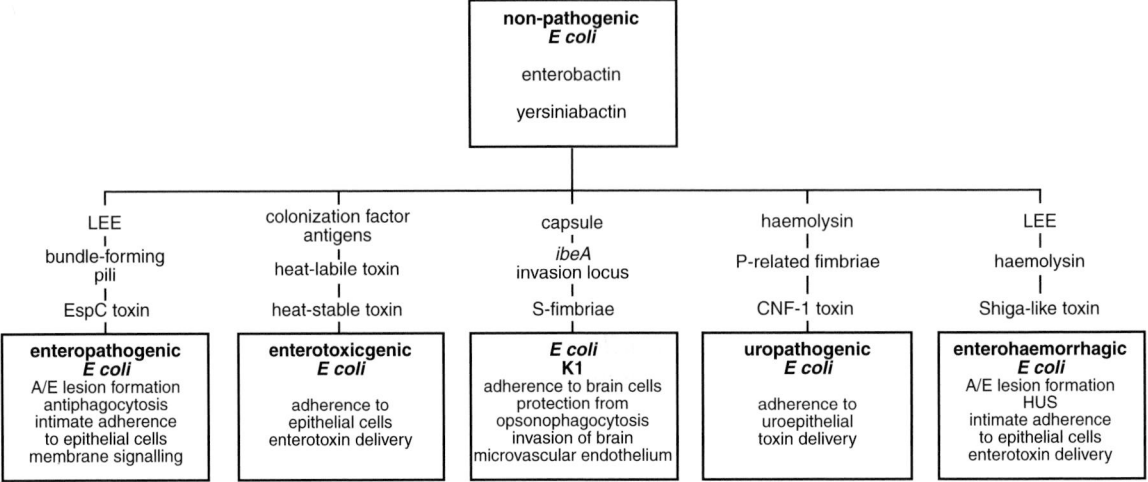

Fig. 12.4 Evolution of *Escherichia coli*. Many *E coli* live as commensals in the gastrointestinal tract and have acquired genomic islands encoding iron-uptake systems. Most pathogenic *E coli* strains appear to have evolved by means of independent acquisitions of pathogenicity islands (PAI) encoding virulence determinants appropriate for particular niches. This has resulted in a broad range of virulence mechanisms and pathogenic lifestyles. (A/E, attaching/effacing lesions; HUS, haemolytic uraemic syndrome; LEE, locus of enterocyte effacement.)

PAI are lost from the chromosome, the resulting strains are unable to cause UTI.[26] Therefore, these PAI are seen to be essential determinants of uropathogenicity.

The pathogenicity of *E coli* strains causing intestinal infections has also been affected by the acquisition of PAI. A phenotype shared by EPEC and EHEC is the ability to adhere tightly to epithelial cells and to induce the formation of attaching and effacing (AE) lesions. These are characterized by loss of microvilli and formation of an actin-rich 'pedestal' upon which the bacteria sit.[48,49] The AE phenotype is dependent on the LEE PAI,[50] which encodes a TTSS and several secreted proteins. As well as mediating the tight intimin–Tir adhesion discussed previously, TTSS-mediated translocation results in the induction of host cell signalling pathways by tyrosine phosphorylation. This stimulates rearrangement of actin filaments and other cytoskeletal elements at the site of bacterial adherence, leading to pedestal formation.[51] Although the LEE is present in more than one pathogenic *E coli* strain, recent phylogenetic analysis showed that at least two different

lineages of *E coli* acquired the LEE on at least two separate occasions.[52] Although AE lesions are central to the virulence of both EPEC and EHEC, the two pathovars cause different diseases due to the presence of other horizontally transmitted elements. EHEC has acquired a bacteriophage encoding a Shiga-like toxin, thought to cause haemolytic uraemic syndrome, and a plasmid-encoded haemolysin, whereas EPEC strains contain a different plasmid, encoding bundle-forming pili required for production of diarrhoea in human volunteer studies.[53]

The insertion site of PAI I (encoding haemolysins) in UPEC chromosomal DNA is identical to that of the LEE in EPEC, so the identity of the PAI inserted at this site helps to determine whether *E coli* strains are entero- or uropathogens.[5] The LEE is also an example of the ability of horizontal transfer to generate new pathovars in a single step. Introduction of this PAI into a benign strain of *E coli* conferred the ability to form AE lesions and, thus, would presumably increase its pathogenicity.[49] It therefore seems that any strain of *E coli* has the potential to become a pathogen, simply by the acquisition of new virulence determinants by horizontal transfer. This has happened independently several times, resulting in a variety of strains with different pathogenic potential (Fig. 12.4).

4.2 *Salmonella enterica*

The species *S enterica* includes a number of strains of clinical importance. *Salmonella enteritidis* and *S typhimurium* are important causes of gastroenteritis, while *S typhi* and *Salmonella paratyphi* are the aetiological agents of typhoid fever. Whereas many *E coli* isolates are non-virulent, essentially all salmonellae are pathogenic. The evolution of virulence in these pathogens, in contrast to that of *E coli*, appears to have followed a relatively linear progression. A large number of horizontally transmitted virulence factors have been identified in *Salmonella* spp, including a virulence plasmid, at least five major PAI and a large number of smaller pathogenicity 'islets', each carrying a handful of virulence genes (Table 12.3).[54] The sequential acquisition of several PAI seems to have played a major role in the transition from gastrointestinal commensal to intracellular pathogen (Fig. 12.5).[54]

Adherence to and invasion of epithelial cells is the basic virulence mechanism of the genus *Salmonella*, which allows the bacteria to escape from the competitive environment of the intestinal lumen and involves many genetic loci.[54] These include two operons, *lpf* and *fim*, encoding fimbrial adhesins, and the TTSS encoded on the SPI-1 PAI. Proteins injected by this secretion system into epithelial cells have at least two roles. Firstly, rearrangements of the actin cytoskeleton are triggered, directing the uptake of the bacteria into normally non-phagocytic cells.[31] Secondly, several SPI-1-secreted proteins trigger host cell pathways leading to apoptosis in macrophages.[23,55,56] It appears that originally unrelated virulence factors have been incorporated into the repertoire of SPI-1 TTSS translocated proteins and that these induce distinct effects on the host cell. Both invasion of epithelial cells and induction of macrophage apoptosis require injection

of toxins across a host plasma membrane, and the SPI-1 TTSS can fulfil this for both sets of translocated toxins.

Some *Salmonella* strains also cause systemic disease, which involves replication within phagocytic cells, dissemination from the intestinal epithelium to the reticuloendothelial system, and replication in the liver and spleen. A number of genetic loci have been identified as essential for the systemic phase of disease in an *S typhimurium* murine infection model.[57] These include genes encoded by the *Salmonella* virulence plasmid and genes under control of the regulators PhoP/PhoQ and OmpR/EnvZ.[58,59]

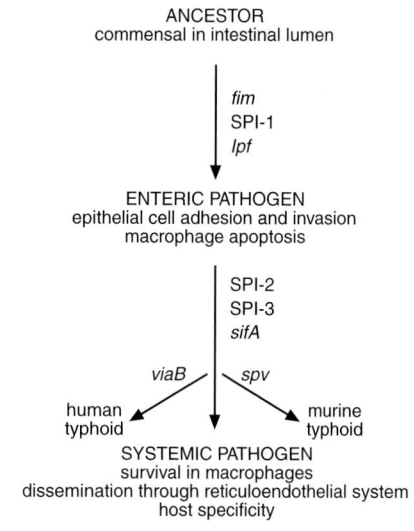

Fig. 12.5 Evolution of *Salmonella*. The common ancestor of the salmonellae is proposed to have been a commensal inhabitant of the intestinal lumen. All modern salmonellae have acquired pathogenicity islands (PAI) conferring the ability to adhere to and invade intestinal epithelial cells. This transition from commensal to pathogen was followed by the acquisition of further PAI, which enabled *Salmonella* to replicate and disseminate systemically within macrophages. The ability of *Salmonella* strains to cause systemic infection is often extremely host specific. This could be a result of further horizontal transfer events, such as the acquisition of the virulence plasmid carrying the *spv* ADP-ribosylating toxin by pathovars causing murine typhoid, or the *viaB* PAI encoding Vi capsule biosynthetic machinery by pathovars causing human typhoid.

Table 12.3 *Salmonella typhimurium* horizontally transferred virulence determinants

Region	Virulence determinant	Function
PAI and pathogenicity islets		
SPI-1	TTSS, secreted proteins	Epithelial cell invasion, macrophage apoptosis
SPI-2	TTSS, secreted proteins	Intramacrophage survival
SPI-3	MgtB, MgtC	Intramacrophage survival, magnesium transport
SPI-4	Type I secretion system	Intramacrophage survival
SPI-5	SopB inositol phosphate phosphatase (SPI-1 secreted)	Intestinal fluid secretion/enteropathogenesis
sifA islet	SifA (SPI-2 secreted)	Tubular structures in epithelial cells, maintenance of intracellular vacuole
slrP islet	SlrP (SPI-1/SPI-2 secreted)	Colonization of murine Peyer's patches
fim operon	Type I fimbriae	Adherence to epithelial cells
lpf operon	Long polar fimbriae	Entry into murine Peyer's patches
Bacteriophages		
Gifsy-3Φ	PagJ, SspH1 (SPI-1/SPI-2 secreted)	Calf enteropathogenesis
SopEΦ	SopE (SPI-1 secreted)	Epithelial cell invasion
Plasmid-borne virulence determinants		
spv operon	ADP-ribosylating toxin	Systemic infection of mice

PAI, Pathogenicity islands; TTSS, type III secretion system.

In addition, SPI-2 encodes a TTSS, which is essential for systemic disease in mice and for bacterial replication within macrophages.[60–62] The distribution of this PAI is restricted to those strains which cause systemic infection.[63,64] The secretion system seems to become active once *Salmonella* is within the phagocytic vacuole of the macrophage and injects proteins into the host cell from this location. Thus, this second *Salmonella* TTSS is a delivery system for a different subset of secreted toxins to those of the SPI-1 TTSS. Many other horizontally acquired genes appear to have important roles in intracellular survival and replication. For example, SPI-3 and SPI-4 both contain genes required for bacterial growth within macrophages.[65–67]

It is interesting that both gastrointestinal and systemic infection by *Salmonella* requires protein export by TTSS. Both TTSS inject proteins encoded within their PAI and elsewhere on the chromosome, often within other horizontally transmitted elements. The acquisition of these two secretion systems seems to have provided a means for the delivery into host cells of separately acquired toxins. SPI-1 is expressed in conditions of high osmolarity, such as would be found in the intestinal lumen.[68] Conversely, conditions favouring expression of SPI-2 genes include magnesium starvation and low pH, as might be found intracellularly.[69] The differential regulation of SPI-1 and SPI-2 gene expression restricts the activities of the TTSS and their associated toxins to different stages in the disease process, therefore preventing possible disadvantageous effects of delivering a toxin to inappropriate targets.

4.3 *H pylori*

The role of the major virulence factors of *H pylori* in causing gastritis and peptic ulcer disease remains unclear, but a PAI is thought to play an important part.[70] Two main classes of *H pylori* strains are distinguished, with type I strains associated with more serious disease.[71] These strains possess the 40 kb Cag PAI encoding the cytotoxin-associated antigen (CagA), which is translocated into gastric epithelial cells by a TFSS also encoded on the PAI.[19,72] This PAI appears to be highly unstable. It is deleted from natural populations, even within a single individual, and it has been interrupted by a 20 kb insertion sequence or partially deleted in some isolates.[71] Phenotypes associated with the Cag PAI include the formation of pedestals on epithelial cell surfaces, tyrosine phosphorylation of host proteins, and activation of host cell transcription factors and signalling cascades.[72–75] At present, it is not known which bacterial proteins are directly responsible for these effects, but some are likely to be substrates of the TFSS. Although a clear picture of the role of the PAI-encoded virulence factors in pathogenesis is not yet available, it is known that type II strains of *H pylori*, which do not possess the Cag PAI, are less likely to be isolated from patients with severe disease.[71]

5. PAI OF GRAM-POSITIVE BACTERIA

Although the PAI of Gram-negative bacteria have been the most intensively studied, some PAI have also been found in Gram-positive species. PAI of Gram-positive bacteria do not usually conform well to the definition of classical PAI. For example, they do not appear to be bordered by specific junction sites such as direct repeats or tRNA genes. This has perhaps made their identification more difficult.[9] One rare exception is the 15 kb PAI of *S aureus*, which possesses many features common to Gram-negative PAI and encodes TSST-1.[15]

Other Gram-positive pathogens possess groups of virulence determinants which bear some similarity to PAI and have been called pathogenicity gene clusters (Table 12.4).[10] For example, pathogenic species of *Listeria* possess a 10 kb region encoding listeriolysin O and regulatory proteins, required for escape from the phagosome into the macrophage cytoplasm, which appears to have been acquired by bacteriophage transduction.[76,77] Some strains of *Clostridium difficile* harbour a 19 kb cluster encoding two toxins, TcdA and TcdB, responsible for causing pseudomembranous colitis.[78] A further possible example of a horizontally acquired region is the *S pyogenes* M protein and M-related proteins, which are encoded by a 6 kb cluster.[79] As more bacterial genomes are fully sequenced, more putative PAI and clusters may be found in Gram-positive pathogens. This may allow the identification of specific features common to horizontally transferred virulence determinants of Gram-positive pathogens.

Table 12.4 Pathogenicity islands and gene clusters of Gram-positive organisms

Organism	PAI/cluster	Virulence determinants	Function
Staphylococcus aureus	SaPI	TSST-1	Superantigen
Listeria monocytogenes	PrfA cluster	Listeriolysin O, PlcA/B	Lysis of phagocytic vacuole
Clostridium difficile	Pathogenicity locus	TcdA, TcdB	Enterotoxins
Streptococcus pyogenes	*vir* regulon	M-protein, ScpA	Antiphagocytic surface protein, C5a peptidase
Streptococcus pneumoniae	PPI-1	Pit2 ABC transporter	Iron uptake

6. REGULATION OF PAI GENES

For horizontally acquired genes to confer a fitness advantage, their expression must be regulated appropriately. The importance of this is illustrated by the listeriolysin O pathogenicity gene cluster. Listeriolysin-O-mediated escape from phagocytic vacuoles into the macrophage cytosol is essential for *Listeria* virulence.[80] Surprisingly, the listeriolysin O cluster is also present in non-pathogenic *Listeria seeligeri*,[76] but it appears that the genes within the PAI are not expressed to a significant level in this species. Introduction of a *Listeria monocytogenes* transcriptional activator to *L seeligeri* induces intracellular expression of the listeriolysin O gene and confers upon this species the ability to escape from the phagosome.[81] Therefore, the inability of *L seeligeri* to adopt a pathogenic lifestyle appears to be solely due to inappropriate regulatory control over horizontally acquired virulence determinants.

Genes with regulatory functions may be located within a PAI. SPI-2 of *S typhimurium* encodes a two-component regulatory system, SsrAB.[69] SsrB is a transcriptional activator not only of genes within SPI-2 but also of at least 10 other loci within the *Salmonella* genome, all of which appear to have been horizontally acquired.[82] Upon introduction into a bacterial genome, genes within a PAI may also be assimilated into existing regulatory circuits. For example, the expression of SsrAB is, in turn, regulated by the OmpR/EnvZ system, which responds to osmotic stress.[59] Components of the independently acquired SPI-1 and SPI-3 pathogenicity islands of *S typhimurium* are regulated by the PhoPQ wide domain regulatory system.[58,83] This system regulates the expression of a large number of loci in response to magnesium concentration, including both housekeeping and virulence genes.[58]

Expression of genes within PAI may also be affected by elements surrounding the integration site. For example, PAI II of *E coli* is situated downstream of the tRNA^{leuX} gene, which regulates the expression of a large number of virulence determinants including type I fimbriae, flagellae, the iron chelator enterobactin and factors involved in serum resistance.[84,85] Loss of tRNA^{leuX} by mutation results in loss of virulence of UPEC strains in a mouse model.[86]

7. ACQUISITION OF PAI

7.1 Horizontal gene transfer in prokaryotes

In contrast to eukaryotes, where the main route of horizontal transfer of genetic information is by sexual processes and may only occur within or between closely related species, prokaryotes are able to integrate non-homologous DNA from distantly related species. This allows for extremely rapid generation of new variants by the incorporation of large novel genetic units into the bacterial genome, rather than the more limited shuffling of homologous DNA to which eukaryotes are restricted.

Several conditions must be fulfilled for successful horizontal DNA transfer to occur.[87] First, the DNA must be taken up successfully by the recipient cell through transformation, transduction or conjugation (Table 12.5). Secondly, foreign DNA must survive the defence mechanisms of the recipient cell. Bacteria possess restriction-modification systems whose function is to recognize and degrade foreign DNA. Pathogenic enterobacteria often carry defects in the *mutS* gene, which reduce the efficiency of DNA repair and thus increase the likelihood of mismatches during genome replication, favouring the integration of novel DNA.[88] Thirdly, new genetic information must adopt a form allowing its inheritance. The DNA must be incorporated into a plasmid or become integrated into the bacterial chromosome to be replicated prior to cell division. As well as by homologous recombination, DNA integration events may be mediated by several classes of mobile genetic elements.[87] Transposable elements do not require large stretches of homologous sequence for their insertion, so can act as vectors carrying new genes between distantly related strains.

Finally, newly acquired genetic information must be maintained at the level of the bacterial population. Plasmids need to be under continuous selective pressure in order to be maintained, as they can be easily lost through segregation at

Table 12.5 Bacterial DNA uptake

Method of uptake	Description
Transformation	Some bacterial species are naturally able to take up free DNA at some point in their life cycle, including *Neisseria gonorrhoeae*, *Haemophilus influenzae*, *Helicobacter pylori* and *Streptococcus pneumoniae*
Conjugation	A plasmid, chromosomal fragment or conjugative transposon is transferred through a specialized organelle from donor to recipient cell
Transduction	Transfer of bacterial DNA mediated by viruses (bacteriophages). The bacteriophage replicates within a donor cell, and may package some of the donor's DNA into new virus particles along with its genome

cell division. On the chromosome, such a great degree of selective pressure is not required, but genes which are detrimental to the survival of the recipient would rapidly be lost. Genetic information neutral to the bacterium carrying it may also be lost by deletion of a large DNA segment or the gradual accumulation of mutations. However, newly acquired genes providing benefits for the recipient are likely to be maintained in the bacterial population because of the growth advantage conferred upon recipients. Selection pressure for the loss of non-beneficial DNA has probably favoured the incorporation of related virulence genes into physically linked genetic units under the control of conserved regulatory systems. These would be immediately functional upon their acquisition,[87] whereas sequential acquisition of several separate genes to create a new virulence function would be unlikely.

7.2 Mechanisms of acquisition of PAI

PAI often contain features which indicate possible mechanisms of acquisition. Many PAI are flanked by direct repeat sequences, usually between 16 and 20 base pairs in length, which were probably generated during insertion of bacteriophages, plasmids or transposons into the genome. These short repeats may represent target sequences for site-specific recombinases. Other features characteristic of mobile genetic

elements are often present, including origins of plasmid replication and transposon or phage genes such as recombinases or integrases. It is worth noting that because PAI appear to be hotspots for recombination and insertion of mobile genetic elements, some mobility features present on PAI could have been acquired after the initial PAI integration.[10]

A number of PAI are associated with complete bacteriophages, including PAI harbouring toxin genes of *Corynebacterium diphtheriae*, *S aureus*, *Pseudomonas aeruginosa*, *V cholerae* and *E coli*. Some of these remain capable of excising from the genome, such as the *V. cholerae* pathogenicity island (VPI), which can be mobilized between strains of *V cholerae* by phage transduction.[89] However, the phages associated with other PAI are reduced to defective remnants. For example, the SaPI PAI of *S aureus* contains a defective phage, that can only be mobilized by infecting bacteria with a 'helper' virus to provide the missing functions in *trans*.[15]

Movement, rearrangement and deletion of PAI may occur naturally, mediated by the mobility factors present within the island or elsewhere in the bacterial genome. The Cag PAI of *H pylori* appears to undergo extensive rearrangement and deletion even within infected individuals. The high-pathogenicity island of *Yersinia pseudotuberculosis* contains phage integrase genes and can be mobilized between three different *asn*-specific tRNA genes, which represent specific recombination sites for the phage.[90,91] PAI I and II of UPEC both contain defective phage integrase genes but remain unstable. They are probably deleted with the help of functional recombinase/integrase genes encoded elsewhere in the genome.[10,25]

Phage or transposon integration occurs at specific sites within the genome. Hence, PAI do not insert randomly but rather at specific sites. PAI of Gram-negative pathogens are frequently located downstream of tRNA genes (Table 12.6),[9] possibly because tRNA loci are known to be integration target sites of several phages and plasmids.[92–94] Interestingly, the tRNA *selC* locus is the site of at least four different PAI.[25,27,42,66] The insertion site of each of these PAI is identical and probably represents a hotspot for the integration of certain transposable elements.

7.3 Where do PAI come from?

There has been no example of the clear identification of the original source of a PAI and, in many cases, the donor may well be unculturable or extinct. Some PAI appear to consist of a 'mosaic' of fragments with different origins.[95] The origins of some virulence factors can be traced back to related genes found in non-pathogens. For example, the TTSS and TFSS found in many Gram-negative pathogens are homologous to the export and assembly machinery for flagellae and conjugative pili, respectively.[16,18] Even some eukaryotic genes appear to have been incorporated into bacterial PAI. An example is YopH, a secreted tyrosine phosphatase of *Yersinia*, which has greater similarity to eukaryotic tyrosine phosphatases than those of other bacteria.[96]

8. FUTURE DIRECTIONS

8.1 Vaccine development and drug discovery

The range of antimicrobial therapy available for the treatment of bacterial infections has become increasingly limited in recent years, as multidrug resistance has continued to spread.[97] Furthermore, some bacterial diseases, such as tuberculosis, which were once thought to be under control, are re-emerging as serious public health threats.[98] These problems have led to an intensified search for new drugs and vaccines, and increased research in the rapidly expanding field of microbial pathogenesis, over the past few decades.

The identification of conserved 'families' of virulence genes, such as the TTSS and TFSS, opens up the possibility of developing drugs to inhibit these virulence mechanisms.[99] These types of drug would have a number of advantages over current antimicrobial agents. They could be active against a range of pathogens without having any effect on the normal flora. In addition, many antibiotic-resistant genes are thought to have originated as self-protection mechanisms for antibiotic-producing microbes, such as *Streptomyces*, and are already present in bacteria within the normal human commensal population. However, it is unlikely that resistance mechanisms to antivirulence drugs would occur naturally. Furthermore, as drugs targeting pathogen-specific gene products would not affect non-pathogenic bacteria, there would be no selective pressure favouring the spread of resistance genes among commensal organisms,

Table 12.6 Examples of pathogenicity island (PAI) insertion sites		
Site	**PAI**	**Organism**
tRNA genes		
selC	LEE	EPEC
selC	PAI I	UPEC
selC	SPI-3	Salmonella typhimurium
selC	SHI-2	Shigella flexneri
leuX	PAI II	UPEC
valV	SPI-2	S typhimurium
Other RNA genes		
ssrA	VP1	Vibrio cholerae
Other locations		
glr	Cag PAI	Helicobacter pylori
potABCD	sifA	S typhimurium

EPEC, Enteropathogenic *Escherichia coli*; LEE, Locus of enterocyte effacement; UPEC, uropathogenic *E coli*.

which is thought to be an important factor in the rapid spread of antimicrobial resistance.[100]

It is difficult to produce a live attenuated vaccine strain (traditionally by repeated laboratory passage or deletion of housekeeping genes) which is sufficiently attenuated but persists well enough in the body to generate a good immune response. PAI may be good candidates for deletion to produce safely attenuated, but potentially immunogenic, strains. For example, PAI encoding toxins could be removed without affecting a strain's ability to colonize epithelial surfaces. There is also considerable interest in utilizing bacterial strains as epitope delivery systems. Use of TTSS and TFSS to deliver these epitopes to different intracellular locations could allow modulation of the type of immune response generated by a vaccine.[101]

A new and interesting field arising from our increased knowledge of bacterial virulence determinants is the therapeutic use of modified pathogenic bacteria to treat other diseases. For example, some bacteria appear to target and multiply preferentially in solid tumours. Administration of attenuated bacteria alone prolonged survival in a range of animal tumour models, but the tumours eventually resumed growth.[102] In the future, it might be possible to improve this type of treatment by exploiting bacterial virulence mechanisms. For example, TTSS and TFSS are precise intracellular delivery systems, and could be used to inject prodrugs directly into target cells. Expression of a particular combination of adhesins may allow targeting of particular cell types, thus enhancing the specificity of the treatment so that more powerful drugs could be delivered without harming other cells in the body.

8.2 Diagnostic applications

PAI are, by definition, unique to specific pathogens. With the advent of faster, cheaper DNA analysis methods, such as array technology and real-time polymerase chain reactions (PCR), the possibility of simultaneously analysing samples for presence of many PAI sequences as a diagnostic tool is fast becoming available. This type of analysis would not only

identify pathogens more quickly than traditional diagnostic laboratory methods, but could also give indications of the expected course of disease and possible complications, depending on the virulence determinants detected.

8.3 Pathogen genome sequencing projects

The genome sequences of a large number of microbial pathogens, and their non-pathogenic relatives, are currently either completed or in progress (see Websites). The increasing power of bioinformatic approaches makes it possible to search, annotate and compare this genome information. By using experimental approaches to find defining characteristics of virulence genes and PAI, it should be possible to identify new candidate pathogenicity determinants from the sequence data. This might include genes in unculturable organisms or those with intractable genetic systems which are not amenable to study in the laboratory. By providing a source of candidate virulence genes for investigation, thus furthering our understanding of bacterial pathogenesis, bioinformatics may also prove to be a valuable method for the development of antibacterial drugs and vaccines.

NOTE ADDED IN PROOF

Since this manuscript was written in 2001, a number of significant papers have been published, particularly on the subject of PAIs of Ciran-positive pathogens.

ACKNOWLEDGEMENTS

We thank C Beuzon, J Brown and C Tang for critical review of the manuscript. Work in DWH's laboratory is supported by grants from the MRC (UK) and the Wellcome Trust.

REFERENCES

Websites

Microbial genome sequencing projects:
http://www.sanger.ac.uk/Projects/Microbes/
http://genome.wustl.edu/gsc/Projects/bacteria.shtml

Scientific papers

1. Davies J. Bacteria on the rampage. *Nature* 1996; **383**: 219–20.
2. Hacker J, Knapp S, Goebel W. Spontaneous deletions and flanking regions of the chromosomally inherited hemolysin determinant of an *Escherichia coli* 06 strain. *J Bacteriol* 1983; **154**: 1145–52.
3. Waldor MK, Mekalanos JJ. Emergence of a new cholera pandemic: molecular analysis of virulence determinants in *Vibrio cholerae* O139 and development of a live vaccine prototype. *J Infect Dis* 1994; **170**: 278–83.
4. de la Cruz I, Davies I. Horizontal gene transfer and the origin of species: lessons from bacteria. *Trends Microbiol* 2000; **8**: 128–33.
5. Groisman EA, Ochman H. Pathogenicity islands; bacterial evolution in quantum leaps. *Cell* 1996; **87**: 791–4.
6. Lipsitch M, Moxon ER. Virulence and transmissibility of pathogens: what is the relationship? *Trends Microbiol* 1997; **5**: 31–7.
7. Lan R, Reeves PR. Gene transfer is a major factor in bacterial evolution. *Molec Biol Evol* 1996; **13**: 47–55.
8. Morschhauser J, Kohler G, Ziebuhr W et al. Evolution of microbial pathogens. *Philos Trans R Soc Lond B Biol Sci* 2000; **355**: 695–704.
9. Hacker J, Blum-Oehler G, Muhldorfer I et al. Pathogenicity islands of virulent bacteria: structure, function and impact on microbial evolution. *Molec Microbiol* 1997; **23**: 1089–97.
10. Hacker J, Kaper JB. Pathogenicity islands and the evolution of microbes. *Annu Rev Microbiol* 2000; **54**: 641–79.
11. Beuzón CR, Méresse S, Unsworth KE et al. *Salmonella* maintains the integrity of its intracellular vacuole through the action of SifA. *EMBO J* 2000; **19**: 3235–49.
12. Janakiraman A, Slauch JM. The putative iron transport system SitABCD encoded on SPII is required for full virulence of *Salmonella typhimurium*. *Molec Microbiol* 2000; **35**: 1146–55.
13. Mills DM, Bajaj V, Lee CA. A 40 kb chromosomal fragment encoding *Salmonella typhimurium* invasion genes is absent from the corresponding region of the *Escherichia coli* K-12 chromosome. *Molec Microbiol* 1995; **15**: 749–59.
14. Zhou D, Hardt WD, Galan JE. *Salmonella typhimurium* encodes a putative iron transport system within the centisome 63 pathogenicity island. *Infect Immunol* 1999; **67**: 1974–81.
15. Lindsay JA, Ruzin A, Ross HF et al. The gene for toxic shock toxin is carried by a family of mobile pathogenicity islands in *Staphylococcus aureus*. *Molec Microbiol* 1998; **29**: 527–43.
16. Hueck CJ. Type III protein secretion systems in bacterial pathogens of animals and plants. *Microbiol Molec Biol Rev* 1998; **62**: 379–433.
17. Nguyen L, Paulsen IT, Tchieu J et al. Phylogenetic analyses of the constituents of Type III protein secretion systems. *J Molec Microbiol Biotechnol* 2000; **2**: 125–44.
18. Christie PJ, Vogel JP. Bacterial type IV secretion: conjugation systems adapted to deliver effector molecules to host cells. *Trends Microbiol* 2000; **8**: 354–60.
19. Odenbreit S, Puls J, Sedlmaier B et al. Translocation of *Helicobacter pylori* CagA into gastric epithelial cells by type IV secretion. *Science* 2000; **287**: 1497–500.
20. Bik EM, Bunschoten AE, Gouw RD et al. Genesis of the novel epidemic *Vibrio cholerae* O139 strain: evidence for horizontal transfer of genes involved in polysaccharide synthesis. *EMBO J* 1995; **14**: 209–16.
21. Kaper JB, Morris JG, Levine MM. Cholera. *Clin Microbiol Rev* 1995; **8**: 48–86.
22. Henderson IR, Czeczulin J, Eslava C et al. Characterization of *pic*, a secreted protease of *Shigella flexneri* and enteroaggregative *Escherichia coli*. *Infect Immunol* 1999; **67**: 5587–96.
23. Hersh D, Monack DM, Smith MR et al. The *Salmonella* invasin SipB induces macrophage apoptosis by binding to caspase-1. *Proc Natl Acad Sci USA* 1999; **96**: 2396–401.
24. Collazo CM, Galan JE. The invasion-associated type III system of *Salmonella typhimurium* directs the translocation of Sip proteins into the host cell. *Molec Microbiol* 1997; **24**: 747–56.
25. Blum G, Ott M, Lischewski A et al. Excision of large DNA regions termed pathogenicity islands from tRNA-specific loci in the chromosome of an *Escherichia coli* wild-type pathogen. *Infect Immunol* 1994; **62**: 606–14.
26. Hacker J, Bender L, Ott M et al. Deletions of chromosomal regions coding for fimbriae and hemolysins occur *in vitro* and *in vivo* in various extraintestinal *Escherichia coli* isolates. *Microb Pathog* 1990; **8**: 213–25.
27. McDaniel TK, Jarvis KG, Donnenberg MS et al. A genetic locus of enterocyte effacement conserved among diverse enterobacterial pathogens. *Proc Natl Acad Sci USA* 1995; **92**: 1664–8.
28. Kenny B, De Vinney R, Stein M et al. Enteropathogenic *E. coli* (EPEC) transfers its receptor for intimate adherence into mammalian cells. *Cell* 1997; **91**: 511–20.

29. Stins MF, Prasadarao NV, Ibric L et al. Binding characteristics of S fimbriated *Escherichia coli* to isolated brain microvascular endothelial cells. *Am J Pathol* 1994; **145**: 1228–36.

30. Morschhauser J, Vetter V, Emody L et al. Adhesin regulatory genes within large, unstable DNA regions of pathogenic *Escherichia coli*: cross-talk between different adhesin gene clusters. *Molec Microbiol* 1994; **11**: 555–66.

31. Galán JE, Zhou D. Striking a balance: modulation of the actin cytoskeleton by *Salmonella*. *Proc Natl Acad Sci USA* 2000; **97**: 8754–61.

32. Kaniga K, Trollinger D, Galan JE. Identification of two targets of the type III protein secretion system encoded by the *inv* and *spa* loci of *Salmonella typhimurium* that have homology to the *Shigella* IpaD and IpaA proteins. *J Bacteriol* 1995; **177**: 7078–85.

33. Kaniga K, Tucker S, Trollinger D et al. Homologs of the *Shigella* IpaB and IpaC invasins are required for *Salmonella typhimurium* entry into cultured epithelial cells. *J Bacteriol* 1995; **177**: 3965–71.

34. Hardt WD, Chen LM, Schuebel KE et al. *S. typhimurium* encodes an activator of Rho GTPases that induces membrane ruffling and nuclear responses in host cells. *Cell* 1998; **93**: 815–26.

35. Lesser CF, Scherer CA, Miller SI. Rac, ruffle and rho: orchestration of *Salmonella* invasion. *Trends Microbiol* 2000; **8**: 151–2.

36. Méresse S, Steele-Mortimer O, Moreno E et al. Controlling the maturation of pathogen-containing vacuoles: a matter of life and death. *Nat Cell Biol* 1999; **1**: E183–E188.

37. Garcia-Del Portillo F. Pathogenic interference with host vacuolar trafficking. *Trends Microbiol* 1999; **7**: 467–9.

38. Goebel W, Kuhn M. Bacterial replication in the host cell cytosol. *Curr Opin Microbiol* 2000; **3**: 49–53.

39. Uchiya K, Barbieri MA, Funato K et al. A *Salmonella* virulence protein that inhibits cellular trafficking. *EMBO J* 1999; **18**: 3924–33.

40. Bearden SW, Fetherston JD, Perry RD. Genetic organization of the yersiniabactin biosynthetic region and construction of avirulent mutants in *Yersinia pestis*. *Infect Immunol* 1997; **65**: 1659–68.

41. Moss JE, Cardozo TJ, Zychlinsky A et al. The *selC*-associated SH1-2 pathogenicity island of *Shigella flexneri*. *Molec Microbiol* 1999; **33**: 74–83.

42. Vokes SA, Reeves SA, Torres AG et al. The aerobactin iron transport system genes in *Shigella flexneri* are present within a pathogenicity island. *Molec Microbiol* 1999; **33**: 63–73.

43. Brown JS, Gilliland SM, Holden DW. A *Streptococcus pneumoniae* pathogenicity island encoding an ABC transporter involved in iron uptake and virulence. *Molec Microbiol* 2001; **40**: 572–85.

44. Salyers A, Whitt D. *Bacterial Pathogenesis: A Molecular Approach*. Washington: ASM Press, 1994.

45. Perna NT, Plunkett G, Burland V et al. Genome sequence of enterohaemorrhagic *Escherichia coli* O157:H7. *Nature* 2001; **409:** 529–33.

46. Blum G, Falbo V, Caprioli A et al. Gene clusters encoding the cytotoxic necrotizing factor type 1, Prs-fimbriae and alpha-hemolysin form the pathogenicity island II of the uropathogenic *Escherichia coli* strain J96. *FEMS Microbiol Lett* 1995; **126**: 189–95.

47. Swenson DL, Bukanov NO, Berg DE et al. Two pathogenicity islands in uropathogenic *Escherichia coli* J96: cosmid cloning and sample sequencing. *Infect Immunol* 1996; **64**: 3736–43.

48. Moon HW, Whipp SC, Argenzio RA et al. Attaching and effacing activities of rabbit and human enteropathogenic *Escherichia coli* in pig and rabbit intestines. *Infect Immunol* 1983; **41**: 1340–51.

49. McDaniel TK, Kaper JB. A cloned pathogenicity island from enteropathogenic *Escherichia coli* confers the attaching and effacing phenotype on *E. coli* K-12. *Molec Microbiol* 1997; **23**: 399–407.

50. Elliott SJ, Wainwright LA, McDaniel TK et al. The complete sequence of the locus of enterocyte effacement (LEE) from enteropathogenic *Escherichia coli* E2348/69. *Molec Microbiol* 1998; **28**: 1–4.

51. Vallance BA, Finlay BB. Exploitation of host cells by enteropathogenic *Escherichia coli*. *Proc Natl Acad Sci USA* 2000; **97**: 8799–806.

52. Reid SD, Herbelin CJ, Bumbaugh AC et al. Parallel evolution of virulence in pathogenic *Escherichia coli*. *Nature* 2000; **406**: 64–7.

53. Bieber D, Ramer SW, Wu CY et al. Type IV pili, transient bacterial aggregates, and virulence of enteropathogenic *Escherichia coli*. *Science* 1998; **280**: 2114–18.

54. Baumler AJ. The record of horizontal gene transfer in *Salmonella*. *Trends Microbiol* 1997; **5**: 318–22.

55. Chen LM, Kaniga K, Galan JE. *Salmonella* spp. are cytotoxic for cultured macrophages. *Molec Microbiol* 1996; **21**: 1101–15.

56. Monack DM, Raupach B, Hromockyj AE et al. *Salmonella typhimurium* invasion induces apoptosis in infected macrophages. *Proc Natl Acad Sci USA* 1996; **93**: 9833–8.

57. Groisman EA, Ochman H. How *Salmonella* became a pathogen. *Trends Microbiol* 1997; **5**: 343–9.

58. Groisman EA. The ins and outs of virulence gene expression: Mg2+ as a regulatory signal. *Bioessays* 1998; **20**: 96–101.

59. Lee AK, Detweiler CS, Falkow S. OmpR regulates the two-component system *ssrA–ssrB* in *Salmonella* pathogenicity island 2. *J Bacteriol* 2000; **182**: 771–81.

60. Hensel M, Shea JE, Gleeson C et al. Simultaneous identification of bacterial virulence genes by negative selection. *Science* 1995; **269**: 400–3.

61. Ochman H, Soncini FC, Solomon F et al. Identification of a pathogenicity island required for *Salmonella* survival in host cells. *Proc Natl Acad Sci USA* 1996; **93**: 7800–4.

62. Shea JE, Beuzón CR, Gleeson C et al. Influence of the *Salmonella typhimurium* pathogenicity island 2 type III secretion system on bacterial growth in the mouse. *Infect Immunol* 1999; **67**: 213–19.

63. Ochman H, Groisman EA. Distribution of pathogenicity islands in *Salmonella* spp. *Infect Immunol* 1996; **64**: 5410–12.

64. Shea JE, Hensel M, Gleeson C et al. Identification of a virulence locus encoding a second type III secretion system in *Salmonella typhimurium*. *Proc Natl Acad Sci USA* 1996; **93**: 2593–7.

65. Blanc-Potard AB, Groisman EA. The *Salmonella selC* locus contains a pathogenicity island mediating intramacrophage survival. *Eur Molec Biol Org J* 1997; **16**: 5376–85.

66. Blanc-Potard AB, Solomon F, Kayser J et al. The SPI-3 pathogenicity island of *Salmonella enterica*. *J Bacteriol* 1999; **181**: 998–1004.

67. Wong KK, McClelland M, Stillwell LC et al. Identification and sequence analysis of a 27-kilobase chromosomal fragment containing a *Salmonella* pathogenicity island located at 92 minutes on the chromosome map of *Salmonella enterica* serovar Typhimurium LT2. *Infect Immunol* 1998; **66**: 3365–71.

68. Bajaj V, Lucas RL, Hwang C et al. Co-ordinate regulation of *Salmonella typhimurium* invasion genes by environmental and regulatory factors is mediated by control of *hilA* expression. *Molec Microbiol* 1996; **22**: 703–14.

69. Deiwick J, Nikolaus T, Erdogan S et al. Environmental regulation of *Salmonella* pathogenicity island 2 gene expression. *Molec Microbiol* 1999; **31**: 1759–73.

70. Graham DY, Yamaoka Y. Disease-specific *Helicobacter pylori* virulence factors: the unfulfilled promise. *Helicobacter* 2000; **5(Suppl 1)**: S3–S9; discussion S27–S31.

71. Covacci A, Telford JL, Gel Giudice G et al. *Helicobacter pylori* virulence and genetic geography. *Science* 1999; **284**: 1328–33.

72. Censini S, Lange C, Xiang Z et al. *cag*, A pathogenicity island of *Helicobacter pylori*, encodes type I-specific and disease-associated virulence factors. *Proc Natl Acad Sci USA* 1996; **93**: 14,648–53.

73. Segal ED, Lange C, Covacci A et al. Induction of host signal transduction pathways of *Helicobacter pylori*. *Proc Natl Acad Sci USA* 1997; **94**: 7595–9.

74. Tummuru MK, Sharma SA, Blaser MJ. *Helicobacter pylori picB*, a homologue of the *Bordetella pertussis* toxin secretion protein, is required for induction of IL-8 in gastric epithelial cells. *Molec Microbiol* 1995; **18**: 867–76.

75. Yamaoka Y, Kita M, Kodama T et al. Induction of various cytokines and development of severe mucosal inflammation by *cagA* gene positive *Helicobacter pylori* strains. *Gut* 1997; **41**: 442–51.

76. Gouin E, Mengaud J, Cossart P. The virulence gene cluster of *Listeria monocytogenes* is also present in *Listeria ivanovii*, an animal pathogen, and *Listeria seeligeri*, a nonpathogenic species. *Infect Immunol* 1994; **62**: 3550–3.

77. Chakroborty T, Hain T, Domann E. Genome organization and the evolution of the virulence gene locus in *Listeria* species. *Int J Med Microbiol* 2000; **290**: 167–74.

78. Braun V, Hundsberger T, Leukel P et al. Definition of the single integration site of the pathogenicity locus in *Clostridium difficile*. *Gene* 1996; **181**: 29–38.

79. Podbielski A, Woischnik M, Pohl B et al. What is the size of the group A streptococcal *vir* regulon? The Mga regulator affects expression of secreted and surface virulence factors. *Med Microbiol Immunol* 1996; **185**: 171–81.

80. Camilli A, Goldfine H, Portnoy DA. *Listeria monocytogenes* mutants lacking phosphatidylinositol-specific phospholipase C are avirulent. *J Exp Med* 1991; **173**: 751–4.

81. Karunasagar I, Lampidis R, Goebel W et al. Complementation of *Listeria seeligeri* with the *plcA–prfA* genes from *L. monocytogenes* activates transcription of seeligerolysin and leads to bacterial escape from the phagosome of infected mammalian cells. *FEMS Microbiol Lett* 1997; **146**: 303–10.

82. Worley MJ, Ching KH, Heffron F. *Salmonella* SsrB activates a global regulon of horizontally acquired genes. *Molec Microbiol* 2000; **36**: 749–61.

83. Behlau I, Miller SI. A PhoP-repressed gene promotes *Salmonella typhimurium* invasion of epithelial cells. *J Bacteriol* 1993; **175**: 4475–84.

84. Ritter A, Blum G, Emody L et al. tRNA genes and pathogenicity islands: influence on virulence and

metabolic properties of uropathogenic *Escherichia coli*. *Molec Microbiol* 1995; **17**: 109–21.

85. Susa M, Kreft B, Wasenauer G et al. Influence of cloned tRNA genes from a uropathogenic *Escherichia coli* strain on adherence to primary human renal tubular epithelial cells and nephropathogenicity in rats. *Infect Immunol* 1996; **64**: 5390–4.

86. Dobrindt U, Cohen PS, Utley M et al. The *leuX*-encoded tRNA5(Leu) but not the pathogenicity islands I and II influence the survival of the uropathogenic *Escherichia coli* strain 536 in CD-1 mouse bladder mucus in the stationary phase. *FEMS Microbiol Lett* 1998; **162**: 135–41.

87. Arber W. Evolution of prokaryotic genomes. *Gene* 1993; **135**: 49–56.

88. LeClerc JE, Li B, Payne WL et al. High mutation frequencies among *Escherichia coli* and *Salmonella* pathogens. *Science* 1996; **274**: 1208–11.

89. Karaolis DK, Somara S, Maneval DR et al. A bacteriophage encoding a pathogenicity island, a type-IV pilus and a phage receptor in cholera bacteria. *Nature* 1999; **399**: 375–9.

90. Buchrieser C, Brosch R, Bach S et al. The high-pathogenicity island of *Yersinia pseudotuberculosis* can be inserted into any of the three chromosomal *asn* tRNA genes. *Molec Microbiol* 1998; **30**: 965–78.

91. Rakin A, Noelting C, Schropp P et al. Integrative module of the high-pathogenicity island of *Yersinia*. *Molec Microbiol* 2001; **39**: 407–15.

92. Inouye S, Sunshine MG, Six EW et al. Retronphage phi R73: an *E. coli* phage that contains a retroelement and integrates into a tRNA gene. *Science* 1991; **252**: 969–71.

93. Alegre MT, Cournoyer B, Mesas JM et al. Cloning of *Frankia* species putative tRNA(Pro) genes and their efficacy for pSAM2 site-specific integration in *Streptomyces lividans*. *Appl Environ Microbiol* 1994; **60**: 4279–83.

94. Hayashi T, Matsumoto H, Ohnishi M et al. Molecular analysis of a cytotoxin-converting phage, phi CTX, of *Pseudomonas aeruginosa*: structure of the *attP-cos-ctx* region and integration into the serine tRNA gene. *Molec Microbiol* 1993; **7**: 657–67.

95. Hensel M, Nikolaus T, Egelseer C. Molecular and functional analysis indicates a mosaic structure of *Salmonella* pathogenicity island 2. *Molec Microbiol* 1999; **31**: 489–98.

96. Guan KL, Dixon JE. Protein tyrosine phosphatase activity of an essential virulence determinant in *Yersinia*. *Science* 1990; **249**: 553–6.

97. Walsh C. Molecular mechanisms that confer antibacterial drug resistance. *Nature* 2000; **406**:775–81.

98. Cohen ML. Changing patterns of infectious disease. *Nature* 2000; **406**: 762–7.

99. Stephens C, Shapiro L. Bacterial protein secretion – a target for new antibiotics? *Chem Biol* 1997; **4**: 637–41.

100. Chopra I, Hodgson J, Metcalf B et al. New approaches to the control of infections caused by antibiotic-resistant bacteria. An industry perspective. *J Am Med Assoc* 1996; **275**: 401–3.

101. Russmann H, Shams H, Poblete F et al. Delivery of epitopes by the *Salmonella* type III secretion system for vaccine development. *Science* 1998; **281**: 565–8.

102. Sznol M, Lin SL, Bermudes D et al. Use of preferentially replicating bacterial for the treatment of cancer. *J Clin Invest* 2000; **105**: 1027–30.

Glossary

ADCC	antibody-dependent cell-mediated cytotoxicity	COX	cyclooxygenase
AE	attaching and effacing	CR1	complement receptor 1
AICD	activation-induced cell death	CrmA	cytokine response modifier A
AIDS	acquired immunodeficiency syndrome	CRP	C-reactive protein
		CSF	colony-stimulating factor
AIg	immunoglobulin aggregates	CTL	cytotoxic T-lymphocytes
ALG	anti-lymphocyte globulin	DM	diabetes mellitus
ALPS	autoimmune lymphoprolifera-tive syndrome	dsDNA	double-stranded DNA
		DST	donor-specific (blood) transfusion
ANA	anti-nuclear antibodies	DTH	delayed-type hypersensitivity
ANCA	anti-neutrophil cytoplasmic antibody	EAE	experimental allergic encephalomyelitis/autoimmune
AOP	aminooxypentane	EBNA	Epsein-Barr virus nuclear antigen
AP	adaptor protein		
APC	antigen-presenting cells	EBV	Epstein-Barr virus
ARDS	adult respiratory distress syndrome	ECM	extracellular matrix
		EHEC	enterohaemorrhagic *Escherichia coli*
ARE	AU-rich elements		Encephalitis
AS	ankylosing spondylitis	EP	endogenous pyrogen
(₂-GPI	(₂-glycoprotein I	EPEC	enteropathogenic *Escherichia coli*
BCR	B-cell receptor	EPO	erythropoietin
BF	blastogenic factor	ER	endoplasmic reticulum
BLC	B-lymphoctye chemokine	ERGIC	endoplasmic reticulum Golgi intermediate compartment
BLyS	B-lymphocyte stimulator		
BM	basement membrane	ESR	eythrocyte sedimentation rate
BMT	bone marrow transplantation	EU	exposed uninfected
BPV	bovine papillomavirus	FACS	fluorescence activated cell sorter
BSA	bovine serum albumin		
CD	cluster domain	FasL	Fas ligand
cDNA	complementary DNA	FcR	Fc receptors
CFTR	cystic fibrosis transmembrane regulator	FADD	Fas-associated death domain
		FFP	fresh frozen plasma
CLR	collagen-like region	FGF	fibroblast growth factor
CNS	central nervous system	FLS	fibroblast-like synoviocytes
COP	coated protein		

FMLP	formyl methionyl leucyl phenylalanine	kb	kilobases
FMP	familial Mediterranean fever	LAF	lymphocyte activation factor
GAD	glutamic acid decarboxylase	LD	linkage disequilibrium
GAG	glucosaminoglycans	LDL	low-density lipoprotein
GALT	gut-associated lymphoid tissue	LEE	locus of enterocyte effacement
GBM	glomerular basement membrane	LIF	leukaemia inhibitory factor
GM-CSF	granulocyte—macrophage colony-stimulating factor	LIR	leucocyte immunoglobulin-like receptor
gp	glycoprotein	LKM	liver kidney microsomal
GPI	glucose-6-phosphate isomerase	LMF	lymphocyte mitogenic factor
GvHD	graft versus host disease	LMP	latent membrane protein
GvL	graft versus leukaemia	LPS	lipopolysaccharide
HAART	highly active antiretroviral therapy	LRR	leucine-rich repeats
		LT	lymphotoxin
HbsAg	hepatitis B surface Ag	MAPK	mitogen-activated protein kinase
HCMV	human cytomegalovirus	MASP	MBL-associated serine protease
HHV	human herpesvirus	MBL	mannose-binding lectin
HIV	human immunodeficiency virus	MBP	myelin basic protein
		MCMV	mouse cytomegalovirus
HLA	human leucocyte antigen	MCP	monocyte chemoattractant protein
HPI	high-pathogenicity island	MCV	*Molluscum contagiosum*
HPLC	high-performance liquid chromatography	MHC	major histocompatibility complex
HPV	human papillomavirus	MIP	macrophage inflammatory protein
HSP	heat-shock protein		
HSV	herpes simplex virus	MMP	matrix metalloproteinases
HUS	haemolytic uraemic syndrome	MOG	myelin oligodendrocyte
HVS	herpes virus saimiri	MS	multiple sclerosis
IC	immune complexes	MT-MMP	membrane-bound type matrix metalloprotein
ICAM	intercellular adhesion molecule		
ICE	interleukin-1(converting enzyme	NeF	nephritic factor
ICP	infected cell protein	NF-κB	nuclear factor of *kappa* B
IDDM	insulin-dependent diabetes mellitus	NFAT	nuclear factor for activation of T-cells
IDO	indoleamine-2,3-dioxygenase	NK	natural killer
IE	immediate–early	NKT	natural killer T-cells
IFN	interferon	NOD	non-obese diabetic
Ig	immunoglobulin	NSI	non-syncytium inducing
IGF	insulin-like growth factor	OA	osteoarthritis
Ii	invariant chain	OR	odds ratio
IL	interleukin	ORF	open reading frame
IMP	inflammation modulatory protein	*P*	probability
		PAI	pathogenicity islands
ITAM	immunoreceptor tyrosine-based activating motif	PAMP	pathogen-associated molecular patterns
ITIM	immunoreceptor tyrosine-based inhibitory motif	PCP	*Pneumocystis carinii* pneumonia
		PCR	polymerase chain reaction

PCV	packed cell volume	TB	tuberculosis
PDGF	platelet-derived growth factor	TBI	total body irradiation
PG	proteoglycan	TCR	T-cell receptor
PGE_2	prostaglandin E_2	TD antigens	T-dependent antigens
PLP	proteolipoprotein	TFSS	type IV secretion systems
PMN	neutrophil	TGF	transforming growth factor
pp	phosphoprotein	TGN	trans-Golgi network
PRR	pattern recognition receptors	Th	helper T-cell
RA	rheumatoid arthritis	TI antigens	T-independent antigens
RANTES	regulated-upon-activation, normal T expressed and secreted	TIMP	tissue inhibitors of matrix metalloproteinases
RCA	regulators of complement activation	TIR domain	Toll- and interleukin-1-related domain
RCT	randomized controlled trial	Tir	translocated intimin receptor
RID	receptor internalization and degradation	TLR	Toll-like receptors
RR	relative risk	TNF	tumour necrosis factor
RSV	respiratory syncytial virus	TNFR	tumour necrosis factor receptor
SDF	stromal cell-derived factor	TPA	tissue plasminogen activator
SEREX	serological identification of antigens	Tr	regulatory T-cell
sHEL	soluble hen egg lysosyme	TRADD	tumour-necrosis-factor-receptor-associated death domain
SI	syncytium inducing	TT	tetanus toxoid
SIV	simian immunodeficiency virus	TTSS	type III secretion systems
SLE	systemic lupus erythematosus	uPA	urokinase-type plasminogen activator
SNP	single nucleotide polymorphisms	UPEC	uropathogenic *Escherichia coli*
SPI-1	*Salmonella* pathogenicity island 1	US	unique short
ssDNA	single-stranded DNA	UTI	urinary tract infection
sTNFR	soluble tumour necrosis factor receptor	UTR	3′ untranslated region
		v	viral
TACE	tumour necrosis factor-alpha converting enzyme	VCAM	vascular cell adhesion molecule
		VEGF	vascular endothelial growth factor
TAP	transporters associated with antigen processing	vFLIP	viral FLICE inhibitory protein
		VPI	*V. cholerae* pathogenicity island

Index